Kidney Failure and the Federal Government

Richard A. Rettig and *Norman G. Levinsky, Editors*

Committee for the Study of the Medicare
End-Stage Renal Disease Program

Division of Health Care Services

INSTITUTE OF MEDICINE

NATIONAL ACADEMY PRESS
Washington, D.C. 1991

NATIONAL ACADEMY PRESS · 2101 Constitution Avenue, N.W. · Washington, D.C. 20418

NOTICE: The project that is the subject of this report and its technical appendixes was approved by the Governing Board of the National Research Council, whose member are drawn from the councils of the National Academy of Sciences, the National Academy of Engineering, and the Institute of Medicine. The members of the committee responsible for this report were chosen for their special competencies and with regard for appropriate balance.

The Institute of Medicine was chartered in 1970 by the National Academy of Sciences to enlist distinguished members of the appropriate professions in the examination of policy matters pertaining to the health of the public. In this, the Institute acts under both the Academy's 1863 congressional charter responsibility to be an adviser to the federal government and its own initiative in identifying issues of medical care, research, and education.

This study was supported by the Health Care Financing Administration, U.S. Department of Health and Human Services, under Cooperative Agreement No. 14-C-99338/3-02.

Library of Congress Cataloging-in-Publication Data

Institute of Medicine (U.S.). Committee for the Study of the Medicare
ESRD Program.
   Kidney failure and the federal government / Committee for the
Study of the Medicare ESRD Program, Division of Health Care
Services, Institute of Medicine ; Richard A. Rettig and Norman G.
Levinsky, editors.
      p. cm.
   Includes bibliographical references and index.
   ISBN 0-309-04432-4
   1. United States. Medicare Bureau. End-Stage Renal Disease
Program. 2. Chronic renal failure—Government policy—United
States. 3. Medicare. I. Rettig, Richard A. II. Levinsky, Norman
G. (Norman George), 1929- . III. Title.
   [DNLM: 1. Health Policy—United States. 2. Kidney Failure,
Chronic—economics—United States. 3. Kidney Failure, Chronic—
therapy. 4. Medicare—economics. WJ 342 I593k]
   RA645.K5157 1991
   362.1'9614'00973—dc20
   DNLM/DLC   91-15611
   for Library of Congress   CIP

Printed in the United States of America

The serpent has been a symbol of long life, healing, and knowledge among almost all cultures and religions since the beginning of recorded history. The image adopted as a logotype by the Institute of Medicine is based on a relief carving from ancient Greece, now held by the Staat-lichemussen in Berlin.

Study Staff

Division of Health Care Services

KARL D. YORDY, Director
RICHARD A. RETTIG, Study Director
JOEL H. BROIDA (1989)
YEN-PIN CHIANG, Research Associate
ANNE PAGE CHIAPELLA, Research Associate
DIANE B. MURDOCK, Research Associate
GREGORY P. YOUNG, Research Associate
DOUGLAS JOHNSON, Research Assistant
NAOMI H. HUDSON, Project Secretary
BRENDA A. PATTERSON, Project Secretary

Acknowledgments

This report results from the deliberations of the Institute of Medicine Committee for the Study of the Medicare End-Stage Renal Disease Program and its recommendations reflect the judgments of the committee.

The actual preparation of the report under the direction of the committee has been accomplished by the collective efforts of committee members, staff, and other contributors. The committee wishes to acknowledge its gratitude for these various contributions.

The committee thanks the authors of the commissioned papers and contract reports for their invaluable input to the deliberations of the committee and to its report. These experts include: William Amend, Marjorie A. Cahn, Harold I. Feldman, Richard N. Fine, Jose R. Garcia, Daniel S. Gaylin, Frank A. Gotch, Victor M. Hawthorne, Philip J. Held, Prakash Keshaviah, Michael J. Klag, Susan L. Laudecina, Bernard Lo, Nathan W. Levin, Edith T. Oberley, Mark V. Pauly, Anna Pesce, Victor E. Pollack, Drummond Rennie, Ash Seghal, Jonathan Showstack, and Constance S. Thomas. Their specific papers and reports are listed in Appendix C. In particular, it thanks Robert A. Wolfe for his essay, "Survival analysis methods for the End-Stage Renal Disease (ESRD) program of Medicare," published as Appendix D.

The committee expresses its appreciation to those individuals and organizations who testified before its two public hearings (Appendixes E and F), to the participants in the three workshops on ESRD staffing, kidney transplantation, and black and nonwhite renal failure patients (Appendixes G, H, and I), and to the participants in the patient focus groups (Appendix J).

The committee benefited from the work of the following consultants: Marcia F. Clark, Betty C. Crandall, John G. Eresian, Judith R. Lave, Dale Lupu, Naomi Naierman, and Winfred W. Williams.

The committee wishes to acknowledge the specific contributions of the

v

following individuals to the particular chapters of the report. The study director, Richard A. Rettig, had primary responsibility for preparation of the report. He and the committee chairman, Norman G. Levinsky, edited the entire document and prepared the Summary and Chapter 1. The other contributors to specific chapters were: Chapter 2, Gregory P. Young and Edith T. Oberley; Chapter 3, Christine K. Cassel, Alvin W. Moss, Richard A. Rettig, and Norman G. Levinsky; Chapter 4, Anne P. Chiapella, with the assistance of Paul W. Eggers; Chapter 5, Anne P. Chiapella; Chapter 6, Yen-Pin Chiang and Gregory P. Young; Chapter 7, Gregory P. Young and Yen-Pin Chiang; Chapter 8, Richard A. Rettig, Gregory P. Young, and Douglas Johnson; Chapter 9, Diane B. Murdock and Yen-Pin Chiang; Chapter 10, Richard A. Rettig and Yen-Pin Chiang; Chapter 11, Diane B. Murdock and Yen-Pin Chiang; Chapter 12, Richard A. Rettig, Sheldon Greenfield, John H. Sadler, and Klemens B. Meyer; Chapter 13, Richard A. Rettig; and Chapter 14, Richard A. Rettig and Anne P. Chiapella.

Several members of the Institute of Medicine's professional staff contributed to this report. Karl D. Yordy, as Director of the Division of Health Care Services, provided valuable guidance over the duration of the project. Marilyn J. Field made very useful comments on a draft of Chapters 9, 10, and 11. Similarly, Kathleen N. Lohr reviewed a draft of Chapter 12 and, during the time the two projects overlapped, kept us informed of the progress of the Institute of Medicine's study of quality assurance in the Medicare program.

The study and the resulting report would not have been possible without the dedicated support of the IOM staff, including Naomi Hudson, project secretary in 1990; Brenda Patterson, project secretary in 1989; H. Donald Tiller, administrative assistant; and Lisa Chimento and Nina Spruill, financial specialists. Wallace Waterfall provided helpful editorial advice.

Finally, support for this study was provided by the U.S. Department of Health and Human Services, Health Care Financing Administration, through a cooperative agreement (No. 14-C-99338/3-02). At HCFA, we thank Charles Booth and Bernadette Schumaker, Bureau of Policy Development; Paul Mendelsohn and Suzanne Rohrer, Health Standards and Quality Bureau; Kathy Sagel and Roger Milam, Bureau of Data Management and Strategy; and Paul W. Eggers and Joel Greer, Office of Research. Our special thanks go to Carl Josephson, project officer, Office of Research.

Contents

List of Tables and Figures ix

PART I   Overview

Summary.. 3
1 Introduction 23

PART II   Patients and Providers

2 Perspectives of ESRD Patients 39
3 Ethical Issues 51
4 The Patient Population 62
5 The ESRD Patient Population: Special Groups 85
6 Structure of the Provider Community....................... 110

PART III   Access

7 Access Problems of ESRD Patients 135
8 Access to Kidney Transplantation......................... 167

PART IV   Reimbursement and Quality

9 Medicare ESRD Payment Policy............................ 191
10 Reimbursement Effects on Quality 212
11 Outpatient Dialysis Reimbursement Issues 236
12 Quality Assessment and Assurance......................... 274

PART V Data and Research

13 Data Systems 315
14 Research Needs 328

APPENDIXES

A Glossary 335
B Acronyms and Initialisms.................................. 347
C Commissioned Papers and Contractor Reports 351
D Survival Analysis Methods for the End-Stage Renal
       Disease (ESRD) Program of Medicare, Robert A. Wolfe 353
E Institute of Medicine ESRD Study Committee
       Public Hearing, May 5, 1989, Chicago, Illinois 401
F Institute of Medicine ESRD Study Committee
       Public Hearing on "Issues in Dialysis Reimbursement
       Rate-Setting," February 15, 1990, Washington, D.C........... 403
G Institute of Medicine ESRD Study Committee
       Workshop on ESRD Staffing, November 3, 1989,
       Washington, D.C. 405
H Institute of Medicine ESRD Study Committee
       Workshop on Kidney Transplantation, December 13,
       1989, Washington, D.C. 406
I Institute of Medicine ESRD Study Committee
       Workshop on Black and Other Nonwhite ESRD
       Patients, May 15, 1990, Washington, D.C. 408
J Institute of Medicine ESRD Study Committee
       ESRD Patient Focus-Group Participants 409

Index 411

List of Tables and Figures

TABLES

1-1 Incidence and Prevalence of Patients in Medicare End-Stage Renal Disease (ESRD) Program, 1974-89, 28

1-2 New Elderly and Diabetic End-Stage Renal Disease (ESRD) Patients as a Percentage of New Medicare ESRD Patients, 29

1-3 Projections of Medicare End-Stage Renal Disease (ESRD) Patients to the Year 2000, 30

1-4 Cumulative Percentage Change in Medicare End-Stage Renal Disease (ESRD) Benefit Payments, 1974-88 Nominal and Real-Dollar Payments, 30

1-5 Growth of End-Stage Renal Disease (ESRD) Program: Patient Growth Versus Real-Dollar Benefit Payment Growth, 31

1-6 End-Stage Renal Disease (ESRD) Benefit Payments by Type of Service, 1988, 32

1-7 Medicare End-Stage Renal Disease (ESRD) Benefit Payments, 1974-88, 32

1-8 End-Stage Renal Disease (ESRD) Expenditures in Department of Veterans Affairs, 1984-89 (millions of dollars), 33

4-1 Age of New Dialysis Patients, 1960-67, 65

4-2 1967 Projections of New End-Stage Renal Disease (ESRD) Patients, 1968-77, 66

4-3 New End-Stage Renal Disease (ESRD) Patients by Age, Gender, Race, and Primary Diagnosis, 1978-89, 67

4-4 New End-Stage Renal Disease (ESRD) Patients per Million Population by Age, Gender, and Race, 1987, 68

4-5 New End-Stage Renal Disease (ESRD) Patients per Million Population by Primary Diagnosis, Gender, and Race, 1988, 69

4-6   Prevalent End-Stage Renal Disease (ESRD) Patients by Age, Gender, Race, and Primary Diagnosis, 1978-89, 70

4-7   Gross and Unadjusted One-Year Mortality for All End-Stage Renal Disease (ESRD) Patients, 1978-88, 73

4-8   Mortality for Medicare End-Stage Renal Disease (ESRD) Patients (ever entitled) Adjusted for Age, Race, Gender, and Primary Diagnosis, 1978-88 Patient Cohorts, 75

4-9   One-Year Mortality (percent) for All End-Stage Renal Disease (ESRD) Patients, at Year of Incidence, by Age, Gender, Race, and Primary Diagnosis, 1978-88, 76

4-10   One-Year Mortality (percent) for Dialysis Patients at Year of Incidence by Age, Gender, Race, and Primary Diagnosis, 1978-88, 78

4-11   Five-Year Survival of Dialysis Patients by Country and Diagnosis of Diabetes, 81

4-12   Medicare End-Stage Renal Disease (ESRD) Population Projections, Year 2000, 82

5-1   Incidence and Prevalence of Pediatric End-Stage Renal Disease (ESRD) Patients, 1978 and 1987, 86

5-2   Percentage of Pediatric End-Stage Renal Disease (ESRD) Patients with Functioning Graft, 1978 and 1987, 87

5-3   Pediatric End-Stage Renal Diseases (ESRD) Patient Survival (percent) at One Year by Year of Incidence and Age Group, 1978 and 1987, 88

5-4   New End-Stage Renal Disease (ESRD) Patients in 1978 and 1988, by Age Group, 91

5-5   Patients with Diabetic Kidney Disease as a Percentage of Total End-Stage Renal Disease (ESRD) Patients, by Age Group, 93

5-6   Percentage of U.S. Population with Definite Hypertension, 1976-80, 96

5-7   Incidence of Treated Hypertensive End-Stage Renal Disease (ESRD) per 10 Million Population by Age Group for Blacks and Whites in 1988, 98

5-8   End-Stage Renal Disease (ESRD) Treatment Modalities (percent) for Blacks and Whites on December 31, 1980, 1984, and 1988, 104

5-9   Survival of Black Versus Other Dialysis Patients by Year of Incidence, 104

6-1   Growth of Outpatient Dialysis Providers, 1980-88, 112

6-2   Definitions of Dialysis Unit Size, Demand, Capacity, and Utilization, 113

6-3   Outpatient Dialysis Providers, Independent Versus Hospital-Based, 1980-88, 117

6-4   Outpatient Dialysis Providers, For-Profit Versus Not-For-Profit, 1980-88, 120

6-5   Outpatient Dialysis Providers, by Profit Status and Type of Facility, 1980-88, 121

6-6 Outpatient Dialysis Providers, by Facility Size, 1980-88, 125

6-7 Outpatient Dialysis Providers, by Type of Facility, Profit Status, and Size, 1980-88, 127

6-8 Hemodialysis Stations, by Type of Facility, Profit Status, and Size, 1980-88, 128

7-1 Medicare Eligibility Status of Dialysis Patients, 1980-89, 138

7-2 Percentage of Non-Medicare Patients Among Total Dialysis Patients, by State and Year, 1980-89, 139

7-3 Percentage of Non-Medicare Patients Among Total Dialysis Patients, by City Versus State, and Year, 1980-87, 141

7-4 Services of State Kidney Programs, 144

7-5 Trends in State Kidney Program Expenditures, 145

7-6 Department of Veterans Affairs (DVA) Expenditures for Dialysis Patients, 1980-89, 147

7-7 ESRD Facility Capacity and Utilization, 1984 and 1988, 159

7-8 Connecticut ESRD Patient Log, 161

7-9 Percentage of Non-Medicare Total Dialysis Patients by State and Year, 1980-89, 162

Appendix: Estimated Additional Program Expenditures Required for Universal Entitlement of Medicare ESRD Program, 1990-95, 166

8-1 Number and Type of Kidney Transplant Procedures (Medicare and Non-Medicare), by Donor Type, 1980-89, 169

8-2 One-Year Survival of Kidney Transplant Patients 1980, 1984, and 1988, 170

8-3 Distribution of Kidney Transplants (percent) by Age and Type of Transplant, 1989, 175

8-4 Percentage of Responses to Organ Transplantation/Donation Surveys, 1983, 1984, and 1987, 181

Appendix: Estimated Additional Medicare ESRD Program Expenditures Required for Removing the 3-Year Eligibility Limit of Transplant Patients and the 1-Year Limit on Payment for Immuno-suppressive Drugs, 1990-95, 187

9-1 Comparison of the Inpatient Hospital Prospective Payment System (PPS) and ESRD Outpatient Dialysis Payment Policy, 194

9-2 Medicare Payment for Facility Outpatient Dialysis Services, 196

9-3 Medicare ESRD Benefit Payments, by Type of Service, 1974-87 (in millions of dollars and as percent of total), 206

10-1 Outpatient Dialysis Units: Staff Hours per Patient-Week, 1982 and 1987, 219

10-2 Staffing Changes, 1986-1990: North Central Dialysis Centers, Chicago, Illinois, 220

11-1 Injections for Per Year Complex Medications, Hemodialysis Outpatients, University of Cincinnati Medical Center and Dialysis Clinic, Inc.-Cincinnati, 1978-1989, 240

11-2 Outpatient Dialysis Facilities, 1985: Distribution of Differences (in dollars) Between Facility-Specific Composite Rates and Audited Costs, 246

11-3 Outpatient Dialysis Facilities, 1985: Distribution of Differences (in dollars) Between Facility-Specific Composite Rates and Reported (unaudited) Costs, 248

11-4 Outpatient Dialysis Facilities, 1985: Comparison of Differences Between Reported (unaudited) and Audited Costs (in dollars), 250

11-5 Results of Alternative Scenarios for Rebasing and Updating the ESRD Composite Rate for All Dialysis Facilities, 254

12-1 Conditions of Coverage for ESRD Providers, 289

13-1 Medicare Data Sources and Data Files for ESRD Patients and Providers, 317

D-1 Death Rates and Age Among All Black ESRD Patients in 1988, 385

D-2 Survival Probabilities for ESRD Patients Incident in 1979, 387

FIGURES

1-1 Medicare ESRD Benefit Payments, 31

4-1 Number of ESRD Patients by Age Group, 1978-88, 64

4-2 Number of ESRD Patients by Primary Diagnosis, 1978-88, 64

4-3 Number of ESRD Patients, Actual and Projected, 1974-2000, 83

5-1 ESRD Patients: Treatment Modality by Age Group, 1988, 92

5-2 Age Distribution of New ESRD Patients, by Race, 1988, 100

5-3 Distribution of Primary Diagnosis Leading to ESRD, by Race, 1986-88, 101

5-4 ESRD Patients, by Race, 1978-88, 103

5-5 Two-Year Survival of Transplanted Cadaver Kidneys, by Race, 1978-88, 105

6-1 Outpatient Dialysis Units, 1980-88: Independent Versus Hospital-Based, 118

6-2 Outpatient Hemodialysis Stations, 1980-88: Independent Versus Hospital-Based Units, 119

6-3 Outpatient Hemodialysis Units, 1980-88: For-Profit Versus Not-For-Profit, 123

6-4 Outpatient Hemodialysis Stations, 1980-88: For-Profit Versus Not-For-Profit Units, 123

6-5 Outpatient Dialysis Units, by Size, 1980-88, 126

8-1 Kidney Transplantation Procedures and ESRD Patients on Waiting Lists, 1980-88, 171

9-1 Outpatient Dialysis Reimbursement Rates for Independent Units, 1973-89 (current and constant dollars), 198

12-1 Conceptual Framework of the Medical Outcomes Study, 278

Kidney Failure
and the
Federal Government

PART I
Overview

This part of the report includes the Summary and Chapter 1. The former summarizes the report and presents the recommendations of the committee. Chapter 1 introduces the report and indicates how it is organized.

Summary

THE CONGRESSIONAL CHARGE TO
THE INSTITUTE OF MEDICINE

In the Social Security Amendments of 1972, Congress created an entitlement to Medicare for all persons with a diagnosis of permanent kidney failure who were fully or currently insured or eligible for benefits under Social Security, and for spouses or dependent children of such persons. The End-Stage Renal Disease (ESRD) program thus established has been very successful, saving several hundred thousand Americans from premature death and giving hope to individuals who once faced certain death. At present, over 150,000 ESRD patients receive Medicare services, including inpatient and outpatient care, from both physicians and treatment units, for dialysis, kidney transplantation, and other medical services.

The ESRD program is unique within Medicare. It is the only case in which the diagnosis of a categorical disease provides the basis for an entitlement for persons of all ages. In addition, both ESRD patients and providers depend on Medicare reimbursement policy to a greater extent than in any other domain of medicine. Its highly visible status has led Congress to request studies of various aspects of the program from time to time.

In the Omnibus Budget Reconciliation Act of 1987 (OBRA 1987),[1] Congress asked the Institute of Medicine (IOM) to study the ESRD program with respect to the following issues:

- major epidemiological and demographic changes in the ESRD patient population that may affect access to treatment, quality of care, or the resource requirements of the program (Chapters 4 and 5),
- access to treatment by persons with chronic kidney failure, both those eligible and those not eligible for Medicare benefits (Chapters 7 and 8),

• the quality of care provided to ESRD beneficiaries, as measured by clinical indicators, functional status of patients, and patient satisfaction (Chapter 12),
• the effect of reimbursement on quality of care (Chapters 9, 10, and 11), and
• the adequacy of existing data systems to monitor these matters on a continuing basis (Chapter 13).

The IOM convened an expert committee to conduct the study; this report constitutes its response.[2] The committee also examined patient perspectives (Chapter 2), ethical issues (Chapter 3), the structure of the provider community (Chapter 6), and ESRD research needs (Chapter 14).

BASIC ASSUMPTIONS

The committee believes that people with permanent renal failure should be the primary concern of Medicare ESRD policy. This emphasis is reflected in the chapters that deal with patient perspectives, ethical issues, and the epidemiology of the patient population, as well as in the committee's concern with access, quality, and reimbursement.

Some recommendations of this committee would entail increased funding. The committee recommends (in Chapters 7 and 8) that Congress extend the Medicare entitlement for ESRD treatment to all Americans, remove the three-year limit on Medicare eligibility of successful transplant recipients, and pay for immunosuppressive drugs for the period of a transplant patient's entitlement. It proposes these as ways to improve an already successful program by increasing the equitable treatment of all ESRD patients and promoting improved patient outcomes.

The committee was not asked to address, nor has it considered, the broader health needs of the American people or the relation of expenditures for ESRD patients relative to other deserving claimants. However, the committee recognizes that Congress must weigh the recommendations that involve increased funding against competing uses of resources and must make the appropriate and equitable decisions regarding the allocation of scarce resources. The committee is quite aware of the fact that the continuing annual federal budget deficits and increasing health care costs make such decisions very difficult.

The IOM committee, therefore, endorses the following objectives for the Medicare ESRD program: to guarantee access to treatment for all for whom it is medically appropriate; to provide care of high quality that achieves desirable health outcomes consistent with patient health status and current professional knowledge; to develop policies that steadily improve patient well-being and patient outcomes; and to manage the program prudently at the lowest cost compatible with adequate care.

ESRD PATIENTS AND THEIR TREATMENT

The number of patients under treatment for ESRD has grown substantially over time, increasing from approximately 10,000 beneficiaries when the entitlement became effective in 1973, to over 150,000 dialysis and transplant patients today. In the year 2000, it is projected that a quarter of a million patients will be enrolled in the ESRD program.

The ESRD patient population is highly diverse in age, sex, race, and primary diagnosis and has changed greatly over time. For example, those 65 years and older increased from 5 percent of the total Medicare ESRD population in 1973 to 27 percent in 1988, and accounted for 38 percent of all new patients in 1988. The major diseases causing kidney failure are glomerulonephritis, diabetes, and hypertension. The proportion of ESRD patients with a primary diagnosis of diabetes mellitus increased from about 13 percent in 1980 to 24 percent in 1988; this diagnosis accounted for 31 percent of all new patients in 1988. Those with a primary diagnosis of hypertension increased from about 20 percent in 1980 to 24 percent in 1988; they constituted 27 percent of new patients in 1988.

Kidney failure is nearly four times as frequent among blacks as in whites. In the late 1960s, black patients constituted 10 percent of the treated ESRD patient population; today they represent 29 percent of the total population and 28 percent of all new patients. Several studies suggest that renal failure in the growing Hispanic population also is substantially higher than in the white population. These trends—more elderly, more diabetic and hypertensive patients, and disproportionate representation of minorities—have characterized the ESRD program in the 1980s and will continue to do so in the 1990s.

The ESRD patient population, as of December 31, 1988, is distributed by treatment modality as follows: 60 percent, hemodialysis; 10 percent, peritoneal dialysis; 25 percent, transplantation; and 5 percent, unknown. Even though dialysis is the major ESRD treatment modality, kidney transplantation is clearly the treatment of choice for the great majority of renal failure patients in the committee's view. Kidney transplants increased from almost 3,200 in 1974 to almost 9,000 in 1986. The number of Medicare ESRD beneficiaries with functioning transplanted kidneys was 30,000 at the end of 1989; another 10,000 individuals with functioning transplants are estimated to have left the Medicare rolls after reaching the three-year limit on eligibility for benefits. The outcome of both living related and cadaver donor transplants, as measured by survival of the recipient and the transplanted kidney, has improved markedly during the past decade largely because of improved ways to prevent kidney rejection. The total number of transplants performed, however, has leveled off since 1986 due to a shortage of kidneys.

A major challenge of ESRD treatment, for both individuals and society, is its cost. Based on 1987 cost data provided by the Health Care Financing

Adminstration (HCFA), the annual Medicare expenditure for a dialysis patient was $32,000. First-year expenditures for a successful transplant patient were $56,000, but were only $6,000 in each subsequent year. These costs are not atypical for patients with serious, chronic diseases. Medicare, of course, does not cover all costs either for dialysis or transplant patients: premiums, deductibles, and copayments must be met from other sources.

Although total ESRD program costs are high, cost control for dialysis has been impressive. The initial reimbursement rates for outpatient dialysis were established in 1973 and remained unchanged until 1983. They were lowered in 1983 and again in 1986. During this time, no adjustment was made for inflation. In real dollars, payment rates per dialysis treatment have fallen steadily over the program's history. The outpatient dialysis reimbursement rate was $138 in 1974 and $125 in 1989. *When adjusted for inflation by the GNP price deflator, the 1989 reimbursement rate was less than $54 in 1974 dollars, a 61 percent reduction over this period.*

In 1988, Medicare spent $3.0 billion ($1.3 billion in 1974 dollars) for ESRD beneficiaries. (A recent estimate by HCFA, using a new methodology, places 1988 expenditure at $3.7 billion.) Total national expenditures for ESRD patients from all sources are estimated at $5.4 billion in 1988. The total cost of the program has grown primarily because the number of patients has increased steadily over time. It has been controlled by progressively lower real costs per dialysis treatment, by the beneficial cost effects of successful transplantation, and by some shifting of payment responsibility to private payers.

ACCESS

The kidney provision of the Social Security Amendments of 1972 removed most of the financial barriers to ESRD treatment for the vast majority of U.S. citizens. However, it did not establish a universal benefit, a fact not widely appreciated. From the outset of the program through 1986, Medicare-certified dialysis facilities reported 6-7 percent of the ESRD dialysis patients as not eligible for benefits; this proportion increased to 7.2 percent in 1987 and 7.5 percent in 1989. The absolute number of such patients has been growing, and substantial variation exists among states and major cities.

The major non-Medicare sources for financing ESRD treatment are not adequate to meet the needs of the unentitled patients. The Department of Veterans Affairs dialysis program is shrinking, the Indian Health Service faces many other demands on its limited resources, and the 19 state kidney disease programs have benefits that vary and budgets that are not increasing. State Medicaid programs, therefore, represent the only payer for many ESRD patients who are not eligible for Medicare. Although Medicaid ESRD benefits appear to be adequate in many states, in others they are not, as eligibility criteria and covered benefits vary widely according to state discretion. Moreover, as state Medicaid programs consume a rapidly increasing proportion of state government budgets, they will be closely scrutinized by governors and legislatures and are unlikely to receive more resources for ESRD services.

Practically speaking, eligibility for Medicare ESRD coverage is a function of Social Security insured status.[3] Those ineligible include some federal, state, and local government employees,[4] domestic, farm and all other workers in covered occupations but who may not have applied for benefits, and those who have never worked, such as young, nonworking mothers, many welfare mothers, and their children. Persons in most of these categories are disproportionately concentrated among the poor and minorities.

The available evidence on ESRD patients who are reported as not eligible for Medicare coverage is sparse. No information is available about their demographic, health status, and socioeconomic characteristics nor about the effects of their noneligible status on the receipt or denial of treatment. Clearly, information on these matters should be obtained. However, the committee does not believe that access to life-saving dialysis and transplantation should depend on the precise number of ESRD patients not eligible for Medicare. Limiting Medicare ESRD eligibility to those with Social Security insured status places some excluded persons at risk of death.

> **As a matter of equitable treatment of all individuals with end-stage renal disease, the committee finds no justifiable basis for restricting Medicare eligibility other than citizenship or resident alien status. It recommends that Congress modify the Medicare eligibility criteria for individuals with ESRD and extend the entitlement to all United States citizens and resident aliens.**

Kidney transplant patients face two major restrictions on access. First, their Medicare eligibility is limited to a three-year period following a successful transplant. Second, they are eligible for only a single year of reimbursement for expensive immunosuppressive drugs which they must take on a life-long basis. Transplant patients are not cured: they remain at risk of rejecting the transplanted kidney throughout their lives; the medications they must take to prevent rejection place them at risk of other medical problems. Congress, in various pieces of legislation enacted in 1978, 1984, 1986, 1988, and 1990, has sought to encourage organ transplantation. However, the committee believes that the Medicare limits on eligibility of transplant patients and on payment for immunosuppressive drugs inadvertently tend to discourage kidney transplantation and should be changed to foster this treatment.

> **The committee recommends that Congress eliminate the three-year Medicare eligibility limit for successful transplant patients and thereby authorize a lifetime entitlement comparable to that of dialysis patients.**

The committee also recommends that coverage for payment of immunosuppressive medications for kidney transplant patients be made coterminous with the period of entitlement.

The reasons for the shortage of transplantable kidneys are not well understood. Although several studies suggest that only a fraction of suitable kidneys is made available for renal transplantation, the extent of the gap between potential and actual donors is unclear and effective ways to close this gap are not well understood. When coupled with the rapid annual increase in new ESRD patients, the shortage of kidneys means that dialysis will continue to be the predominant form of ESRD treatment. Because transplantation is generally recognized as the preferred therapy for the great majority of ESRD patients, because kidneys are scarce, and because the long-term cost of transplantation is less than dialysis,

the committee recommends that increasing the donation of kidneys receive very high priority in the coming decade.

ETHICS

Dialysis and transplantation have raised ethical questions since their introduction to clinical practice in the early 1960s. The questions have changed over time as the patient population, treatment, and financing have changed. The committee focused on three major concerns—the acceptance of patients for treatment, the termination of treatment, and ethical questions arising for caregivers who deal with problem patients.

Some concern has been expressed that patient acceptance criteria have expanded since enactment of the Medicare ESRD entitlement, resulting in an increasing number of patients with limited survival possibilities and relatively poor quality of life. *The committee, recognizing this concern, believes that patient acceptance criteria should be medical, not economic, and based on concern for the best interest of individual patients.* Age was considered and explicitly rejected by the committee as a patient acceptance criterion, as it does not measure the ability of an individual to benefit from treatment. Comorbidities—at any age—are the primary determinants of quality of life and of survival.

Decision making about the initiation of treatment should result from informed discussion among the patient, the family, the physician, and other caregivers. ESRD patients usually rate their quality of life higher than do "objective" observers. This emphasizes the need to regard patient preferences very highly in decisions about their care. However, physicians should recognize that the existence of a public entitlement does not mean that they are obligated to treat all patients who present with kidney failure. Clinical judgment and patient-family preferences will sometimes indicate terminal palliative care rather than life-extending care. Thus, the choice is not between treatment and abandonment, but rather between different goals of treatment.

Withdrawal from treatment by competent patients is increasingly reported, especially among the elderly. This should be regarded as a rational decision by an autonomous person who has concluded that the burdens of continuing treatment outweigh the benefits. The termination of treatment of incompetent patients should occur only after full discussion between the patient's family, or other representatives, and the physician.

Three types of patients raise different ethical problems for clinicians today: the noncompliant, self-destructive dialysis patient; the hostile, abusive dialysis patient; and the self-destructive transplant patient. The physician's responsibility is to care for the patient with an understanding of human frailty and the complex psychology of living with chronic illness, to develop and maintain effective communication with them, and to assure continuity of care. The self-destructive transplant patient whose behavior threatens the survival of the transplanted kidney may disqualify himself as a candidate for a subsequent transplant if the current organ fails.

> **The committee recommends that patients, clinicians in adult and pediatric nephrology, and bioethicists develop guidelines for evaluating patients for whom the burdens of renal replacement therapy may substantially outweigh the benefits. These guidelines should be flexible and encourage the physician to use discretion in assessing an individual patient. Guidelines should be developed specifically for children and should describe the role of the parents in the decision-making process.**

> **Nephrologists and other clinicians should discuss with all ESRD patients their wishes about dialysis, cardiopulmonary resuscitation, and other life-sustaining treatments and encourage documented advance directives.**

> **ESRD clinicians should be encouraged to participate in continuing education in medical ethics and health law. Some specialists in the medical ethics of renal disease should be available to educate clinicians, to train members of ethics committees, and to do research on ethical issues in dialysis and transplantation.**

THE PROVIDER COMMUNITY

The organization of the provider community has changed over time. During the past decade, the number of transplant centers increased from 150 to 219. Organ procurement organizations (OPOs) shifted from being hospital-based to being independent entities, and consolidation of OPOs occurred in response to the National Organ Transplant Act of 1986.

Treatment capacity for outpatient dialysis grew from 1980 to 1988: the number of units increased at an annual rate of 7.1 percent, from 1,004 to 1,740 units; the number of approved dialysis stations increased at an average annual rate of 8.1 percent from 12,216 to 22,803.[5] The demand for treatment also grew during this time; outpatient hemodialysis treatments increased at an average annual rate of 9.7 percent from over 5,672,000 in 1980 to 11,866,000 in 1988. The increased demand for treatment outpaced the growth in treatment capacity and resulted in an increased utilization of units and stations at the national level. On empirical grounds, the committee concludes that the rate of growth in outpatient treatment capacity, measured by treatment stations, is not unreasonable in relation to the increased demand for treatment, measured by number of treatments. It further observes that normative criteria relating capacity to demand have not been advanced by either the provider community or HCFA.

Independent rather than hospital-based units accounted for most of the growth in outpatient dialysis facilities. They now account for 70 percent of all dialysis stations. The independents' share of dialysis treatments increased from 40 percent to more than 60 percent between 1980 and 1988. For-profit units, primarily independent, increased more rapidly than not-for-profit units. The committee is not aware of any evidence that shifts among providers from hospital-based to independent and from nonprofit to for-profit dialysis facilities have resulted in access or quality problems.

It recommends, however, that such changes be monitored closely to assess their implications for access and quality.

Differences in growth of dialysis capacity are apparent between states having certificate-of-need (CON) and those without CON. CON states have had much slower increases in the number of units and stations, and thus greater utilization in both treatments and patients per station.

Who benefits from state CON regulations as they are applied to ESRD units? In particular, what are the effects of higher utilization (or productivity) of treatment capacity in CON states? Existing data permit only a limited response. First, higher utilization does not reduce Medicare expenditures, nor does lower utilization in non-CON states involve any additional cost to Medicare. Second, CON confers local monopoly benefits on approved providers, allowing them to reap the economic benefits of increased productivity; the costs of the legal defense of monopoly, moreover, can be absorbed more easily by provider chains than by single-owner facilities. Third, by sanctioning local provider monopoly, CON decreases patient choice of providers and eliminates competition among facilities for patients on the basis of amenities. Fourth, CON provides no assurance of improved quality, for which it was not designed. Finally, in some states it has contributed to serious access problems.

The committee finds no persuasive reason for the application of state certificate-of-need regulations on dialysis treatment capacity that is regulated mainly by the Medicare payment level. The committee strongly favors the elimination of CON as applied to dialysis facilities, but recognizes that this requires state government rather than federal government action. It recommends that HCFA review with each of the relevant states the effect of CON regulations on ESRD patient access to care in light of national data on utilization.

REIMBURSEMENT AND QUALITY

The committee confronted several basic facts as it considered the effects of reimbursement on quality. First, reimbursement rates for outpatient dialysis, in real dollars, have steadily decreased over the 18-year history of the ESRD program, due both to a fixed rate (from 1973 to 1983) that was never adjusted for inflation as well as to explicit rate reductions in 1983 and 1986. No other part of the Medicare program has been subjected to a similar reimbursement policy.

Second, quality has not been systematically measured or monitored by the federal agencies responsible for the ESRD program. HCFA has initiated a quality assurance effort within the past several years, but it currently bears no relationship to reimbursement policy.

Third, HCFA argues that reimbursement rates should be cut still further, although no system exists to monitor the effects of such cuts on quality. On the other hand, many providers, patients, and researchers believe that quality has been adversely affected by the progressive reductions in reimbursement and that further cuts will erode quality dangerously. Regrettably, existing data are inadequate to document adequately whether or how quality has changed over time or to determine whether the present level of quality is reasonable in the context of the patient population and current professional knowledge. Evaluating these divergent views has been a major endeavor of this committee.

Reimbursement Effects on Quality

The committee examined several aspects of the effect of reimbursement on quality: mortality, morbidity (as measured by hospitalization), dialysis unit staffing patterns, and treatment innovation.

The trends in mortality in the ESRD program in the 1980s have received much attention. After a period of stable mortality rates from 1978 to 1982, an abrupt rise in unadjusted ESRD mortality occurred between 1982 and 1983, and gross mortality has increased since then. Interpretation of this rise is complicated by changes in the patient population, treatment patterns, and methodological factors. For example, the incidence and prevalence of elderly and diabetic ESRD patients, who often have other comorbid conditions, have increased. These patients have higher mortality rates than younger patients or those without diabetes. ESRD mortality data, when adjusted for age and primary diagnosis, show stability over time.

The committee examined the question of the effects of reimbursement on mortality, which only two studies have addressed directly. In 1987, an Urban Institute report (Held et al., 1987) found no association between the introduction in 1983 of the composite rate, which reduced reimbursement to most providers, and a change in mortality. In 1990, this study requested the Urban Institute to update its earlier analysis. This more recent analysis, discussed in Chapter 10, suggests, by one approach (a price-level model), an inverse relation between patient mortality and the standardized price (reimbursement rate) received by a dialysis facility. This relation was not statistically supported by a second approach (a first-difference model). The committee regards these results as suggestive but insufficient to establish firmly a direct effect of reimbursement on quality.

An indirect effect of reimbursement changes on mortality is suggested. Treatment times of dialysis patients have become shorter in the past decade, due partly to the pressures to reduce costs by treating more patients in a given nursing shift. Shorter treatment time has been implicated in higher mortality. Although an inverse relation of reimbursement to mortality is not proved directly, decreased reimbursement is associated with shorter treatment time. The committee interprets this possible indirect effect cautiously, since factors such as prevailing clinical opinion and patient preferences appear to have influenced treatment time.

The use of mortality as an outcome measure represents a positive step toward the quantification of outcomes. However, the emphasis on the effect of the 1983 composite rate on mortality may be inappropriate. The changing patient population has been mentioned above, as has the effect of clinical opinion on shorter treatment time. In addition, the reimbursement reduction introduced by the 1983 composite rate was small compared with the unadjusted effects of inflation over a longer time. Finally, physicians and treatment units, confronting reduced reimbursement, tend to adapt in numerous ways that may protect the lives of patients but may result in diminished quality as reflected in increased morbidity, inadequate dialysis, reduced staffing patterns, and lower health status.

The committee examined hospitalization as a measure of morbidity. In 1987, the Urban Institute (Held et al., 1987) found that inpatient stays of a 1984 ESRD patient cohort were higher than those of a 1982 cohort, but did not find an association between the decrease in the payment rate in 1983 and increased inpatient stays in the following year. The 1990 Urban Institute study (Held et al., 1990) provides some evidence that the level of the dialysis price may affect hospital use by ESRD patients. Using a price-level model, the study found a significant inverse correlation between the dialysis price level and hospital admission rates as well as hospital length of stay (days). These results were most conclusive for diabetic patients, who are clinically less stable and often require extra care in management on dialysis. However, when the data were analyzed by a different method in which each facility was used as its own control (first-difference model), there was no correlation between price changes and hospital use. As with mortality, there is the suggestion that there may be an indirect effect mediated by changes in dialysis treatment time. Shorter treatment time, which correlates with reduced reimbursement, also correlates with increased hospitalization. Thus, there is evidence that reimbursement reductions are associated with excess morbidity as measured by hospitalization, but no firm conclusions can be drawn.

Staffing in a treatment unit is a structural measure of quality. There is increasing evidence of staff changes as a result of reimbursement. One study found that units receiving higher payment had more total staffing hours per patient per week and more registered nurses (RNs) available per patient; the converse was true for units receiving a lower payment. Another study showed a reduction of 17 percent in total staff hours per patient per week for hospital-based outpatient units and 11 percent for independent units from 1982 to 1987. Data from several providers also show that staff-to-patient ratios decreased substantially during the 1980s.

The composition of dialysis unit staff has changed as well: in general, the proportion of RNs decreased, that of technicians increased, and licensed practical nurses and nursing assistants show a mixed pattern. Replacement of RNs with technicians decreases the clinical training and skill level of the personnel who directly treat patients.

Staffing by social workers and dietitians also decreased during the 1980s. These professionals are currently responsible for very large numbers of patients; for example, staff-to-patient ratios of 1 to 100 and 1 to 200, respectively, exist in many dialysis units. Consequently, social workers and dietitians may have been reduced to fulfilling minimal routine functions rather than the essential social or nutrition counseling considered optimal for patient care.

ESRD reimbursement policies for outpatient dialysis have resulted in reduced staffing patterns. Although optimal patterns are not known, the professional capability to treat a patient population of increasing complexity has been reduced. However, the effect of these staffing changes on patient outcomes has not been monitored and should be assessed. At minimum, HCFA should recognize the likely impact of any proposed reimbursement reductions on staffing and undertake to monitor the effect of decreased payments on patient management and outcomes.

The committee also considered the effects of reimbursement on innovation. In general, economic discipline has encouraged cost-reducing, quality-enhancing technical change in the competitive equipment and supplies product market. Such economies have reduced the equipment and supply (nonlabor) component of the total cost per dialysis treatment from roughly one-third fifteen years ago to one-fifth or less at present. Further cost-saving technical change, therefore, will afford smaller economic benefits to providers and payers.

Major clinical innovations, such as cyclosporine for preventing rejection of the transplanted kidney and erythropoietin for treating anemia in dialysis patients, have resulted from progress in basic scientific research. The development of such innovations is not likely to be influenced by ESRD reimbursement policy, although their adoption and use by the medical community surely will be.

Some data suggest that decreased reimbursement may increase mortality, directly or indirectly. However, available studies are insufficient to establish either a direct or an indirect effect of reimbursement on mortality conclusively. Similarly, some studies suggest but do not prove a direct or indirect effect of decreased reimbursement on increased morbidity, assessed from hospitalization data.

Data strongly suggest that decreased reimbursement has led to decreased staffing in dialysis units, to shifts from nurses to technicians, and to important reductions in social worker and dietitian staffing. Although there is no evidence that these changes in staffing patterns have affected quality, professional opinion favors this contention.

Dialysis treatment time has decreased in the past decade. Studies indicate that decreased time may have adversely affected mortality and morbidity. The shorter times are attributable in part to economic pressure from decreased reimbursement. However, a clear relation between quality and reimbursement cannot be established because clinical judgment and patient preference also have influenced shortening of dialysis times.

The lack of progressive improvement in age- and diagnosis-adjusted dialysis patient mortality over the past decade suggests that providers may have reached the limits of increasing efficacy in the application of current technology. It is possible that age- and diagnosis-adjusted mortality would have improved over the past decade, as has happened with other medical conditions, had reimbursement not been eroded by reductions and by inflation. Even if prior reductions in reimbursement had had *no* effect, it does not follow logically that further decreases will not increase mortality. We may be at the edge of a "slippery slope," beyond which further cuts will have large effects because the limit of ability of providers to absorb the effects of decreased payment without dangerously eroding quality has been reached. Because dialysis is a life-sustaining treatment, the committee concluded that it must give some weight even to imperfect data that point in the direction of adverse effects.

Taken together, the suggestive evidence deserves attention because all results point in the same direction (decreased reimbursement may have eroded quality). Changes in quality are related temporally to changes in reimbursement, and the underlying behavioral and physiological hypotheses are plausible. Although none of these studies constitute conclusive proof of the adverse effects of prior reductions in reimbursement on patient outcomes, none rule out such an effect. None suggest that such reductions are contributing to improved quality of care.

Outpatient Dialysis Reimbursement Issues

The committee addressed the implications for dialysis reimbursement policy of the information about (1) the effect of reimbursement on quality of care and (2) future needs in the light of projections of growth in the size and diversity of the dialysis patient population over the next decade. It did so (in Chapter 11) with respect to covered services, the rate-setting process, and payment policy for facilities and physicians. Transplant reimbursement issues are treated in Chapter 9.

Covered Services

Two broad approaches to reimbursement policy were considered, which may be termed the "implicit" and the "explicit" approaches. Historical and current policy has taken the implicit approach. Since the inception of the ESRD program, Medicare has defined the set of covered services as "all necessary services" required for dialysis and has listed the items that are included within this framework (as well as separately billable services). These services implicitly reflect what providers do in the dialysis procedure. Rates are determined by what providers actually spend to deliver these dialysis services to patients.

This approach minimizes governmental involvement in clinical practice. Providers are free to use their judgment in deciding how to achieve quality within the limits of their reimbursement rate. Historically, this implicit rate-setting process succeeded in financing adequate care for patients, fostered progressive reduction in costs, promoted technical innovations, and developed a climate in which dialysis capacity grew appropriately to meet increasing patient need.

However, the committee came to believe on the basis of the data assembled in this report that the current reimbursement system needs modification if it is to serve dialysis patients and society well in the future. Concern about the implicit rate-setting method arose primarily because it makes no connection between reimbursement and quality.

In particular, covered services have changed over time without change in reimbursement: some services that were billed separately before 1983 have since been incorporated into the composite rate; in addition, the composite rate now covers some services, such as the labor-intensive administration of complex medications, that were nonexistent in 1983. Although covered services have changed, no explicit analysis has been made to determine how reduced payment levels have influenced what providers do or whether the outcomes of care are altered. Nor have proposed reimbursement changes been made with a prior assessment of their likely quality impacts.

The committee's concern is that implicit rate-setting may have generated a vicious cycle in which rate reductions lead to unmonitored system-wide quality reductions; the lower cost of these inferior services then constitutes the basis in the rate-setting process for a cut in reimbursement.

Two policy options were considered by the committee. First, continue to rely on the implicit definition of covered services that is used by HCFA, i.e., defining covered services in terms of what providers actually furnish to dialysis patients.[6] Second, as some providers recommend, develop a more explicit definition of covered services. Absent data on the effects of reimbursement on patient outcomes to guide an explicit approach, the committee favors continued reliance on the implicit standard. However, the committee is concerned that the services currently provided reflect not only professional judgments but also the effects of prior reductions in reimbursement that may have reduced services below desirable levels. Therefore, it believes that a technical advisory committee should examine covered services on a continuing basis and make judgments about the elements needed for appropriate care and outcomes, ideally based on patient outcomes research.

Rate-Setting and Payment Policy

ESRD providers operate in a system dominated by Medicare. HCFA determines the services that are to be included in the reimbursement rates, the reimbursement rates for these services, and the corresponding audited or allowable "costs" of providing these services. Allowable costs, in turn, provide the basis for rate revision.

Nominally, reimbursement rates for dialysis are based on the audited costs of providers. In fact, the rate-setting process for dialysis facilities, unlike that for the hospital sector under prospective payment, has made no provision for updating rates to reflect the effects of inflation on costs during the time between the year when cost data are collected and the adoption of a new rate. The current rate is based on 1977-79 cost data and has never been updated for inflation.

In principle, rates should be recalculated (rebased) periodically using timely data on audited costs. Rebasing, in effect, adjusts reimbursement to reflect the cost of the services providers actually furnish patients. As noted above, the committee believes that current expenditure levels by providers reflect not only their professional judgment of services needed for adequate care of dialysis patients but also the effects of prior reductions in reimbursement that may have reduced services below desirable levels. Therefore, it seems imprudent to rebase payment now using recent audited provider cost data.

The committee proposes two stages for reimbursement policy. First, for the immediate future, rates should not be decreased. Moreover, until a quality assessment program is in place, annual rates should be adjusted for inflation by some appropriate factor. During this initial phase of the proposed rate-setting policy, the committee believes that a quality assessment and assurance program should be implemented. It notes the research opportunity inherent in the data showing wide variations in costs among dialysis units. Analysis of the relation between cost and quality may reveal that the least costly units have maintained quality or, on the contrary, that low costs have been achieved only at the price of unacceptable decreases in quality.

Second, once a quality assessment program is in place, HCFA may wish to revert to an "implicit" rate-setting process. Should that process lead to rate reductions, HCFA will be in a position to monitor its effects in patients. The committee discussed the alternative of an "explicit" rate-setting process that would specify a detailed "bundle of services" needed for the adequate care of dialysis patients. The sum of the prices of these individual components would constitute the basis for rate-setting. However, the committee decided against this alternative because it would unduly involve government agencies in setting detailed and potentially rigid standards of clinical practice. On the other hand, the committee felt strongly that some mechanism for ongoing review of rate-setting was appropriate. It recommends, therefore, that ProPAC, which has been mandated to review ambulatory care, also review rate-setting in the ESRD program.[7] In addition, the committee recommends that HCFA establish an expert committee to advise it on potential additions to the "bundle of services" needed for dialysis patients as innovations arise and clinical practice changes.

Given a patient population of increasing complexity, suggestive but not conclusive evidence of the erosion of quality, the absence of a system to monitor quality, and the life-saving nature of dialysis treatment,

the committee recommends[8] that Congress and HCFA adopt the following payment policies for dialysis facilities:

Do not reduce the composite rate at this time.

Do not, at present, rebase (recalculate) the rate using recent cost report data because there is reason to believe that current costs reflect prior payment reductions rather than provider decisions about the services needed for appropriate medical care.

Follow general Medicare payment policies in setting dialysis payment policies:

1. Update the rate yearly, as is the practice for the rest of Medicare.
2. Rebase the rate only when HCFA rebases the other parts of Medicare governed by the Prospective Payment System.
3. Ultimately, predicate rebasing of outpatient dialysis reimbursement on efficacy and quality studies that determine the components needed for appropriate dialysis care. Because these components will change as clinical and technical knowledge advance, HCFA should establish an expert advisory body to review periodically the services that Medicare should reimburse.
4. The Prospective Payment Assessment Commission, consistent with its recently expanded charge to examine Medicare outpatient as well as inpatient reimbursement, should periodically review ESRD payment policy.

Adopt the following specific ESRD reimbursement policies:

1. Evaluate the justification for the rate differential between hospital-based and independent facilities, especially in terms of patient complexity, and retain or eliminate the differential based on that analysis.
2. Establish a separate rate for hospital backup units that treat both inpatients and outpatients and that provide support to independent units in the care of complex outpatient cases.
3. Establish a separate rate for ESRD pediatric patients.
4. Evaluate the need for a separate rate for rural facilities.

The committee also recommends that HCFA review the monthly capitation physician payment policy (MCP) in light of its exclusion from the Medicare Fee Schedule regarding the impact of this policy on the quality of care provided.

QUALITY ASSESSMENT AND ASSURANCE

In all areas of medicine, there is increasing emphasis on the need for effective systems for quality assessment and assurance (QA). This is especially true for the ESRD program, which provides life-extending treatment for a large group of patients at high cost. Both patients and policy would benefit from systematic evaluation of the quality of ESRD treatment. Although a number of quality indicators are widely used, no systematic guidelines for evaluating quality have been developed for the ESRD program. Moreover, support for quality assessment research in this area has been very limited.

The ESRD QA function within Medicare involves several elements. Conditions of coverage for ESRD providers, published as regulations in 1976, represent traditional quality criteria and standards. However, these have never been related to outcomes or to all relevant process measures.

The HCFA-funded state surveys of dialysis facilities have potential for effective quality assurance, especially for structural and some process measures of quality. However, this system at present is demoralized by poor support, inadequate training of surveyors, and inconsistent oversight. Its surveys vary so widely in approach, thoroughness, and fairness that they are not accepted as valid by clinicians. State surveys could be an important component, but not the centerpiece, of an integrated ESRD QA system.

The committee recommends that HCFA improve the Medicare ESRD state survey system by developing uniform training and certification requirements for surveyors and integrating the state survey system with other ESRD QA efforts.

The HCFA Health Standards and Quality Bureau (HSQB), working with the ESRD networks, is currently (1990-91) testing the "National Medical Review Criteria Screens" and "Medical Case Review Procedures" to implement certain provisions of OBRA 1986 regarding the quality and appropriateness of patient care. Although the HSQB effort is creditable, it has certain technical limitations, is costly, and implicitly assumes that quality is best assured by a top-down monitoring system.

The committee believes that better methods are available for QA. These include integrated clinical indicators of outcomes and process and the use of functional and health status outcome measures. The report includes an example of the former as applied to the treatment of anemia. Also discussed is the use of continuous quality improvement, which focuses on improving patient management at the treatment-unit level. The report presents three examples of providers using some of these modern QA methods.

The committee also believes that justifiable HCFA QA oversight of ESRD providers could be exercised by coordination within HCFA of all relevant bureaus, linking of existing data bases, and the systematic examination of the relations between cost of treatment and quality of care.

The committee recommends that HCFA:

Evaluate all policies, including reimbursement policies, for their quality impacts on patients.

Provide adequate financial support to facilities for QA by incorporating facility QA costs in reimbursement for both dialysis and transplantation.

Coordinate within the HCFA the efforts of Health Standards and Quality Bureau, Bureau of Policy Development, and Office of Research and Demonstrations; link existing data bases for the development and operation of ESRD QA oversight systems to relate cost of treatment and quality of care; and integrate the ESRD networks and state surveys in a coherent national QA strategy.

Establish an advisory group of nephrology professionals and experts in QA to design and develop ESRD-specific QA systems.

Support the regional and national data systems necessary for an effective QA system.

Support a continuing program of ESRD QA research.

DATA SYSTEMS

The data available for evaluating the ESRD program and for monitoring epidemiology, access, quality, and reimbursement effects on quality are good in some respects and limited in others. The committee considered three major data systems: the HCFA ESRD Program Management and Medical Information System (PMMIS), the United States Renal Data System (USRDS), and the United Network for Organ Sharing (UNOS) data system.

In general, data about the ESRD program are currently more available and of higher quality than ever before, reflecting a decade of substantial accomplishment. HCFA is to be commended for its efforts, National Institute of Diabetes and Digestive and Kidney Diseases (NIDDK) for establishing the USRDS, and UNOS for its new data system.

In the coming decade, HCFA should address itself to these needs: improving data on primary diagnosis of renal failure, including data on insulin-dependent and non-insulin-dependent diabetes mellitus; developing overall measures of patient complexity, including the extent and severity of comorbid conditions; developing measures of functional and health status and other short-term outcomes; collecting information on ESRD patients who are not eligible for Medicare coverage; obtaining better ethnic data on ESRD patients, including those of Hispanic origin; and measuring patient mortality in the first three months of treatment (before Medicare eligibility is established) for patients under 65 years of age. A critical need is for HCFA to link its existing data systems in order to examine the relations among resources, treatment, and patient outcomes.

The committee recommends that HCFA maintain a strong ESRD data acquisition and analysis capability; modify the acquisition of patient information to include the periodic collection of data on comorbid conditions, risk factors, functional status, and other factors bearing on treatment and outcomes; identify data needs for systematically analyzing the relations among resource use, treatment, and patient outcomes; fund research pertinent to these questions; and provide public use tapes for research on all aspects of the ESRD program to the interested research community.

The decision by the NIDDK to develop the epidemiology of kidney disease as an integral part of its research efforts is a welcome step, one taken earlier by the National Institutes of Health dealing with cancer, heart disease, and aging. The NIDDK establishment of the USRDS represents an extremely important initiative in this context. The committee commends NIDDK for this action.

The committee recommends that USRDS be authorized to conduct research linking epidemiologic and economic data on the ESRD patient population and that the special studies approach be exploited to its full potential.

The National End-Stage Renal Disease Registry was authorized by Congress in OBRA 1986. Its mission was (1) to collect and analyze data pertaining to the epidemiology of kidney disease, (2) to conduct cost and cost-effectiveness analyses of treatment modalities, and (3) to analyze trends in mortality and morbidity and develop other indices of quality. The committee finds that the first function is being performed by USRDS, the second function has been the subject of bureaucratic controversy and is not yet implemented, and the third is being implemented mainly in regard to mortality.

The committee recommends that the Secretary of Health and Human Services take all steps necessary to fully implement all functions of the National End-Stage Renal Disease Registry called for in OBRA 1986 within the next two years.

It also recommends that the renal data system be continued another five years when the current USRDS contract expires and that the contract be recompeted at that time.

RESEARCH

The committee believes that a comprehensive program of basic and applied research related to end-stage renal disease is essential. This includes basic research on the diseases that cause ESRD, clinical studies, preventive and epidemiological research, and health services research. Basic research holds great potential for reducing the frequency and severity of ESRD, with both human and economic benefits. At present there is great need for clinical research on dialysis and transplantation, which has the potential to improve patient quality of life and to reduce costs by creating less expensive technology and techniques. Preventive and epidemiologic research also has high clinical and economic potential.

The committee recommends that:

NIDDK expand its support for basic research having the promise to prevent or to reduce the progression of kidney disease that leads to ESRD.

Clinical research on dialysis, supported by NIDDK or HCFA, be resumed.

Epidemiologic research be supported to identify risk factors for ESRD and its clinical outcomes, the value of various interventions to prevent and treat ESRD, and factors influencing access to ESRD care. Special attention should be given to racial and ethnic differences in the incidence and causes of renal failure and in transplantation (access, outcomes, organ donation).

Health services research be supported to determine which components of medical care lead to better outcomes and to identify and validate quality measures for structure, process, and outcomes.

NOTES

1. Section 4036(d), Omnibus Budget Reconciliation Act of 1987 (Public Law 100-203), December 19, 1987.
2. The study was supported by the Health Care Financing Administration (Cooperative Agreement No. 14-C-99338/3-02).
3. Insured status is measured by "quarters of coverage." Fully insured status requires a minimum of 6 quarters of covered employment; 40 quarters of coverage grants permanent status. Currently insured status requires 6 quarters of covered employment in the past three years.
4. State and local government employees have been covered by Social Security on a voluntary basis since 1950 but on a mandatory basis only since 1984.
5. A dialysis station consists of a dialysis machine, a chair or bed, and the associated floor space required to dialyze a single patient.
6. Indeed, some members of the committee believe this is the preferable method in any case because no expert committee can equal or improve on the patterns of services revealed by provider actions.
7. The committee discussed this recommendation during 1989 and 1990. In the Omnibus Budget Reconciliation Act of 1990 [Public Law 101-508, Section 4201(b)], Congress directed ProPAC to "conduct a study to determine the costs and services and profits associated with various modalities of dialysis services provided to end stage renal disease patients" under Medicare. ProPAC was also directed to consider the conclusions and recommendations of this study.
8. One committee member recommends a different payment policy; this is described in Chapter 11.

REFERENCES

Held PJ, Bovbjerg RR, Pauly MV, Garcia JR, Newmann JM. 1987. Effects of the 1983 "Composite Rate" Changes on ESRD Patients, Providers, and Spending. Washington, D.C.: Urban Institute, December 21.

Held PJ, Garcia JR, Wolfe RA, Gaylin DS, Pauly MV, Cahn MA. 1990. Price of dialysis and hospitalization. Paper prepared for the Institute of Medicine ESRD Study Committee. Washington, D.C.: Urban Institute, June 19.

1

Introduction

In the Social Security Amendments of 1972, the U.S. Congress established entitlement to Medicare benefits for people with a diagnosis of permanent kidney failure who were fully or currently insured or eligible for benefits under Social Security, and for their spouses and dependent children. The implementation of this entitlement has come to be known as the End-Stage Renal Disease (ESRD) program of Medicare. Treatments for permanent kidney failure include both dialysis and transplantation; Medicare-covered services for all medical conditions include inpatient and outpatient care from physicians as well as treatment units.

Thirty years ago, individuals who received a diagnosis of ESRD faced near-certain death. Dialysis and kidney transplantation were just then emerging as experimental procedures and were available in only a handful of medical centers. In addition, these treatments were beyond the financial reach of most Americans. The Medicare ESRD program introduced hope where there was none, saving several hundred thousand Americans from premature death by making life-saving treatment financially possible. It has been remarkably successful in fulfilling its intended objectives. Since the program began on July 1, 1973, it has grown from approximately 10,000 to over 150,000 beneficiaries.

THE CONGRESSIONAL CHARGE

The Congress, under OBRA 1987,[1] asked the National Academy of Sciences Institute of Medicine (IOM) to conduct a study of the Medicare ESRD program that would examine the following issues:

1. major epidemiologic and demographic changes in the ESRD patient

23

population that may affect access to treatment, quality of care, or the resource requirements of the program;

2. access to treatment by individuals with chronic kidney failure, whether eligible for Medicare benefits or not;

3. quality of care provided to ESRD beneficiaries, as measured by clinical indicators, functional status of patients, and patient satisfaction;

4. effect of reimbursement on quality of care; and

5. adequacy of existing data systems to monitor these matters on a continuing basis.

The study was supported by the Health Care Financing Administration (HCFA) under Cooperative Agreement No. 14-C-99338/3-02.

BASIC ASSUMPTIONS

The committee believes that people with renal failure should be the primary concern of Medicare ESRD policy. An emphasis on patients and their care underlies both the congressional charge and the committee's concern with the policy issues of access, quality, reimbursement effects on quality, data, and research needs. Consequently, the early chapters of the report (as noted above) deal with patient perspectives, ethics, and the epidemiology of the ESRD patient population.

Some recommendations of this committee would entail increased funding. The recommendations (of Chapters 7 and 8) to extend the Medicare entitlement to all Americans, to remove the three-year limit on Medicare eligibility of successful transplant recipients, and to pay for immunosuppressive drugs for the period of a transplant patient's entitlement are proposed as ways to improve an already successful program by increasing equity, promoting improved patient outcomes, and encouraging the search for means to prevent ESRD. The committee recognizes, however, that Congress must weigh these recommendations against competing uses of resources and make the appropriate allocation decisions.

The IOM committee, therefore, endorses the following objectives for the Medicare ESRD program: to guarantee access to treatment for all for whom it is medically appropriate; to provide care of high quality that achieves desirable health outcomes consistent with patient health status and current professional knowledge; to develop policies that steadily improve patient well-being and patient outcomes; and to manage the program prudently at the lowest cost compatible with adequate care.

CONTEXT OF THIS STUDY

This study of the ESRD program has coincided with an extraordinary amount of ESRD-related activity. OBRA 1986,[2] for example, reorganized the ESRD networks, consolidating them from 32 to 17 (later increased to 18). In addition, OBRA 1986 authorized a National End-Stage Renal Disease Registry, and the U.S. Renal Data System (USRDS) was established in partial response to this legislation. (See Chapter 13.)

OBRA 1986 also called for a study by the IOM of the effects of reductions in reimbursement for physician and facilities services on access to and quality of care. The constraints of time and the narrowness of the question led the IOM to decline to submit a proposal. Subsequently, the Urban Institute conducted that study and submitted a report in December 1987 that HCFA sent to Congress in December 1988 (Held et al., 1987). (See Chapter 10.)

In 1986, Home Intensive Care, Inc. (HIC), a dialysis supplier based in Florida, began providing paid aides for home hemodialysis patients in a way not originally anticipated by Congress. In 1978, Congress had called for a study of paid home aides, but that study had failed to provide HCFA with an adequate justification for adopting such a policy (Orkand Corporation, 1982). HIC billed its carriers for supplies at a rate that allowed it to pay for a home aide without billing directly for that aide. In 1988, HCFA sought to restrict this activity of HIC through an instruction to its financial intermediaries. Litigation before the U.S. District Court of Washington, D.C., however, resulted in a temporary injunction against HCFA's enforcement of this instruction in Florida and Illinois.[3] (See Chapter 9.)

Congress in OBRA 1989[4] limited reimbursement for home dialysis supplies purchased by patients and paid for through Method II to a level not to exceed the facility composite rate (or Method I).[5] The question of how to deal with patients being treated at home with the help of a paid aide, but too ill to travel to facilities or having severe ambulatory problems, was addressed in OBRA 1990 by the authorization of a demonstration project.[6]

Also during the study, the first recombinant DNA-based biological for use by dialysis patients was introduced into clinical practice. In June 1989, the Food and Drug Administration (FDA) approved recombinant human erythropoietin (Amgen Inc.'s Epogen or Epoetin-alfa) for the treatment of anemia in dialysis patients (FDA, 1989). HCFA responded immediately with an affirmative coverage decision and an interim reimbursement policy (HCFA, 1989b). That interim policy is under review by HCFA as data about dosage, response rates, and administration are considered. Reports on the subject have been issued by the Office of Technology Assessment (OTA, 1990) and by the U.S. Department of Health and Human Services (DHHS) (OIG, 1990a). Congress, in OBRA 1990, authorized self-administration of erythropoietin for home patients and also modified reimbursement policy.[7] (See Chapter 9.)

Congress addressed kidney transplantation as well during the study. The National Organ Transplant Act of 1984, which amended the Public Health Service Act and expanded the federal government's interest in whole-organ transplantation beyond kidneys, authorized the creation of the Organ Procurement and Transplantation Network.[8] That law was amended in 1986 and 1988 and was reauthorized in 1990 as this study was nearing completion. In addition, a draft report on access to kidneys for transplantation was issued by the DHHS in August 1990 (OIG, 1990b) as this IOM report was being written. (See Chapter 8.)

Change is occurring across many dimensions, then, within the ESRD program. The patient population continues to grow and to change in composition. Treatment technology in both dialysis and transplantation changes incrementally, punctuated on occasion by major new innovations. Total program expenditures continue to grow, primarily because of growth in the patient population.

STUDY METHODS

The composition of the IOM's End-Stage Renal Disease Study Committee reflected a balance among experts in the treatment of ESRD, including a patient, nephrologists (including a pediatrician) and transplant surgeons, nurses, and a social worker; also included were a sociologist and an economist, both familiar with the ESRD program. In addition, a breadth of perspective was achieved by individuals from internal medicine, epidemiology, quality assessment, ethics, and economics who were not immediately involved with dialysis or transplantation.

The IOM committee held seven 2-day meetings and one 3-day retreat. For the most part, these meetings were open to the public, were attended by a number of observers, and involved a combination of presentations and discussions.

The committee commissioned papers on the following subjects: pediatric renal failure patients; elderly renal failure patients; diabetic renal failure patients; hypertensive renal failure patients; black and other nonwhite renal failure patients; and the effect of reimbursement on innovation. The IOM also contracted for the following activities: three patient focus groups held in Washington, D.C., Los Angeles, and St. Louis; a survey of the state certificate-of-need (CON) programs that affect the ESRD program; a survey of state expenditures for ESRD purposes by state Medicaid programs, state medical assistance programs, and state kidney disease programs; and three analyses of the effects of the 1983 composite rate on mortality, hospitalization, and dialysis unit staffing. A list of authors and titles of these commissioned papers and contractor reports appears in Appendix C.[9]

In addition, a methodological paper on mortality in the ESRD population was prepared by Robert A. Wolfe, University of Michigan, and appears as Appendix D to this report. Finally, a paper on ethics (Cassel and Moss, 1990) was prepared by Christine K. Cassel, a committee member, and Alvin H. Moss, a nephrologist, and used extensively in preparing Chapter 3.

The committee held two public hearings, the first in Chicago in May 1989.

Respondents were invited to comment on the five issues of the congressional charge to the IOM study, and written testimony was a prerequisite for oral testimony. Participants and their affiliations are listed in Appendix E.

The second public hearing, in Washington, D.C., in February 1990, focused on dialysis reimbursement rate-setting. Project staff prepared a draft document that was circulated for comment (Young and Rettig, 1989). Interested parties were invited to comment on this draft, which became the basis for written and oral testimony. The committee received detailed responses to this document. Participants and their affiliations are listed in Appendix F.

HCFA supported this study by a cooperative agreement, and cooperation characterized the working relations with HCFA staff throughout the study. Encouragement and support were provided by the Office of Research and Demonstrations through Carl Josephson, project officer, and Paul W. Eggers. The Bureau of Policy Development supplied audited and unaudited cost data for 1985 and unaudited cost data for 1987 and responded to a number of queries from project staff. In June 1990, the Health Standards and Quality Bureau staff briefed the IOM staff on their quality assurance initiative. The Bureau of Data Management and Strategy made data and analyses available to the study from the Program Management Medical Information System (PMMIS). The IOM project staff also established direct computer access to PMMIS that enabled epidemiologic analyses to be done that would not otherwise have been possible.

Throughout the study, the project staff and committee members interacted with HCFA, congressional staff, the renal provider community, and patients, including attendance at and participation in professional meetings. The committee benefited greatly from this interaction.

THE ESRD PATIENT POPULATION

The ESRD patient population has changed strikingly in numbers, characteristics, and treatment modalities over the history of the program. The increase in new patients (incidence) and the total patient population (prevalence) between 1974 and 1989 are shown in Table 1-1. These incidence and prevalence figures are for treated ESRD patients only and are thus somewhat lower than the true incidence and prevalence of all ESRD patients.

The proportion of new ESRD patients who are elderly grew from 24 percent in 1978 to 38 percent in 1988, while diabetic patients increased from 21 to 35 percent of new ESRD patients, as shown in Table 1-2.

Projections of Medicare ESRD patients through the year 2000 are shown in Table 1-3. These projections, developed by Eggers for this study, are described in Chapter 4. They estimate that nearly one-quarter of a million ESRD patients will be enrolled in Medicare at the end of the decade.

TABLE 1-1   Incidence and Prevalence of Patients in
Medicare End-Stage Renal Disease (ESRD) Program,
1974-89

Year	Incidence[a]	Prevalence[b]
1974	NA	15,993
1975	NA	22,674
1976	NA	28,941
1977	NA	34,778
1978	15,174	44,153
1979	16,937	52,184
1980	18,437	60,053
1981	19,356	67,493
1982	21,927	76,316
1983	25,155	86,354
1984	26,552	95,522
1985	29,419	104,879
1986	31,561	114,659
1987	34,273	125,011
1988	36,743	134,786
1989	40,497	146,657

NOTE: NA = Not available.

[a]New ESRD patients during the reference year.

[b]Figures are for patients currently enrolled in the Medicare ESRD
program as of July 1 for 1974-77 and as of December 31 for 1978-89.

SOURCES: Incidence: HCFA, 1990b; prevalence: 1974-79, Eggers
et al., 1984; 1980-89, HCFA, 1990c.

NATIONAL EXPENDITURES FOR ESRD

Total Medicare expenditures[10] for all ESRD beneficiaries were $229 mil-
lion in 1974, the first full year of the program. Since then, the program has
grown significantly, both in enrollments and in expenditures. By 1988,
total Medicare ESRD expenditures reached $3.0 billion, a 12-fold increase
from 1974 (Table 1-4). Measured in 1974 constant dollars, however, this
increase is less than fivefold, from $229 million to $1.3 billion (Figure 1-1).

The primary contributor to the growth in Medicare ESRD payments has
been the 10-fold increase in beneficiary enrollments from 1974 to 1989
(Table 1-1). This faster growth of patients compared to constant-dollar
expenditures suggests that treatment has become more cost-effective over
time (Table 1-5).

Medicare expenditures for ESRD beneficiaries, moreover, are for all medical
services, not just those related to renal disease. About 36 percent of these

expenditures in 1988 went for inpatient hospital stays. Outpatient services and physician-supplier services accounted for another 40 percent and 23 percent, respectively (Table 1-6). In this context, services covered for ESRD treatment include outpatient hemodialysis and peritoneal dialysis (in-center or at home), inpatient dialysis (hemodialysis and peritoneal dialysis), kidney donor acquisition (cadaver and living donor), transplant procedures, and some medications. Medicare ESRD expenditures as a percentage of total Medicare expenditures grew to 3.4 percent in 1980, declined to 3.0 percent in 1985, and climbed again to 3.4 percent in 1988 (Table 1-7).

Medicare, however, does not cover all costs for either dialysis or transplant patients: premiums, deductibles, and copayments must be met from other sources such as state Medicaid programs, Department of Veterans Affairs (Table 1-8), private insurance companies, and patients. The U.S. Renal Data System 1990 Annual Data Report (USRDS, 1990) has estimated that the total direct medical payment from all sources for Medicare and non-Medicare ESRD patients in 1988 was $5.4 billion.

Based on 1987 cost data provided by HCFA, the annualized Medicare expenditure for a dialysis patient (for renal and nonrenal care) was $32,000. Transplant patients have a first-year per-capita expenditure of $56,000, but they cost Medicare approximately $6,000 on average in succeeding years for successful transplants (P.W. Eggers, unpublished data, 1990).

TABLE 1-2 New Elderly and Diabetic End-Stage Renal Disease (ESRD) Patients as a Percentage of New Medicare ESRD Patients

Year	Over Age 65	Diabetics[a]
1978	24.1	20.6
1979	26.7	21.3
1980	27.8	24.7
1981	27.0	26.1
1982	29.5	26.8
1983	35.3[b]	28.4
1984	34.6	30.7
1985	36.1	31.4
1986	37.5	33.5
1987	38.8	34.0
1988	38.4	34.9

[a]Calculated as a percentage of all patients for whom a diagnosis of diabetes was reported.

[b]The large jump between 1982 and 1983 in the percentage over age 65 may be due to irregularities in data reporting in those years.

SOURCE: HCFA, 1990a.

TABLE 1-3 Projections of Medicare End-Stage
Renal Disease (ESRD) Patients to the Year 2000

Year	Incidence	Prevalence
1989	38,111	141,236
1990	40,375	149,868
1991	42,601	159,047
1992	44,766	168,583
1993	46,844	178,314
1994	48,808	188,099
1995	50,634	197,812
1996	52,298	207,338
1997	53,774	216,563
1998	55,042	225,388
1999	56,082	233,714
2000	56,877	241,452

SOURCE: P.W. Eggers, Health Care Financing Administration,
unpublished data, 1990.

TABLE 1-4 Cumulative Percentage Change in Medicare End-Stage Renal
Disease (ESRD) Benefit Payments, 1974-88 Nominal and Real-Dollar
Payments

Year	Annual ESRD Payments (millions of dollars)[a]	Cumulative Change (%)	GNP Deflator Adj. Payments (1974 dollars)	Cumulative Change (%)
1974	229	—	229	—
1975	361	58	329	44
1976	512	124	438	91
1977	641	180	514	124
1978	800	249	598	161
1979	1,011	341	694	203
1980	1,252	447	789	245
1981	1,477	545	848	270
1982	1,662	626	897	292
1983	1,898	729	986	331
1984	2,003	775	1,003	338
1985	2,128	829	1,035	352
1986[b]	2,423	958	1,148	401
1987[b]	2,702	1,080	1,241	442
1988[b]	3,011	1,215	1,343	466

[a]ESRD figures may underestimate the actual benefit payments. In 1990, HCFA introduced
a new method of calculating expenditures. See note 10.

[b]Data are incomplete because of outstanding bills.

SOURCE: HCFA, 1990c.

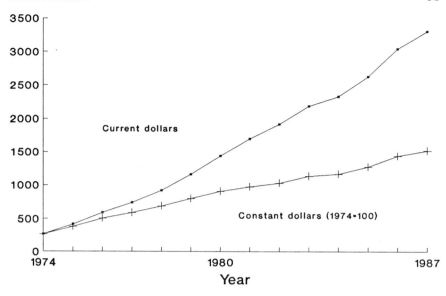

FIGURE 1-1   Medicare ESRD Benefit Payments
NOTE: Adjusted by GNP deflator.   SOURCE: HCFA, 1990.

TABLE 1-5   Growth of End-Stage Renal Disease
(ESRD) Program: Patient Growth Versus Real-Dollar
Benefit Payment Growth

Year	ESRD Annual Patient Growth (%)	ESRD Annual Real-Dollar Expenditure Growth (%)[a]
1974	—	—
1975	41.9	43.7
1976	27.3	33.1
1977	20.4	17.4
1978	27.0	16.3
1979	18.1	16.1
1980	15.1	13.7
1981	9.1	7.5
1982	4.5	5.8
1983	17.5	9.9
1984	9.3	1.7
1985	6.4	3.2
1986	11.6	10.9
1987	9.1	8.1
1988	9.9	8.2

[a]Adjusted by GNP deflator.

SOURCES: Eggers et al., 1984; HCFA, 1990c.

TABLE 1-6   End-Stage Renal Disease (ESRD) Benefit Payments by Type of Service, 1988

	ESRD Payments (millions of dollars)	Each Service as Percentage of ESRD Total
Inpatient	1,084	36.0
Outpatient	1,213	40.3
Physician	691	22.9
Other	23	0.8
Part B only	1,904	63.2
Total payments	3,011	100.0

NOTE: Data are incomplete because of outstanding bills. Data may underestimate actual ESRD benefits payments. See note 10.

SOURCE: HCFA, 1990c.

TABLE 1-7   Medicare End-Stage Renal Disease (ESRD) Benefit Payments, 1974-88

Year	Annual ESRD Payments (millions of dollars)	Total Medicare Payments (millions of dollars)	ESRD as Percentage of Total Medicare
1974	229	12,881	1.8
1975	361	15,742	2.3
1976	512	18,621	2.7
1977	641	22,175	2.9
1978	800	25,756	3.1
1979	1,011	30,221	3.3
1980	1,253	36,484	3.4
1981	1,477	43,541	3.4
1982	1,662	51,301	3.2
1983	1,898	58,579	3.2
1984	2,003	64,329	3.1
1985	2,128	69,924	3.0
1986[a]	2,423	75,389	3.2
1987[a]	2,702	81,511	3.3
1988[a]	3,011	89,300	3.4

NOTE: Data may underestimate actual ESRD benefit payments. See note 10.

[a]Data are incomplete because of outstanding bills.

SOURCE: HCFA, 1990c.

TABLE 1-8 End-Stage Renal Disease (ESRD) Expenditures in Department of Veterans Affairs, 1984-89 (millions of dollars)

Year	Dialysis Expenditures[a]	Transplant Expenditures[a]	Physician Expenditures[b]	Total
1980	—	—	—	104.9
1981	—	—	—	107.9
1982	—	—	—	114.3
1983	—	—	—	120.4
1984	124.1	8.5	—	132.6
1985	141.8	6.6	—	148.4
1986	144.4	6.4	—	150.8
1987	137.7	5.8	—	143.5
1988	123.4	5.7	—	129.1
1989	115.7	6.0	9.0	121.7

[a]Before FY 1984, dialysis and transplant cost accounts were a subset of the regular cost distribution system and did not include all applicable indirect costs.

[b]FY 1989 was the first year in which physician costs were reported as a separate component of the ESRD expenditures.

SOURCE: C.R. Wichlacz, Department of Veterans Affairs, personal communication, July 3, 1990.

ORGANIZATION OF THE REPORT

Part I is an overview of the study and the ESRD program. It contains the Summary and this introductory chapter.

Part II deals with patients and providers. Chapter 2 presents the results of three patient focus groups convened to provide direct access to patient concerns. Chapter 3 addresses ethical issues related to the initiation and termination of treatment and to the problem patient. Chapter 4 includes general background information about the ESRD patient population, a projection of that population to the year 2000, and a discussion of ESRD patient mortality. Chapter 5 discusses special ESRD patient groups: pediatric, elderly, diabetic, hypertensive, and black and nonwhite renal failure patients. Chapter 6 describes the nature and structure of dialysis and transplantation providers (facilities and centers).

Part III deals with access issues. Although eligibility for Medicare coverage for ESRD treatment is estimated to cover over 90 percent of the American people, the entitlement is not universal.[11] Chapter 7 addresses the access problems of individuals with no Medicare eligibility for ESRD treatment,[12] as well as the access problems of Medicare-eligible ESRD patients. Chapter 8 deals with kidney transplantation, focusing on the limits of access to this treatment that stem from policy limits on eligibility and coverage of immunosuppressive drugs and from the shortage of donor organs. Part IV addresses the relationship between reimbursement and quality. Chapter 9 discusses current reimbursement policy for facilities as well as physicians. This partial digression from the congressional charge was deemed necessary in order to deal with the issue of reimbursement effects on quality. Chapter 10 analyzes these effects with respect to mortality and hospitalization (two outcome measures), treatment unit staffing (a structural measure with substantial implications for the process of care), and innovation in treatment technology. Chapter 11 deals with reimbursement policy issues of covered services, rate-setting, and payment structure of the composite rate. Chapter 12 examines the conceptual elements of quality assessment and assurance (QA) as applied in the ESRD area, analyzes how the federal government manages the ESRD QA function, and argues for a treatment-unit QA approach.

Part V on data and research concludes the report. Chapter 13 describes the HCFA, the USRDS, and the United Network for Organ Sharing (UNOS) data systems, analyzes the implementation of the OBRA 1986 provision for the National ESRD Registry, and examines the adequacy of specific features of these data systems. Chapter 14 considers research needed to support the ESRD program, ranging from laboratory studies through clinical studies, epidemiology, and health services research.

NOTES

1. Omnibus Budget Reconciliation Act of 1987, Pub. L. No. 100-203, § 4036(d), (1987).
2. Omnibus Budget Reconciliation Act of 1986, Pub. L. No. 99-509, § 9335, (1986).
3. *National Kidney Patients Association* v. *Otis R. Bowen*, Civ. No. 88-3251 (D.D.C. Dec. 22, 1988).
4. Omnibus Budget Reconciliation Act of 1989, Pub. L. No. 101-239, § 6203.
5. Method I involves payment under the composite rate for home dialysis at the same rate as outpatient center hemodialysis (see Chapter 9). Method II involves direct billing of a fiscal carrier by the patient.
6. Omnibus Budget Reconciliation Act of 1990, Pub. L. No. 101-508, § 4202.
7. OBRA 1990, Pub. L. No. 101-508, § 4201(c) and (d).
8. Pub. L. No. 98-507.
9. Although some IOM studies publish commissioned papers, the ESRD Study Committee has treated these as inputs to its deliberations and has encouraged the authors to publish their work independently.
10. The ESRD Quarterly Statistical Summary, prepared by the Bureau of Data Management and Strategy, HCFA, publishes the only historical ESRD expenditure data series. Expenditure data are also presented in some of the annual HCFA research reports on ESRD (HCFA 1986, 1987, 1990d). The U.S. Renal Data System publishes summary cost data only.

    HCFA (1990d) recently presented expenditure data for 1984-87 that are substantially higher than previously published data. These new expenditure data are shown below in relation to the data presented in Table 1-4 (which are based on the HCFA ESRD Quarterly Statistical Summary):

Year	Millions of Dollars 1988 Report	Quarterly Summary
1984	2,333	2,003
1985	2,629	2,128
1986	3,048	2,423
1987	3,315	2,702

Although the methodology for calculating these data is described at length, HCFA gives no indication that they differ from previously published data. In brief, the new data are derived from the Medicare Automated Data Retrieval System (MADRS), a system for linking 100 percent of each beneficiary's Part A and Part B expenditure records for each calendar year. People identified as ESRD beneficiaries from the ESRD PMMIS are linked with MADRS data to obtain the new expenditure data. This new method of matching ESRD PMMIS enrollment records with MADRS identifies some ESRD patients who were previously not captured by the PMMIS data base and thus results in higher expenditures than previously attributed to the ESRD program.

11. Eligibility depends on a diagnosis of permanent kidney failure, on "fully or currently insured" status regarding Social Security or entitled to or receiving Social Security benefits, and on application for benefits.

12. At any time, ESRD patients will be classified as Medicare eligible, eligibility pending, and not eligible.

REFERENCES

Cassel CK, Moss AH. 1990. An ethical analysis of the End-Stage Renal Disease program with recommendations for physician-patient decision making and appropriate use of dialysis. Paper prepared for the Institute of Medicine ESRD study.

Eggers PW, Connerton R, McMullan M. 1984. The Medicare experience with end-stage renal disease: Trends in incidence, prevalence, and survival. Health Care Financing Rev 5:69-88.

FDA (Food and Drug Administration). 1989. Summary Basis of Approval: Drug License name: Epoetin alfa; Brand name: EPOGEN. June 1.

HCFA (Health Care Financing Administration). 1986. Health Care Financing Research Report: End Stage Renal Disease, 1984. Baltimore, Md.

HCFA. 1987. Health Care Financing Research Report: End Stage Renal Disease, 1985. Baltimore, Md.

HCFA. 1988. Health Care Financing Research Report: End Stage Renal Disease, 1986. Baltimore, Md.

HCFA. 1989a. Health Care Financing Research Report: End Stage Renal Disease, 1987. Baltimore, Md.

HCFA. 1989b. Medicare Provider Reimbursement Manual, Part 1-Chapter 27: Reimbursement for ESRD and transplant services. Medicare Provider Reimbursement Manual: Transmittal No. 11. Baltimore, Md. July.

HCFA. 1990a. ESRD Program Management and Medical Information System, March Update. Baltimore, Md.

HCFA. 1990b. ESRD Program Management and Medical Information System, August Update. Baltimore, Md.

HCFA. 1990c. End Stage Renal Disease Program Quarterly Statistical Summary. September. Baltimore, Md.

HCFA. 1990d. Health Care Financing Research Report: End Stage Renal Disease, 1988. Baltimore, Md.

Held PJ, Bovbjerg RR, Pauly MV, Garcia JR, Newmann JM. 1987. Effects of the 1983 "Composite Rate" changes on ESRD patients, providers, and spending. Washington, D.C.: The Urban Institute. December 21.

OIG (Office of Inspector General, Department of Health and Human Services). 1990a. The Effect of the interim payment rate for the drug Epogen on Medicare expenditures and dialysis facility operations. Draft Report. Washington, D.C.

OIG. 1990b. The Distribution of Organs for Transplantation: Expectations and Practices. Washington, D.C. Draft Report. August.

Orkand Corporation. 1982. Evaluation of the home dialysis aide demonstration: Executive Summary. Silver Spring, Md.

OTA (Office of Technology Assessment, U.S. Congress). 1990. Recombinant erythropoietin: Payment options for Medicare. OTA-H-451. Washington, D.C.

USRDS (U.S. Renal Data System). 1990. Annual Data Report. The National Institute of Diabetes and Digestive and Kidney Diseases, Bethesda, Md.

Young GP, Rettig RA. 1989. Issues in dialysis reimbursement rate-setting. Washington, D.C.: Institute of Medicine.

PART II
Patients and Providers

The IOM committee to study the Medicare ESRD program places great importance on the ESRD patient as the appropriate focal point of policy. In this section, this perspective is expressed in several ways. Chapter 2 reports on the results of three ESRD patient focus groups convened to provide the committee direct access to patient views on their treatment. Chapter 3 addresses several major ethical issues that confront physicians and other caregivers as the patient population grows and changes in composition.

Chapters 4 and 5 deal directly with the epidemiological changes of the patient population. Chapter 4 provides general background and presents projections of the patient population to the year 2000 and analyzes the mortality experience of the ESRD patient population. Special attention is given in Chapter 5 to elderly, pediatric, diabetic, hypertensive, and black and other nonwhite renal failure patients. These chapters reflect the diversity of the ESRD patient population and the way in which it has changed over time.

Finally, in this part, Chapter 6 examines the structure of the ESRD provider institutions: kidney transplantation centers as well as outpatient dialysis units.

2

Perspectives of ESRD Patients

The IOM ESRD Committee believes that people with renal failure should be the primary concern of Medicare ESRD policy. The committee also believes that patients should be encouraged to participate actively in all aspects of their care. Such participation can be aided by providing patients with understandable, timely, and ongoing information about all aspects of treatment; ensuring patient choice of providers through competition among facilities; determining patient preferences for clinical options; and assessing patient satisfaction with the outcomes of care. The committee emphasizes the importance of patients' rights and responsibilities in both the philosophy and the operations of treatment units.

The committee wished to obtain information directly from ESRD patients on their experience. A patient survey was considered but rejected on feasibility grounds. As an alternative approach, the committee held three patient focus groups.[1] The objective of the focus groups was to explore kidney patients' experiences in receiving treatment services and to identify opportunities for improvements in the ESRD program.

The three patient focus groups reflected diversity in age, sex, modality, time on treatment, type of facility, and home setting. Each group included 10 to 15 patient-participants, some of whom had a family member present. Each session lasted between 3 and 4 hours and was taped for later transcription. They were moderated by Edith T. Oberley, President of Medical Media Associates, Inc., who has more than 17 years of experience in the renal field as a professional in medical education/communications and as a home hemodialysis partner.

In an effort to avoid a regional bias, the IOM project staff selected Washington, D.C., Irvine, California, and St. Louis, Missouri, as sites. For each region, physicians, social workers, ESRD network personnel, and leaders of the national organizations were identified and asked to nominate patients who represented a cross-section in terms of treatment modality, ethnicity, length of time on treatment, age, treatment center type, and home setting. Nominations were reviewed by staff of the IOM and Medical Media Associates, and potential participants were contacted to generate a list of 15 participants for each group. Participants received an honorarium of $50 and were reimbursed for travel expenses.

Each focus group addressed two major topics: experiences with renal failure and the economic effects of kidney failure. The experiences with renal failure occupied more than 50 percent of each discussion and encompassed relations between patients, physicians, and staff; patient education; available services; and the effects of erythropoietin (EPO). For each topic, the moderator encouraged participants to reflect on the ideal situation— such as the ideal doctor-patient relationship, the ideal educational program— rather than focusing exclusively on what was lacking. The major findings are outlined below.

EXPERIENCES WITH RENAL FAILURE

Patient Relationships with Physicians and Staff

Kidney failure patients require continuing treatment over their entire lives. Consequently, they spend a lot of time with their physicians and with other medical professionals. Most dialysis patients see health professionals three times each week at a treatment unit where they spend 3 to 4 hours on each visit. Home dialysis patients also have frequent telephone contact with their physician or with a nurse. Individuals wanting a transplant often have to wait for a kidney. They must dialyze while waiting, during which extensive presurgery work-up is conducted. Even a successful transplant often involves extensive telephone contact with the transplant center as well as continued follow-up care from a nephrologist. If a transplant recipient's body attempts to reject a kidney, the clinical management of the rejection process intensifies the interaction between the patient and the health care team. All of these situations add up to a lot of time that patients spend with physicians and staff, and consequently these relationships are a very important part of the treatment process.

The importance of a good patient-physician relationship cannot be overemphasized since it is central to effective treatment. The doctor holds the key to the ongoing provision of life support to the patient, and patients are well aware of this power and the high degree of dependency implicit in the relationship. The doctor is not only "captain" of the treatment team, but also the very key to life support. Participants wanted their physicians to spend more time with them and reassure them as well as provide them with advice, guidance, information, and treatment. The participants reporting a good relationship with their physician were clearly committed to him or her.

Prior to kidney failure, you go to a doctor, and you're choosing this doctor, and he's providing information and a service for the fee, or whatever, and there's no dependency. This is a big difference. Once you go into kidney failure, the doctor holds the key to life. You can't get life support without the doctor, and it becomes a power that is sometimes abused. [Irvine, California]

Normally, I think, in the beginning, a dialysis patient puts his trust in the doctor's hands. It's on the basis of this person's words that our life changes. We trust his word, not only in the diagnosis, but in what's going to happen—prognosis and treatment. [Irvine, California]

Patients described the ideal physician-patient relationship as a caring partnership in which a doctor would discuss the issues and options with them so that a mutual decision could be reached that would help to improve the patient's quality of care. Most patients recognize their dependency on their physicians and make it clear that they don't want this trust abused.

Conflict often exists between a beneficence model of physician behavior, however, and an autonomy model of patient rights as patients attempt to assert control over their lives. Beneficence implies the responsibility of the physician to do what is best for the patient—"do no harm" is its obvious corollary. Patient autonomy, an equally strong value in our society, sometimes conflicts with the physician's view of what is best for the patient. There are constant decisions to be made in ESRD care, both major and minor. Physicians might prescribe behaviors (diet, medication, frequency and duration of dialysis, advisability of transplantation, and others) that are intended to correct the patient's metabolic imbalances and lead to an optimal medical condition. Patients may, at times, prefer less optimal medical conditions to more freedom or control over aspects of their daily lives. Ultimately, an autonomous patient may even choose to terminate dialysis, in contradiction to the physician's beneficent motive of prolonging life.

Some of these conflicts are inevitable and can be handled better if understood on this basis of a conflict or different values. But in many cases, resolution can be achieved through shared decision making and an explicit attitude of respect for the patient's choices and values. Foremost in this process is the need for patient education and for full communication and uncoerced informed consent of the patient concerning changes in therapy and recommendations. Channels of communications must allow questioning of the physician on numerous occasions. Patients' changes of mind must be anticipated as psychological adjustments occur and life changes intervene.

This shared-responsibility model demands time, openness, and flexibility from the health care professional, but its rewards are significantly lessened frustration with patient "noncompliance" and greater personal satisfaction in patient care.

It doesn't matter where he is, or what he has to do, if you ask him a question and it takes him 2 hours to answer it—he'll give you the 2 hours. [Washington, D.C.]

Another thing he does, he takes up time to explain. After examining you, he sits down on a chair and he takes the time. How are you doing? What are you doing? How's your social life, or home life? [Washington, D.C.]

[The doctor] informs you and then you can make the choice. [St. Louis, Missouri]

He provides individualized treatment and is flexible on the basis of my input. He's willing to change a medicine based on my input. [Irvine, California]

In some cases, however, patients expressed strong disappointment or resentment about their interactions with their physician. They spoke of doctors towering over them during rounds rather than pulling up a stool for a face-to-face conversation. Brevity of contact, a lack of physical touching, and a resistance to patient questions about treatment decisions characterized the unsatisfactory relationships.

The doctors never even touched me, and I can't believe that. It's just reassuring that the doctor comes in and puts his arm around you, or holds your hand, or just some kind of touching. The only physical contact I had was with the stethoscope. [Irvine, California]

The general impression I had of the nephrologist—and we've met more than a few—was that they were on automatic pilot. There wasn't an individual response to the person on dialysis. There was a shocking absence of being a patient advocate. [Irvine, California]

My biggest concern is they never slow down long enough to let you even say anything. They are just kind of like jackrabbits. They hit the chart and they start in the room and there are like 16 or 18 patients and they just walk from chart to chart and if you try to say anything, they are gone. They close the book and they are gone before you can open your mouth. [St. Louis, Missouri]

Some patients expressed concern over continuity of care among different physicians, particularly when the patient must be hospitalized.

Just as you seem to get confident with this doctor, he knows how you are acting, what medicines he is putting you on, how you are reacting to them . . . poof, he is gone. And then you get this other guy, and by the time you get him all where you got confidence and you know he knows what he is doing, he's gone [too]. [St. Louis, Missouri]

But if you go to the hospital to the transplant unit, you will see somebody different every time because there are interns in there all the time. They have what they call a "fellow," and he is there. He is working just on kidneys, but there are interns rotating all the time. So I feel very uneasy about that, because every time you go in you start all over from the beginning and say "this is my situation," and I don't like that. [Washington, D.C.]

There is always a different intern there who is not even familiar with what my problems are. [Washington, D.C.]

Patients tended to be highly supportive of their unit's staff. They are aware of the staff's crucial role in administering the ongoing life-giving treatment, as well as the effects of financial pressure, time constraints, and increased turnover on how well they do.

But most everything I do, I go directly to him, the nurse. He is very helpful, very responsive to my needs. [Washington, D.C.]

We have access [to members of the health care team]. And our nurses and technicians are very good. I don't have any problem with them. They are very good. [Washington, D.C.]

At least at my facility, I can say that they have improved, and the progress is in the area that we have talked about—in the area of encouraging patients to talk with other patients, peer group support and everything, and they're very much behind the Patient Advisory Group. [Irvine, California]

I feel the government has to understand that no matter how big the doctors are, we are not being kept alive by these doctors. And the ones who educate us and keep us alive are the [staff at the] units. And with all our heart and soul, if we could get this to be understood, and [staff] could get more money, we would end up [better off]. [Irvine, California]

Patients expressed concern about increasing staff turnover, the nursing shortage, and the increased prevalence of technicians in patient-care functions. Their primary concern is the effect that these trends have on their quality of care. For example, some patients are concerned that the training that technicians receive is not as complete as it should be. Participants also raised concerns about what they perceive as a lack of recognized standards of care. In general, they would like to see an increase in the staff/patient ratio so that staff can return to or adopt a more nurturing role.

I can see newer faces all the time coming in, and the personal relationship between the doctors and the nurses has significantly decreased over that period of time because of the fact that they have more patients to deal with. . . . It seems that the more they have to do, the less that they can relate to you and your problems personally. [Washington, D.C.]

After getting to know a nurse who's good, you start hearing that they're going to quit because of lack of money—it's unnerving. You finally get somebody who can stick you right [with the needles], and the next thing you know, they're looking for another job because of money. [Irvine, California]

If you want to be trained to go home, they tell you they have a shortage of nurses and only one nurse handles it, and that nurse has been out for 3 months, and you have to wait until that nurse comes back. [Washington, D.C.]

Patient Education

Patients generally agreed that education is vital to them at all stages of their treatment. It alleviates fear, offers hope, and gives them the tools they need to take active and effective roles in their treatments. Effective patient education at the time of kidney failure is especially important.

Knowledge can dissipate fear. When you know where you stand, when you know what your options are, when you know what choices you can make, then you can develop your sense of self to know what you're doing. [Irvine, California]

With the education, I think that you become a partner in your healing, in your treatment. You realize that you have some control over what happens. It brings— for me it brought just a cooperative kind of spirit. I mean, I knew I wanted to stay alive, but then it was just a wonderful feeling of support and cooperation and there was material there, and questions and answers. It was like settling in to something, rather than having this big massive unknown out there. [Washington, D.C.]

We have to know right from the outset that we're not going to die, and that there are options and that it's okay to be healthy and it's okay to be functional, and that you can do it. [Irvine, California]

Most participants reported that they had received some kind of written educational information about their condition and treatment. Nearly all ranked information about the details of daily care, nutrition and diet, different treatment modalities, finances and insurance, and family issues as very important. Participants in each group agreed, however, that the information they received was often inadequate.

I didn't have this information when they started with me, but there is a book now that goes from beginning to end. It starts with the different kinds of kidney diseases. It talks about the medication you have to take. It tells you different kinds of treatment like hemo and CAPD, transplant, different options you can have and what is involved in each of those. It talks about personal relationships with family, friends, how they are going to perceive you, what is going on. It also talks about how you can take care of yourself, or if you don't feel you can, the places you can go. I think it is important that they have something comprehensive that covers all of those details, because I did get information, but I didn't get anything like that. [Washington, D.C.]

Participants clearly felt that the unit staff and physicians have responsibility for educating their patients. Participants reported that the physician has a particularly strong influence at early stages.

People who hang out their shingles as caring for patients with end-stage renal disease . . . need to be given the responsibility to educate their patients. [Washington, D.C.]

After he [my doctor] gave me the literature and told me what was actually happening in my body, then I took an interest. [St. Louis, Missouri]

She [the doctor] sat down with us for about 3 hours and explained every little step right down the line and tried to put you at ease to make you realize this is not the end of the world, that you can still live a productive life. [Washington, D.C.]

Focus-group patients contrasted physicians and staff who did not provide educational materials unfavorably to those concerned that patients take active roles in decision making. They wished the doctor and the staff to take an active teaching role, not just give them a brochure or video. Many patients suggested that inadequate education conveys the message that doctors and staff members don't care.

Participants agreed that the setting and format in which educational materials are provided are important.

It was a brand new unit, a marvelous unit. They had printed material and booklets, they had movies, they had people come in. They were wonderful. And I felt that the world had been lifted off my chest, I really did. [Irvine, California]

The timing of educational programs is also important. Some patients prefer information at an early stage, some later in their treatment. Some are eager to receive information even before their first dialysis, others go through a lengthy period of denial and anger. In light of these differences, focus-group participants agreed that information has to be available when an individual is ready to receive it.

I think that it [education] has to be done before, during, and after [beginning] treatment. [Washington, D.C]

I was too shook up to respond too well at the beginning to videos or written material. I had to calm down to absorb that. [Irvine, California]

In my case a lot of that information that I got, it was not to the point. I didn't want it, I was so angry—I'd throw it in the trash. [St. Louis, Missouri]

Education cannot stop once a patient is familiar with the routine of dialysis. Patients want ongoing information about the latest findings that may affect their treatment. High flux, reuse, EPO dosage calculations, antirejection drugs for transplant patients—all are controversial topics in the dialysis field that are of interest to patients as well as professionals. Many focus-group participants were aware of these and other current issues, some through their own efforts to stay informed, others because of a physician or staff commitment to educate them.

Many participants strongly urged that family members be included in the education process, since they are often an integral part of the patient's support.

I think that even children [need information] . . . you don't have to go into deep details, but if you're confused as a patient, they're really confused about what's going on. What's happening to my Dad? What's happening to my Mom? [Irvine, California]

There was a lack of family education. Our children had no idea what was going on. [parent, St. Louis, Missouri]

There should be a program for the whole family including the siblings to learn what these [patients] have to go through. [parent, St. Louis, Missouri]

Many participants emphasized the value of education by other patients, through both individual counseling and self-help groups. Seeing and talking to a knowledgeable patient who is doing well can make all the difference to a new patient. Self-help groups can provide a forum for patient discussions about ongoing research, grievances at the unit, family problems, and other issues. One focus group suggested that a treatment unit should help organize, or at least not hinder, their organization.

If it wasn't for other patients I wouldn't have learned what I learned. [Washington, D.C.]

. . . you get to understand that you are not the only person in the world with this specific problem; that other people from all walks of life have the same type of problem. [Washington, D.C.]

. . . to have someone come out and sit and talk to you at home and explain to you [how you can lead] a very active life on dialysis. Just coming to grips with it would have been a lot easier. [Washington, D.C.]

Patient-Related Services

Kidney failure influences nearly every aspect of a patient's life—from diet to work to family—and the services that patients deem important reflect a need for assistance in all these areas. Among the services that participants reported as most important were education, flexible hours, family counseling, information about finances, transportation, psychological counseling, vocational and occupational training, appropriate isolation of infectious patients, and the availability of peer support groups. Nearly all participants indicated that they were not receiving some service or services that they ranked as very important on the questionnaires.

They will not come to the door to pick the person up. The person has to make his way from his house to the cab or transportation, and then from that door into the unit. They don't help the person. A lot of time these people cannot make it on their own, especially after dialysis, to make it from their ride into their house. They just cannot get in there. That is a major problem that we have no way to know how to solve that at this time. [Washington, D.C.]

I've bled on the subway a few times, fainted on the subway a few times, and I finally learned that I could afford the taxi rather than the embarrassment. But there wasn't any money available, because I wasn't rich enough and I wasn't poor enough. [Washington, D.C.]

I think that vocational and occupational training should be good. Being I just had the transplant, I am really anxious to enter the job market now. There is a lot of resistance on the part of the party who is hiring me because of my condition. The occupation I had previously, I am not really suited for any more. [St. Louis, Missouri]

As it is, patients must be pioneers, finding information in the wilderness. [Services worksheet]

Effect of Erythropoietin

Patients in all three focus groups reported that the effects of EPO in its first year of use had been substantial. Most participants reported an impressive improvement in health and energy as a result of taking EPO, although a few participants had not yet heard of it. Many patients on EPO no longer experience extreme fatigue, and employment becomes a more realistic option for them than ever before. Consequently, many patients expressed the desire to return to work. In fact, some mentioned privately that they were working, but not reporting the income because of fear of losing their Social Security disability payments. Others discussed their current efforts or future plans for job hunting.

I have to honestly say that [EPO] has been a big determining factor in my decision to return to work. I am not sure I could have hung in there before, where now I feel that I can hold a full-time job again. I am not sure 6 months ago that I really could have. [Washington, D.C.]

The introduction of EPO therapy has resulted in substantially higher energy levels for many patients. It may now be appropriate to deal with rehabilitation issues more directly than has been done in the past. EPO may have shifted attention to economic and social barriers to employment and rehabilitation and away from the physical limitations of patients to pursue active, productive lives.

ECONOMIC EFFECTS OF KIDNEY FAILURE

There is inadequate documentation about the extent of the economic effects of kidney failure on patients and their families. The report of Campbell and Campbell (1978), now more than a decade old, is a notable exception. All patients openly discussed the financial hardships experienced since renal failure; most reported a change in occupation and nearly all reported a decrease in personal income—"substantial" in many cases. Kidney failure, it was agreed, had changed their families' ways of handling finances.

Kidney patients acknowledge that they are fortunate enough to have Medicare support for 80 percent of their basic treatment, although some necessary services, such as certain medications and transportation, are not reimbursed. Even so, the financial hardships reported by these participants were serious. Half of the participants reported that out-of-pocket expenses related to their treatment, such as medications (including vitamins) and transportation, were not co-paid by Medicare or insurance. Many also reported difficulty in paying for and/or qualifying for private insurance and indicated that the financial hardship of renal failure was more difficult than the medical hardship.

If you don't do anything, you can get help. But if you want to work and you want to pull your weight, you can't get any help. That is the problem. [Washington, D.C.]

If only I could make at least two-thirds of what I'll be receiving from Social Security disability insurance, I would like to work. [Washington, D.C.]

It takes a tremendous amount of psychological and physical energy to maintain employment. For those who remain on SSI or SSDI, the disincentives to employment are outrageous, so why put forth the energies to get out of dependency. [St. Louis, Missouri]

It's a real Catch-22 because I've got an 11-year-old son and a 13- year-old daughter who are both going to school and the way things work out it's better for me to stay on dialysis and disability than it is to work right now. It would cost me more to hire somebody to come in and watch my kids than I could make going back to work versus what I get on disability. [St. Louis, Missouri]

The major concerns identified by patients as sources of financial difficulty included the following: disincentives to work resulting from Social Security disability regulations; employer reluctance to hire people with a chronic condition; and problems in keeping or obtaining private health insurance. Disability payments are not high enough to support a family. Those who want to return to work often cannot find jobs that bring in more income than their disability, resulting in forced unemployment.

The financial impact on me has been the most debilitating—and stressful. More than losing my kidneys. [Irvine, California]

And then came the dialysis, and I still finished my doctorate and so forth, and after the transplant then when I got well enough to start looking for jobs, whether it's because I'm blind or I've had a transplant—and I happened to be of the group that tell both—I applied for probably 1,000 jobs in this area, or more, probably 2,000 jobs, and I'm still not full-time employed. Right now is when I am receiving the crunch because the student loans are due. . . . Here I am with a doctoral degree from one of the major universities in the area, and a friend has bought my food for 3 months. [Washington, D.C.]

As a parent of a dialysis patient, I have not been able to work until these past few months when my child was actually old enough and mature enough to ride a cab to and from treatments. One income for five people is not enough to make ends meet. [St. Louis, Missouri]

I lost my job, my home. Now I'm trying to raise two kids so I'm really stuck to where I can't work because I've got two kids at home that I'm trying to raise. [St. Louis, Missouri]

I want to go back to work. I feel that I could handle it, but I can't afford to. They told me that if I make more than $741 a month, I lose my MediCal, and then I'm responsible for 20 percent of my payment to the dialysis unit, plus all of my medical expenses, and it ends up not being worth it. [Irvine, California]

What I found out years later [from] the person that was my boss at the time is the insurance company came in and said, "We've spent $100,000 on this guy in the last quarter. We can't drop him off the policy, we're going to drop your whole policy for 100 employees." So guess who left? I spent about a year looking for a job after that and finally gave up. [St. Louis, Missouri]

I think a lot of employers are reluctant to hire people that are disabled. They don't want to add them to their health insurance policies. They don't want people working part-time. They want you either there all the time, or not at all. [Irvine, California]

These findings suggest that the issue in most immediate need of attention is employment. Although some participants in each groups are employed, many others have been prevented from working by a number of barriers— including the economic disincentives to employment imposed by Social Security disability regulations. Although the economic disincentive is the most frustrating for patients, there are other barriers to employment, including the lack of flexible dialysis hours in many units, the shortage of useful vocational and occupational training programs, problems of obtaining and maintaining health insurance, and the inaccessibility of education and support services.

Nearly all participants expressed frustration at the limitations imposed on earnings by the Social Security disability programs. With the advent of EPO, patients are finding that fatigue is not the barrier to work that it used to be. The real disincentive, participants reported, is economic. More than half reported that limits on earnings imposed by Social Security disability regulations had influenced their decisions about working; half also said that they would return to work if these regulations were changed.

CONCLUSIONS

The focus groups were intended to obtain information directly from patients on their experiences with renal failure and to identify opportunities for improvements from their viewpoint. The quotes of patients speaking for themselves accomplish this. They reveal that patients value effective relationships with their physicians very highly and place great emphasis on continuing education about their disease and its management, as a mechanism for participating in clinical decision making and means for alleviating fear and enhancing interactions with their families and with health professionals. These statements by patients also indicate that they can serve as a key source of information on the systems of care and on how federal regulations affect patients' lives.

The economic effects of kidney failure on the lives of patients and their families are substantial, a feature common to patients with chronic diseases. Although poorly understood, these effects should be acknowledged and policies developed to address them. In particular, ESRD focus-group participants identified employment opportunities and problems, difficulties associated with private health insurance, the frequent dependence of ESRD patients on Social Security disability, and the disincentives that system raises to pursuing employment as matters of great concern.

The barriers to rehabilitation—physical, economic, and social—are important to patients. Ways should be sought to restore patients to good functional and health status and, wherever possible, to provide incentives to encourage them to return to work and to productive social activity. The policy options to address the unintended interactions of Medicare and Social Security disability policies have begun to be addressed by Congress, appropriately in the context of disability and chronic disease. Given the impact of EPO on patients' energy levels, it may be quite timely to address rehabilitation afresh. The committee believes that this set of issues deserves renewed attention.

Many of the issues discussed by the patient focus groups are addressed in various sections of this report. Not all were addressed by the committee, however, because they did not bear directly on its charge and to do justice to them would have required a substantially greater effort. They clearly deserve extended examination.

NOTE

1. A focus group is a structured discussion led by a moderator and designed to elicit information from participants, who interact with each other. Although focus groups cannot provide data that are generalizable to the entire population, they allow researchers to identify attitudes, collect information, and generate hypotheses that may later guide quantitative research, such as surveys.

REFERENCE

Campbell JD, Campbell AR. 1978. The social and economic costs of end-stage renal disease. N Engl J Med 299:386-392.

3

Ethical Issues

Dialysis and transplantation have raised ethical questions since their introduction to clinical practice in the early 1960s. The questions have changed over time, however, as the patient population, treatment, and financing have changed. In the 1960s, the discussion focused on the criteria for access to treatment as a function of financial resources and other characteristics of patients. The Seattle experience, using medical judgments and "social worth" criteria applied by an anonymous lay committee, is widely known (Alexander, 1962). Other treatment facilities also found it necessary to limit access to care on similar grounds before the 1972 Medicare ESRD entitlement.

The 1972 statute, however, provided relief to physicians, federal and state government officials, and members of Congress from the need to ration access on the basis of financial resources of patients. The primary policy concern became making treatment available to those who needed it.

Congress obliquely addressed the matter of appropriate use in the 1972 statute when it directed the Secretary of DHHS to include in the reimbursement regulations a requirement for "a medical review board to screen the appropriateness of patients for the proposed treatment procedures." It did not define appropriateness or provide any clarifying legislative history.[1] Neither legislators nor physicians wished the government to determine patient selection (Rettig, 1991).

When the Medicare entitlement was passed, moreover, the likely beneficiaries were thought to be relatively young, employed, taxpaying members of society, whom treatment would rehabilitate and return to work (Fox and Swazey, 1978). Congress did not foresee a patient population whose average age would increase to 60 years, or one with substantial comorbid conditions other than renal disease. But it did not seek to constrain growth along these lines.

A different set of ethical issues will be raised in the next decade as the ESRD patient population continues to grow and includes a greater proportion of elderly patients and those with comorbid conditions beyond their renal disease. These features of the ESRD population, and its cost, intersect with a general concern for the level and rate of increase of health care expenditures and the now-extensive discussions of the rationing of health care (Aaron and Schwartz, 1984; Callahan, 1987, 1990; Freeman, 1987; OTA, 1987).

The committee, conscious of substantial interest in these issues, focused on three major concerns as they apply to ESRD patients: the acceptance of patients for treatment, the termination of treatment, and ethical questions arising for caregivers who deal with problem patients. Its recommendations emphasize patients' wishes and best interests as well as the appropriate use of the expensive, life-sustaining therapies of dialysis and transplantation.

The committee believes that the ethical issues addressed here are properly the domain of patients, families, and physicians and other caregivers. They deserve thorough, open, and extended discussion. They are not, however, issues of public policy until and unless the federal government undertakes explicit rationing of beneficial care. The committee sees no role for federal statutory or regulatory action.

PATIENT ACCEPTANCE CRITERIA

Since the ESRD program began, nephrologists have seen chronic dialysis treatment as a tremendous success (Lowrie and Hampers, 1981). This view is based largely on the personal satisfaction of being able to provide life-sustaining treatment to patients who would otherwise die. The changing composition of the patient population, however, has resulted in a different treatment population in 1990 than existed nearly 20 years ago (see Chapters 4 and 5). The number of new patients has increased steadily, as has the median age of dialysis patients and the number of dialysis patients with a serious, chronic primary diagnosis such as diabetes (USRDS, 1990). This change occurred in part because physicians, as they gained experience treating older patients and patients with greater medical complications, achieved successful outcomes.

Concern has been expressed by some observers that patient acceptance criteria have expanded since enactment of the Medicare ESRD entitlement to include an increasing number of patients with limited survival possibilities and relatively poor quality of life. In its deliberations on this matter, *the committee concluded that patient acceptance criteria should be based on the medical assessment of the benefits and burdens of treatment and on the best interests of individual patients, not on economic objectives of cost containment.*

The committee also distinguished between the criteria of age and comorbid conditions. Chronological age was considered and explicitly rejected by the committee as a criterion for patient acceptance, since it does not measure the ability of an individual to benefit from treatment. Comorbidities—at any age—are the primary determinants of quality of life and of survival.

The President's Commission for the Study of Ethical Problems in Medicine and Biomedical and Behavioral Research recommended that life-sustaining treatment should be evaluated in terms of both life extension and the quality of the life extended. They concluded that patients are not obligated to undergo life-sustaining treatment (President's Commission, 1983). Others have also observed that the prolongation of life may not always be a benefit that outweighs all burdens (Landau and Gustafson, 1984; McCormick, 1974). The burdens of pain, suffering, loss of body control or integrity, and loss of privacy, independence, and dignity may outweigh the benefit of life prolongation. This view was held *In the Matter of Conroy* [486 A.2d 1209 (N.J. 1985); Lo et al., 1990].

Virtually all nephrologists recognize that dialysis treatment is not always the best choice for every ESRD patient (Cummings, 1989) and that the expected benefits are marginal for some categories of patients. Virtually all would agree that life-sustaining dialysis treatment should not be used just because it is available or reimbursed, that the existence of a public entitlement does not obligate them to treat all patients who present with kidney failure.

The question of the appropriateness of dialysis arises, then, for ESRD patients who have major comorbidities and a limited life expectancy. These include patients with serious comorbidities such as atherosclerotic, cardiac, and peripheral vascular disease, chronic pulmonary disease, cancer, or AIDS, and who are close to death and whose course cannot be interrupted by dialysis treatment. A second group are some patients whose neurologic status renders them unable to relate to others, such as those in a persistent vegetative state or with severe dementia or cerebrovascular disease. These patients are also significantly more likely to withdraw from dialysis than those without these diagnoses (Neu and Kjellstrand, 1986; Port et al., 1989; Rodin et al., 1981). In one major study, neurologic disease (dementia and acute cerebrovascular accident) was the most common complication leading to the withdrawal of dialysis (Neu and Kjellstrand, 1986). In another, 76 percent of dialysis patients and 55 percent of the dialysis staff thought it was reasonable to discontinue dialysis in a patient who became severely demented (Kaye and Lella, 1986). These findings were confirmed in a recent national survey in which internists and nephrologists considered neurologic impairment the most important factor in deciding to limit the use of dialysis (Foulks et al., 1989).

Nephrologists have a professional responsibility to deal with the issues of initiation and termination of treatment. Their training and experience equip them to assess which patients are likely to benefit from dialysis and which from transplantation. They should use this knowledge to make treatment recommendations to patients, including the recommendation that dialysis not be initiated. Coupled with patient and family preferences, a recommendation may indicate that terminal palliative rather than life-extending care be given to allow a peaceful death from uremia (Roy et al., 1990). Thus the choice is not between treatment and abandonment, but rather between different goals of treatment.

For a particular patient, the physician should follow a process that involves a careful clinical assessment of the patient and of all treatment options, including no dialysis. The clinical evaluation provides the initial basis for discussion. Decisions about initiating treatment should then result from full, open, and compassionate discussion with the patient and his or her family. The fact that ESRD patients consistently rate their quality of life higher than "objective" observers rate it (Evans et al., 1985) underlines the need to weigh patient preferences very highly in decision making. The patient and family (or guardians, where appropriate), when fully informed of the benefits and burdens of treatment, should evaluate the proposed treatment in terms of their personal values and accept or reject the physician's recommendation.

Quality-of-life measures, developed as research tools for assessing populations and individual patients, including ESRD patients, have not been used for decision making about the initiation or termination of treatment. These measures may generate information that helps the physician assess a patient, but they should not be used as the primary basis of a decision to treat. No quantitative measure can fully evaluate the specificity of each patient's situation.

Commentators on life-sustaining therapies have called for the development of guidelines to assist patients, families, and physicians who must make decisions about the use of any life-sustaining therapy (Hastings Center, 1987a; Landau and Gustafson, 1984; Lynn and Childress, 1986; Miles and Gomez, 1989). An open discussion involving the nephrology community and experts in medical ethics could lead to the development of guidelines for the use of dialysis. Criteria for these guidelines should include predicted survival and patient functional status. These guidelines could help make explicit the evaluation of patients for whom dialysis would only prolong the dying process or continue a life in which the burdens of treatment outweigh the benefits. They would support nephrologists in not offering dialysis to patients for whom such an intervention would be disproportionately burdensome.

Caring for ESRD patients who are dying because dialysis has been withheld or withdrawn may require an adjustment for some nephrologists. For such patients, the nephrologist, the nurse, and the social worker have to shift from providing life-sustaining dialysis to basically giving hospice care and allowing death to occur naturally. They should comfort the dying patient, ensure the company of his or her family at the moment of death (Ramsey, 1970), and maintain the continuity of caregivers and familiar surroundings in the patient's final days of life. It should not be necessary to transfer dying patients to another physician or facility such as a hospice, although the same principles for palliative care apply.

WITHDRAWAL FROM TREATMENT

Guidelines

A widespread consensus exists that supports the right of competent, informed patients to choose or forgo life-sustaining treatments [AMA, 1989; Hastings Center, 1987b; Jonsen et al., 1986; President's Commission, 1983; *Satz* v. *Perlmutter*, 379 So. 2d 359 (Fla. 1980)]. The termination of treatment of incompetent patients, by contrast, should occur only after full discussion between the patients' family, or other representatives, and the physicians. Withdrawal from dialysis treatment by competent ESRD patients is increasingly reported, especially among the elderly. Such choices may be regarded as rational decisions by autonomous individuals who have concluded that the burdens of continuing treatment outweigh the benefits.

Nephrologists should be open to permitting dialysis to stop when it no longer benefits the patient. The discussion of the decision to stop dialysis might be initiated by the patient for whom the burdens have come to outweigh the benefits or by the physician who recognizes that the treatment goals are no longer achievable.

The general guidelines discussed above could guide physicians as well as treatment units. Dialysis units, in addition, should adopt their own policies for the withdrawal of dialysis which ensure that the patient has been fully evaluated and counseled before stopping dialysis. A psychiatric evaluation to rule out treatable depression should be part of the process.

The guidelines suggested above could also help nephrologists determine that dialysis should be discontinued in some patients. When decisions to withhold or withdraw dialysis are considered in individual patients, there is the potential for disagreement within the health care team, between the health care team and the patient (and family), and within the patient and family circle. There should be a means for conflict resolution available to the health care team, the patient, and the family short of resorting to the court system.

Hospital ethics committees serve this function, as well as the usual range of other hospital purposes, and are available to hospital-based dialysis units (Fost and Cranford, 1985). It is appropriate that freestanding dialysis units have access to an ethics committee, perhaps through their ESRD network, for this purpose. Such committees should be available to review decisions to withhold or withdraw dialysis at the request of the patient, the incompetent patient's family, or any member of the health care team. They could also foster education of all dialysis personnel about the ethical issues in dialysis care and draft policies for units on such issues as withdrawal of dialysis, Do Not Resuscitate status, limited-treatment plans, and time-limited trials. These committees should be composed of members of the health care team: physicians, nurses, social workers, dietitians, and administrators, and other patient advocates, such as clergy, ethicists, and lay representatives.

In situations where the expected benefit to the patient is not clear but the patient (and/or family) wants treatment, a time-limited trial of dialysis of 1 to 3 months satisfies two ethical tenets. First, the patient will have a better understanding of the treatment after the trial and will be able to give consent or refusal that is more informed. Second, the physician will have had a chance to observe the patient's response to dialysis and will be able to evaluate more clearly the benefit to the patient. Prior to the initiation of the trial, there should be carefully delineated parameters of what outcomes of dialysis therapy justify continuation so that at the conclusion of the trial, a decision regarding further dialysis can be made.

Advance Directives

At some point, dialysis patients may become incompetent as a consequence of kidney failure or dialysis treatment. To protect their values and ensure self-determination in their health care, they should execute advance directives[2] (Hastings Center, 1987b; New York State Task Force, 1987). Legal instruments that document the patients' wishes in advance are the living will and the durable power of attorney for health care. Physicians may also document patients' advance directives in patients' charts after a witnessed discussion. Patients should read and sign these chart notes to be sure their physician has understood their preferences.

Since there is a presumption in favor of continued life-sustaining treatment for patients who cannot and have not expressed their wishes, the patient's right to forgo dialysis in certain situations is usually difficult to achieve unless patients have explicitly stated their preferences in advance or named a proxy to speak on their behalf (Hackler, 1989). Nephrologists and other health care professionals who work with dialysis patients should discuss the circumstances under which patients would want to stop dialysis and forgo cardiopulmonary resuscitation, and they should encourage their patients to complete advance directives and appoint a proxy so that their wishes can be followed even when they are unable to participate in decision making.

The number of elderly people on dialysis is rapidly growing. Two studies have documented that 40 percent and 56 percent of the deaths of patients over the age of 70 and 85 years, respectively, are due to withdrawal from dialysis (Husebye and Kjellstrand, 1987; Port et al., 1989). It is particularly important, therefore, for health care professionals in dialysis units to discuss with elderly patients and their families their wishes for future care under a variety of contingencies and to encourage them to complete living wills and durable powers of attorney for health care.

Patients' wishes regarding dialysis and other life-sustaining therapies may change over time. The review of the dialysis patient care plan every 6 months provides an opportunity to review the patient's wishes and to update advance directives.

TREATING THE PROBLEM PATIENT

All physicians encounter problem patients. The difficulties these patients present are related to their specific kinds of disorders and treatments. This is particularly true in ESRD practice, and dealing with such patients presents a constant challenge to ESRD providers. Three types of patients raise ethical problems for ESRD caregivers today: the noncompliant, self-destructive dialysis patient; the hostile, abusive dialysis patient; and the self-destructive transplant patient.

In all cases, the physician's responsibility is to care for the patient with an understanding of human frailty and the complex psychology of living with chronic illness, to make efforts to develop effective communication, and to ensure continuity of care. Legal contracts between patients and health professionals may be necessary in some cases to specify mutual rights and responsibilities. Courts, of course, remain arbiters of conflicts that can be resolved in no other way.

There is substantial literature in internal medicine, family medicine, and psychiatry on dealing with the problem patient, or even the hateful patient (Groves, 1978), which could be productively applied to these problems as they arise in the context of ESRD.

In the context of dialysis, noncompliant, self-destructive patients are those who do not routinely keep their dialysis appointments, do not adhere to diet, and do not generally behave in accordance with medical guidelines for their life-threatening disease. They seem to act out a distinct ambivalence about the value of continued life to them and thus do not behave in a way that facilitates the delivery of care. The psychological complexities of living with a chronic disease such as ESRD, of course, put many pressures on people, and every effort must be made to develop effective communication, support, counseling, and even psychiatric treatment when that is indicated (Landsman, 1975).

When none of these is effective or possible, however, authorities agree that the responsibility of the physician is to care for the patient and to continue patiently to try to deal with him or her in a nonjudgmental fashion. It is not enjoyable or particularly gratifying to care for those who reject one's help (Groves, 1978), yet that is not an ethical justification for withdrawing from the care of such patients (Papper, 1970). If the physician and the patient develop differences that prevent a successful relationship, the physician (with the patient's agreement) should arrange for the transfer of the patient's care to another physician (ACP, 1989). Continuity of care must be ensured because of the life-sustaining nature of the therapy.

When the hostile, abusive patient's actions are destructive to others, the balancing of moral responsibilities becomes more complex. In the event that a patient poses a threat to other patients in a dialysis unit (for example, by hostile behavior of any sort), the physician's or nurse's responsibility to the other patients may outweigh their responsibility to that patient. Hostile, abusive dialysis patients have been found by the courts not to have a right to demand treatment from nephrologists if the nephrologists take care to avoid abandonment. However, dialysis units, because of the scarce and life-saving nature of the treatment they provide, have been found to have a collective responsibility, if not an individual one, to provide dialysis to these patients. The sharing of such a disruptive patient by a network of dialysis units has been the proposed solution in one case [*Payton* v. *Weaver*, 182 Cal. Rptr. 225 (Calif. 1981)].

If a patient is abusive only to staff and not to other patients, then every effort should be made to understand and deal effectively with the underlying psychosocial determinants of that patient's behavior (Groves, 1978). A contract between such a patient and the health care team can be very helpful if it outlines the rights and responsibilities of each, sets limits, and describes consequences of unacceptable behavior. This approach may improve the relationship of the patient to the treating nephrologists and the dialysis unit personnel.

Although the complexity and frailty of human existence must be acknowledged, and physicians cannot insist that patients adhere to strict rules in order to be eligible for care, a different consideration occurs in the case of a transplant patient than for a dialysis patient. Transplanted kidneys have to be viewed as absolutely scarce resources for which there is a substantial waiting list. Thus, a patient who receives a kidney transplant and then engages repeatedly in behavior that threatens the survival of that kidney may disqualify himself or herself as a candidate for a subsequent transplant if the current one fails. This area has not been well described in the ethics literature, although surgeons often report it informally as a difficult issue.

CONCLUSIONS AND RECOMMENDATIONS

The growing public and professional discourse about ethical issues in health care creates an atmosphere in which the special issues in ESRD treatment can be addressed openly. Advances in medical technology and the ensuing health policy debates ensure that value conflicts and ethical dilemmas will continue to arise in all areas of health care, including ESRD. Thus, our recommendations address current and specific issues as well as the need for ongoing education in ethics to provide the language and conceptual framework necessary to ensure the optimal approach to patient care in the future.

The committee recommends that patients, professionals in adult and pediatric nephrology, and bioethicists develop guidelines for evaluation of patients for whom the burdens of renal replacement therapy may substantially outweigh the benefits. These guidelines should be flexible and should encourage the physician to use discretion in the assessment of the individual patient.

Any guidelines for children should be child-specific and should describe the role of the parents in the decision-making process.

Renal professionals should discuss with ESRD patients their wishes for dialysis, cardiopulmonary resuscitation, and other life-sustaining treatments and encourage documented advance directives.

ESRD health care professionals should be encouraged to participate in continuing education in medical ethics and health law.

There is a need for some specialists in the medical ethics of renal disease to educate health care providers, to train members of ethics committees, and to do research on ethical issues in dialysis and transplantation.

NOTES

1. Congress, in 1978, directed the ESRD networks to "evaluate the procedure" by which appropriateness was assessed but did not clarify the basic term.
2. In the Omnibus Budget Reconciliation Act of 1990, Pub. L. No. 101-508, Congress enacted advance directives legislation. Section 4206 applies to Medicare and Section 4751 to Medicaid. As a condition of participation in the Medicare program, hospitals, skilled nursing facilities, home health agencies, and hospice programs are required to establish and maintain written policies regarding advance directives for all adult individuals receiving medical care from such organizations; to provide written information to each such individual regarding their rights to accept or refuse treatment and to formulate advance directives; to document in the individual's medical record whether or not an advance directive has been executed; and "not to condition the provision of care or otherwise discriminate against an individual based on whether or not the individual has executed an advance directive."

Outpatient dialysis units were not specifically included among the organizations to which this legislation pertains, an apparent legislative oversight. Nevertheless, the legislation points to the importance of advance directives for dialysis patients as well and provides a strong reason for nephrologists, other caregivers, and dialysis unit representatives to address this matter.

REFERENCES

Aaron HJ, Schwartz WB. 1984. The Painful Prescription—Rationing Hospital Care. Washington, D.C.: The Brookings Institution.

ACP (American College of Physicians). 1989. American College of Physicians ethics manual. Part 1: History; the patient; other physicians. Ann Intern Med 111:245-252.

Alexander S. 1962. They Decide Who Lives, Who Dies. Life 53 (November 9):102-104.

AMA (American Medical Association). 1989. Current Opinions: The Council on Ethical and Judicial Affairs of the American Medical Association, Vol. 13. Chicago, Ill.

Callahan D. 1987. Setting Limits: Medical Goals in an Aging Society. New York: Simon and Schuster.

Callahan D. 1990. What Kind of Life: The Limits of Medical Progress. New York: Simon and Schuster.

Cummings NB. 1989. Social, ethical and legal issues involved in chronic maintenance dialysis. In: Maher JF, ed. Replacement of Renal Function by Dialysis, 3d ed. Dordrecht, The Netherlands: Kluwer Academic Publishers, 1141-1158.

Evans RW, Mannien DL, Garrison LP, Jr., et al. 1985. The quality of life of patients with end-stage renal disease. N Engl J Med 312:553-559.

Fost N, Cranford RE. 1985. Hospital ethics committees. JAMA 253:2687-2692.

Foulks C, Holley J, Moss AH. 1989. Unpublished data.

Fox RC, Swazey JP. 1978. The Courage to Fail: A Social View of Organ Transplantation and Dialysis, 2d ed. Chicago: University of Chicago Press, 367-375.

Freeman RB. 1987. Renal dialysis decision-making. In: Life-Sustaining Technologies and the Elderly Working Papers, vol. 1: The Technologies, Part 1. Washington, D.C.: Office of Technology Assessment, 650-684.

Groves J. 1978. Taking care of the hateful patient. N Engl J Med 298:883-887.

Hackler C. 1989. Advance directives and the refusal of treatment. Law 7:457-465.

Hastings Center. 1987a. Guidelines on the Termination of Life-Sustaining Treatment and the Care of the Dying. Bloomington: Indiana University Press.

Hastings Center. 1987b. Part three: Prospective planning. Guidelines on advance directives. In: Guidelines on the Termination of Life-Sustaining Treatment and the Care of the Dying. Bloomington: Indiana University Press, 77-84.

Husebye DG, Kjellstrand CM. 1987. Old patients and uremia: Rates of acceptance to and withdrawal from dialysis. Int J Artif Organs 10:166-172.

Jonsen AR, Siegler M, Winslade WJ. 1986. Clinical Ethics, 2d ed., New York: MacMillan, 11-12.

Kaye M, Lella JW. 1986. Discontinuation of dialysis therapy in the demented patient. Am J Nephrol 6:75-79.

Landau RL, Gustafson JM. 1984. Death is not the enemy. JAMA 252:2458.

Landsman MK. 1975. The patient with chronic renal failure: A marginal man. Ann Intern Med 82:268-270.

Lo B, Rouse P, Dornbrand L. 1990. Family decision making on trial: Who decides for incompetent patients. N Engl J Med 322:1228-1232.

Lowrie EG, Hampers CL. 1981. The success of Medicare's end-stage renal disease program. N Engl J Med 305:434-438.

Lynn J, Childress JF. 1986. Must patients always be given food and water? In: Part II

Considerations in Formulating a Moral Response. By No Extraordinary Means: The Choice to Forgo Life-Sustaining Food and Water. Bloomington: Indiana University Press, 47-60.

McCormick RA. 1974. To save or let die: The dilemma of modern medicine. JAMA 229:172-176.

Miles OH, Gomez CF. 1989. Protocols for Elective Use of Life-Sustaining Treatments. New York: Springer.

Neu R, Kjellstrand CM. 1986. Stopping long-term dialysis: An empirical study of withdrawal of life-supporting treatment. N Engl J Med 314:14-20.

New York State Task Force on Life and Law. 1987. Life-Sustaining Treatment: Making Decisions and Appointing a Health Care Agent. New York: The Task Force.

OTA (Office of Technology Assessment, U.S. Congress). 1987. Life-Sustaining Technologies and the Elderly. OTA-BA-306. Washington, D.C.: U.S. Government Printing Office.

Papper S. 1970. The undesirable patient. J Chronic Dis 22:777-779.

Port FK, Wolfe RA, Hawthorne VM, Ferguson CW. 1989. Discontinuation of dialysis therapy as a cause of death. Am J Nephrol 9:145.

President's Commission for the Study of Ethical Problems in Medicine and Biomedical and Behavioral Research. 1983. Deciding to Forego Life-Sustaining Treatment. Washington, D.C.: U.S. Government Printing Office.

Ramsey P. 1970. The Patient as a Person. New Haven, Conn.: Yale University Press, 113-164.

Rettig RA. 1991. Origins of the Medicare kidney disease entitlement: The Social Security Amendments of 1972. In Hanna K, ed. Biomedical Politics. Washington, D.C.: National Academy Press, 176-208.

Rodin GM, Chmara J, Ennis, J, et al. 1981. Stopping life-sustaining medical treatment: Psychiatric considerations in the termination of renal dialysis. Can J Psychiat 26:540-544.

Roy AT, Johnson LE, Lee DBN, Brautbar N, Morley JE. 1990. Renal failure in older people: UCLA Grand Rounds. J Am Geriatr Soc 38:239-253.

USRDS (U.S. Renal Data System). 1990. Annual Data Report. National Institute of Diabetes and Digestive and Kidney Diseases. Bethesda, Md.

4

The Patient Population

The congressional charge for the study of the Medicare ESRD program included the study of major epidemiologic and demographic changes in the ESRD patient population that may affect access to treatment, quality of care, or the resource requirements of the program. Chapters 4 and 5 address this charge.

This chapter presents data on trends in ESRD incidence, prevalence, and mortality in terms of age, gender, race, and primary diagnosis of the cause of renal failure (as reported by the patient's physician). These data include only treated ESRD patients, not all those reaching permanent renal failure; the difference between "treated" and "total" is not known. Mortality data are presented for this population and for various patient subgroups. The chapter also includes projections of incidence and prevalence of treated ESRD patients to the year 2000. Chapter 5 deals with the special needs and problems of pediatric, elderly, diabetic, hypertensive, and minority ESRD patients.

The data presented in these chapters are drawn primarily from the HCFA Program Management Medical Information System (PMMIS) files and the United States Renal Data System (USRDS) 1990 Annual Data Report. PMMIS and USRDS are described in detail in Chapter 13. In this report, patients are included in the data base from the time of diagnosis of ESRD rather than from the beginning of Medicare entitlement. This is consistent with the USRDS reports but differs from most HCFA reports. For incidence and prevalence, for example, HCFA usually counts patients only during their Medicare entitlement. For survival analyses, however, both HCFA and USRDS usually include patients from the time of diagnosis of ESRD.

Incidence is defined as new ESRD patients entering treatment during a given year. Incidence data are useful when considering issues of access, patterns of referral to treatment, and disease prevention. Prevalence is defined as the total number of ESRD patients present in the population at a specific time; period prevalence refers to an interval, usually a year; point prevalence refers to the population on a given date, usually December 31. Prevalence data are useful for evaluating the health effects of the disease on society, estimating the costs of providing health care services, and determining what resources and manpower are necessary to provide these services.

INCIDENCE AND PREVALENCE

The incidence and prevalence of Medicare ESRD patients have increased dramatically from the start of the Medicare ESRD program (Table 1-1), and this pattern is projected to continue through the 1990s (Table 1-3). The highest rates of increase are among the aged (Figure 4-1) and diabetic (Figure 4-2) populations.

In 1967, the Report of the Committee on Chronic Kidney Disease estimated that a maximum of 700 to 1,000 patients started hemodialysis between March 1960 and March 1967. The age distributions of 247 patients in Public Health Service (PHS)-funded units who started dialysis during this period and of 231 Veterans Administration (VA) patients who began treatment during 1963-67 are shown in Table 4-1. Nearly three-quarters of the PHS patients and over 90 percent of the VA patients were 25-54 years old. Virtually no patients were under 15 or over 65 years of age.

By the early 1970s, the numbers of new patients had reached several thousand per year, the vast majority of whom were still between 25 and 55 years old. Although the rate of increase was dramatic—over 10-fold during this period—the absolute number of new patients was modest.

The Committee on Chronic Kidney Disease (1967) estimated the number of patients with renal failure who would be considered appropriate candidates for renal replacement therapy for the period from 1968 to 1977, based on the then-current criteria for acceptance into renal replacement treatment. Most eligible patients were in the 15- to 54-year age range. The projected population was expected to increase sharply during the early 1970s and then become relatively stable. The report estimated that the most probable level of new patients in 1977 would be about 8,400 and the total dialysis population about 40,000.

It was predicted, however, that as therapy became more readily available, acceptance criteria would be liberalized. In addition, the prevention of early death from diabetes and other diseases would probably lead to increased numbers of renal failure patients. After adjustment for age changes, a 5 percent increase in incident cases of chronic uremia was predicted for the end of the 1970s. The upper, lower, and most likely estimates are shown in Table 4-2.

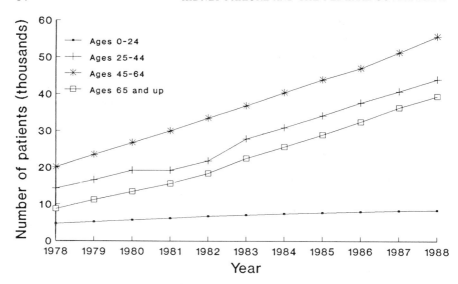

FIGURE 4-1   Number of ESRD Patients by Age Group, 1978-88
NOTE: As of December 31.
SOURCE: USRDS, 1990.

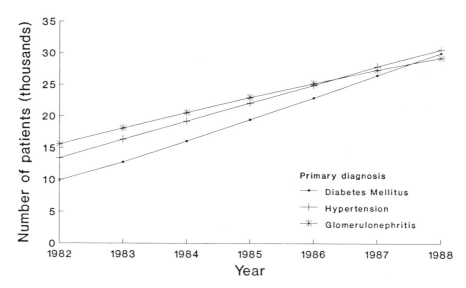

FIGURE 4-2   Number of ESRD Patients by Primary Diagnosis, 1978-88
NOTE: As of December 31.
SOURCE: USRDS, 1990.

TABLE 4-1   Age of New Dialysis Patients, 1960-67

Age Group (years)	Public Health Service		Veterans Administration	
	Number	%	Number	%
Under 15	3	1.2	0	0.0
15-24	42	17.0	8	3.5
25-34	69	27.9	54	23.4
35-44	61	24.7	99	42.8
45-54	52	21.1	62	26.8
55-64	18	7.3	8	3.5
Over 65	2	0.8	0	0.0
TOTAL	247	100.0	231	100.0

NOTE: These data represent an estimated one-half to two-thirds of all new ESRD patients who were treated during 1960-67.

SOURCE: Committee on Chronic Kidney Disease, 1967, pp. 49 and 51.

What actually happened? After the introduction of the Medicare ESRD program in 1973, the number of newly treated patients increased dramatically. The age distribution of new patients began to shift upward; the proportion of new ESRD patients with chronic diseases such as diabetes mellitus and hypertensive vascular disease also began shifting upward. Before 1973, patients were disproportionately white, middle-class men with high educational status. After 1973, the proportion of women and racial minorities increased, and the distribution of patients tended to follow more closely the demographic features of the American population (Evans et al., 1981). The actual number of new Medicare ESRD patients in 1977 (USRDS, 1990) was 15,832 (estimated to be 90 to 93 percent of the total), or almost twice that projected by the Committee on Chronic Kidney Disease (1967).

COMPOSITION OF THE ESRD POPULATION

Not only has the size of the incident population increased over time, but the characteristics of the population also have changed. As mentioned above, the number and proportion of ESRD patients who are elderly have increased dramatically. Between 1978 and 1988, new Medicare ESRD patients over age 65 increased from 3,637 to 13,866 (USRDS, 1990), or from 24 percent to 38 percent of all new patients. In this same period, new patients over age 75 increased from 799 to 5,061, or from 5.4 percent to 14.0 percent of the total; those over age 85 increased from 54 to 531, or from 0.3 percent to 1.5 percent of the total. Table 4-3 shows these trends.

TABLE 4-2   1967 Projections of New End-Stage Renal Disease (ESRD) Patients, 1968-77

Year	Lower Limit	Most Probable	Upper Limit
1968	5,978	6,958	8,152
1969	6,104	7,105	8,324
1970	6,233	7,255	8,499
1971	6,364	7,408	8,678
1972	6,498	7,564	8,861
1973	6,635	7,723	9,048
1974	6,775	7,886	9,239
1975	6,918	8,052	9,434
1976	7,065	8,222	9,633
1977	7,214	8,395	9,836

SOURCE: Committee on Chronic Kidney Disease, 1967, pp. 125-127.

More liberal acceptance criteria and possibly decreased death rates from nonrenal complications have led to a notable increase in the diabetic and hypertensive ESRD population. Between 1982[1] and 1988, the reported number of new Medicare ESRD patients with diabetes as the primary cause of renal failure increased from 5,019 to 11,034 per year (USRDS, 1990), an increase from 23 percent to 31 percent of all new patients.

The incidence of black patients increased at a greater rate than that of whites; between 1978 and 1988, incidence increased an average of 10 percent per year for blacks compared to 8 percent per year for whites. The incidence of Native Americans and Asians/Pacific Islanders increased more rapidly, with average yearly increases of 19 percent and 25 percent, respectively, between 1981 and 1988. Before 1981, reporting for the racial groups Native Americans and Asians was highly incomplete.

More men than women are patients, and the proportions have remained fairly stable between 1978 and 1988.

Incidence *rates*, defined as the number of newly treated ESRD patients per million population, after adjustment for age, show differences between blacks and whites and between men and women that cannot be seen in the unadjusted data (Table 4-4). In all age groups, except 0-5 years, blacks have higher rates of treated ESRD than do whites. Starting in the teenage years, rates among blacks increase rapidly with age. By age 40, the incidence of ESRD among blacks of both sexes is up to four times greater than that of whites.

For both races, men have higher rates than women, with the exception that among blacks aged 55-84 years, rates of men and women are similar. Among whites of all ages, incidence rates for males are higher than those

TABLE 4-3 New End-Stage Renal Disease (ESRD) Patients by Age, Gender, Race, and Primary Diagnosis, 1978-89

	Year											
	1978	1979	1980	1981	1982	1983	1984	1985	1986	1987	1988[a]	1989[a]
AGE GROUP (years)												
0-4	37	39	60	77	101	99	110	120	116	122	115	112
5-14	288	279	307	262	314	281	317	296	309	305	285	273
15-24	1,101	1,112	1,080	1,108	1,164	1,103	1,159	1,186	1,181	1,231	1,254	1,267
25-34	1,763	1,851	2,086	2,178	2,460	2,466	2,624	2,707	2,975	2,837	3,052	3,286
35-44	2,038	2,080	2,240	2,368	2,601	2,838	3,017	3,382	3,647	3,959	4,287	4,615
45-54	2,842	3,116	3,172	3,241	3,546	3,755	3,877	4,222	4,422	4,834	5,318	5,758
55-64	3,464	3,951	4,378	4,737	5,292	5,773	6,283	6,902	7,099	7,733	8,227	8,671
65-74	2,850	2,267	3,785	4,006	4,631	6,067	6,190	7,078	7,703	8,606	9,028	10,272
75-84	748	1,074	1,239	1,310	1,644	2,519	2,696	3,166	3,695	4,167	4,624	5,520
85 & up	56	83	100	101	170	250	275	347	407	474	543	702
GENDER												
Male	8,522	9,462	10,332	10,779	12,139	13,863	14,719	16,047	17,356	18,634	19,998	22,063
Female	6,669	7,494	8,120	8,612	9,788	11,292	11,833	13,372	14,205	15,639	16,745	18,434
RACE												
Native American	37	40	70	131	196	260	265	271	335	345	450	486
Asian	31	41	59	133	312	306	384	507	508	556	644	683
Black	3,920	4,591	4,862	5,064	5,976	7,074	7,491	8,284	8,728	9,666	10,412	11,425
White	10,431	11,417	12,528	13,295	15,260	17,132	18,200	20,098	21,577	23,194	24,588	26,981
Other/unknown	772	867	933	768	183	273	212	259	413	512	649	922
PRIMARY DIAGNOSIS												
Diabetes	1,430	1,635	2,258	3,649	5,050	5,913	7,112	8,192	9,290	10,234	11,247	12,610
Glomeruloneph.	1,918	2,116	2,244	3,500	5,118	5,480	5,775	6,181	6,263	6,500	6,560	6,577
Hypertension	1,845	2,042	2,528	3,965	5,404	5,791	6,459	7,362	7,772	8,829	9,725	10,801
Missing	6,931	7,802	7,802	3,729	1,691	2,897	1,852	1,894	2,239	2,315	2,806	4,271
Other	1,737	1,918	2,125	2,881	3,229	3,642	3,853	4,615	4,393	4,564	4,652	4,764
Unknown	1,330	1,443	1,495	1,667	1,460	1,432	1,501	577	1,604	1,831	1,753	1,474
TOTAL	15,191	16,956	18,452	19,391	21,927	25,155	26,552	29,419	31,561	34,273	36,743	40,497

[a]Data incomplete for this year. SOURCE: HCFA, 1990b.

TABLE 4-4 New End-Stage Renal Disease (ESRD) Patients per Million
Population by Age, Gender, and Race, 1987

Age Group (years)	Men Blacks	Whites	Women Blacks	Whites
Under 5	6 (1+)	6 (1+)	4 (1+)	3 (1+)
5-14	16 (1.9)	10 (1)	9 (1.2)	7 (0.8)
15-24	71 (1.6)	28 (1.2)	55 (1.5)	23 (1.2)
25-34	196 (1.2)	60 (1.2)	105 (1.2)	42 (1.1)
35-44	527 (1.5)	100 (1.3)	232 (1.4)	65 (1.3)
45-54	843 (1.6)	164 (1.4)	564 (1.5)	119 (1.5)
55-64	1,059 (1.6)	304 (1.8)	1,131 (1.8)	214 (1.8)
65-74	1,253 (2.0)	487 (1.9)	1,396 (2.2)	317 (2.2)
75-84	1,138 (3.1)	575 (2.6)	1,133 (3.3)	267 (3.0)
85 and up	696 (5.4)	(3.2)	414 (4.4)	85 (4.2)
TOTAL	335 (1.7)	130 (1.7)	308 (1.9)	94 (1.8)

NOTE: The ratio of the 1987 rate to the 1980 rate is shown in parentheses.

SOURCE: HCFA, 1990a.

for females: after age 75, the incidence among white men is more than
twice that of white women between ages 75 and 85, and four times greater
after age 85.

The incidence of the underlying cause of ESRD also differs substantially
among the principal gender-race subgroups (Table 4-5).[2] Among white men,
ESRD rates attributed to diabetes mellitus and hypertension are quite similar, with these two diagnoses accounting for the majority of patients. Diabetes mellitus is the most frequently reported underlying cause of ESRD
among white women, with incidence rates nearly as high as among white
men. Hypertension and glomerulonephritis contribute about 60 percent and
40 percent as many patients, respectively, as diabetes.

For each diagnosis, incidence rates are higher among blacks than among
whites. Hypertension accounts for nearly half of all ESRD cases among
black men, and the rate of hypertensive ESRD is more than five times
higher among black than white men. Compared to white men, black men
have over twice the incidence of ESRD due to diabetes and glomerulonephritis,
respectively. Compared to white women, black women have incidence rates
seven, four, and three times higher for ESRD attributed to hypertension,
diabetes, and glomerulonephritis. Among the races, Native Americans have
the highest rates of ESRD attributed to diabetes and glomerulonephritis;
nearly two-thirds of ESRD among Native Americans is attributed to diabetes. Clearly, the rates and causes of ESRD differ substantially between the
races, and the burden of ESRD falls more heavily on blacks and Native
Americans than on whites.

TABLE 4-5 New End-Stage Renal Disease (ESRD) Patients per Million Population by Primary Diagnosis, Gender, and Race, 1988

Primary Diagnosis	Men		Women	
	Blacks	Whites	Blacks	Whites
Diabetes	109	37	131	32
Hypertension	187	35	123	18
Glomerulonephritis	52	22	32	12
Other	35	23	30	17
Unknown	71	19	43	11

NOTE: Age adjusted.

SOURCE: USRDS, 1990.

The distribution of prevalent treated ESRD patients generally resembles that of incident patients (Table 4-6). However, because of considerably higher mortality rates among elderly and diabetic ESRD patients compared to other age and diagnostic groups, both represent a considerably smaller proportion of the prevalent compared to the incident population. For example, in 1988 the incidence rate of diabetic ESRD was over twice that of glomerulonephritic ESRD, but the prevalence was very similar. Similarly, in 1988, those over age 65 accounted for 38 percent of the incident population but only 26 percent of the December 31 prevalent population.

MORTALITY ISSUES

The mortality experience of the ESRD program, as a matter of clinical, epidemiologic, and policy concern, raises three basic issues: First, has ESRD mortality changed over time? Second, what factors are causally related to observed patterns of mortality? Third, what are the clinical and policy implications of the first two issues. This section addresses mainly the first and second issues; Chapter 10 deals with the third issue.

HCFA is the primary source of mortality data in the ESRD program. The annual HCFA research report on ESRD presents patient survival data that are generally grouped by age, gender, race, and primary disease. The methods of analysis of these data have changed over time, reflecting a continuing search for improved ways to analyze and present the data (HCFA, 1986, 1987, 1988, 1989). The USRDS, in its first two annual data reports, published extensive summaries of HCFA ESRD data (USRDS, 1989, 1990). The second report made several methodological changes to improve its reporting of the data. Other analyses of ESRD mortality have been published, including analysis of gross mortality (Hull and Parker, 1990) and regional and local analyses (Acchiardo et al., 1983; Blagg et al., 1983; Collins et al.,

TABLE 4-6 Prevalent End-Stage Renal Disease (ESRD) Patients by Age, Gender, Race, and Primary Diagnosis, 1978-89

	Year											
	1978	1979	1980	1981	1982	1983	1984	1985	1986	1987	1988[a]	1989[a]
AGE GROUP (Years)												
0-4	57	68	87	130	175	214	241	274	284	301	309	301
5-14	736	817	913	951	1,079	1,167	1,254	1,303	1,391	1,484	1,551	1,624
15-24	3,937	4,349	4,722	5,095	5,157	5,686	5,922	6,067	6,308	6,460	6,591	6,704
25-34	6,990	8,231	9,627	10,890	12,193	13,382	14,569	15,730	16,959	17,832	18,757	19,752
35-44	7,906	9,029	10,196	11,501	13,136	15,002	16,886	18,986	21,248	23,417	25,731	28,394
45-54	10,105	11,510	12,715	13,953	15,311	16,605	18,157	19,730	21,275	23,331	25,802	28,404
55-64	10,935	12,940	14,937	16,883	19,018	21,063	26,061	24,964	26,547	28,739	30,715	32,903
65-74	7,147	8,937	10,565	12,075	13,986	16,617	18,594	20,616	22,888	25,230	27,226	30,009
75-84	1,567	2,232	2,836	3,441	4,221	5,613	6,682	7,827	9,065	10,427	11,622	13,334
85 & up	86	140	204	261	367	499	602	759	884	1,128	1,327	1,592
GENDER												
Male	27,732	32,477	37,199	41,672	46,983	52,891	58,533	64,038	69,658	75,688	81,700	88,941
Female	21,734	25,776	29,603	33,508	37,960	42,957	47,435	52,319	57,191	62,661	67,931	74,076
RACE												
Native American	102	137	201	320	482	686	856	985	1,144	1,291	1,507	1,729
Asian	102	143	202	333	598	848	1,102	1,424	1,708	2,013	2,353	2,717
Black	12,979	15,616	18,021	20,419	23,480	27,061	30,350	33,683	36,784	40,356	43,972	47,918
White	33,956	39,562	45,176	50,718	57,319	64,303	70,879	77,572	84,456	91,765	98,574	106,858
Other/unknown	2,327	2,795	3,202	3,390	3,064	2,950	2,781	2,693	2,757	2,924	3,225	3,795
PRIMARY DIAGNOSIS												
Diabetes	3,113	3,861	2,258	7,120	9,938	12,743	16,073	19,457	22,969	26,567	30,265	34,611
Glomeruloneph.	8,670	9,991	2,244	13,844	17,454	20,946	24,297	27,609	30,479	33,151	35,538	37,746
Hypertension	5,229	6,424	2,528	10,242	13,431	16,373	19,189	22,099	24,883	27,827	30,679	33,854
Other/unknown	32,454	37,977	7,802	43,974	44,120	45,786	46,409	47,192	48,518	50,804	53,149	56,806
TOTAL	49,466	58,253	66,802	75,180	84,943	95,848	105,968	116,357	126,849	138,349	149,631	163,017

[a]Data incomplete for this year. SOURCE: HCFA, 1990b.

1990; Degoulet et al., 1982; Lowrie and Lew, 1990; Parker et al., 1983; Shapiro and Umen, 1983; Wolfe et al., 1990).

Various factors complicate the discussion of mortality trends. First, data accuracy and completeness have varied over time. However, HCFA has steadily improved its data collection procedures, and current data are more reliable than those available in the 1970s and early 1980s. These problems limit the ability to compare the mortality experience between time periods.

Second, differences in methodology among analysts and over time for a given analyst make the interpretation of mortality complex. In particular, no standard convention or protocol is used for calculating ESRD mortality rates. For example, such calculations may or may not adjust for differences in the composition of the patient population, such as age or race, even though adjustment provides a more appropriate basis for comparing rates between different populations. In addition, populations may be variously described as all patients present at a point in time (point-prevalent population), in a time period (period-prevalent population), or new patients during a time interval (incident cohort). Mortality rates also differ as a function of the method of calculating mortality. Consequently, the study commissioned a paper by Robert A. Wolfe (see Appendix D of this report) to clarify methodological issues and recommends the formation of a technical working group (Chapter 14) related to ESRD patient mortality.

Third, it is necessary to differentiate between mortality *rates* for an entire patient population (unadjusted as well as adjusted mortality) and the *risk* of death attributable to various patient or treatment characteristics such as age, gender, race, diagnosis leading to ESRD, treatment modality, or treatment year. The former may be increasing at the same time that the latter is stable or decreasing.

Fourth, three current hypotheses of major factors causing changes in mortality rates in the ESRD patient population are patient characteristics (e.g., increasing age and complexity), treatment characteristics (e.g., inadequate dialysis), and eroding quality of care resulting from reimbursement reductions. Although it is difficult to distinguish among these factors in most analyses, the practical importance of the conclusions about the causes of mortality varies greatly between providers and the government. This tends to infuse the technical discussions with subjective considerations.

The Medicare ESRD program mortality experience can be summarized as follows:

• The unadjusted mortality (or gross mortality) rate, defined as the rate of death in all patients treated for ESRD during a year, has been increasing over time.

• Unadjusted mortality rates *in incident cohorts*, however, were stable during 1978-82, jumped upward from the 1982 to the 1983 incident cohort, and have remained fairly stable since then.

• Mortality for the 1978-88 incident and prevalent cohorts, *when adjusted for age, gender, race, and primary diagnosis*, has been quite stable.[3]

• Analyses of subgroups of the ESRD patient population show the mortality of some groups decreasing (i.e., survival improving), some stable, and some increasing.

• International data show that the United States has higher gross mortality and adjusted mortality rates than some European countries, although these data must be interpreted cautiously because cross-national comparisons have substantial limitations.

Unadjusted Mortality

This section presents data for annual incident and prevalent cohorts of ESRD patients and discusses the effect of increasing incidence on temporal trends of unadjusted mortality. The following section deals with mortality adjusted for various patient characteristics. The purpose of the discussion is to clarify various published analyses of temporal changes in mortality within the program.

In the literature, ESRD patients have been categorized in several ways for mortality analysis. These include the mortality of all patients treated during a given year, often referred to as gross mortality (Hull and Parker, 1990),[4] the mortality of incident patient cohorts (HCFA, 1986, 1988, 1989; USRDS, 1989, 1990), and the mortality of those patients who have survived at least one year of ESRD treatment (HCFA, 1987). Each method provides a different result for the Medicare ESRD program mortality experience. The importance of these differences will be explored.

Unadjusted annual mortality of the prevalent ESRD population, also referred to as gross mortality, may be defined as the rate of death among all ESRD patients treated during a year. It has been increasing over time as shown in Table 4-7 for the period 1978-88.[5] This trend is in the same direction, although not as large, as that shown by Hull and Parker (1990) for all *dialysis* patients (Medicare plus non-Medicare).

Various patient characteristics contribute to higher unadjusted or gross mortality, including increasing age of the patient population and more severe illness (e.g., diabetes and other comorbid conditions). The age effect is clear: As with mortality in general, the mortality of ESRD patients increases with age. Increased severity of illness also contributes directly to mortality risk. The increase in many comorbid conditions, although not well documented, has been reported in several studies (Collins et al., 1990; Kjellstrand et al., 1990).

Trends in unadjusted mortality of annual *incident patient* cohorts are shown in Table 4-7. Mortality of incident patient cohorts is commonly reported in the literature (Disney, 1990; Eggers, 1990; HCFA, 1986, 1988,

TABLE 4-7   Gross and Unadjusted One-Year Mortality for All End-Stage Renal Disease (ESRD) Patients, 1978-88

Year	Gross Mortality[a] (%)	Prevalent Cohort Unadjusted Mortality[b] (%)	Incident Cohort Unadjusted Mortality[c] (%)
1978	14.0	11.8	18.8
1979	13.7	11.8	19.1
1980	14.2	12.2	18.8
1981	14.0	12.5	18.6
1982	13.8	12.1	18.8
1983	14.2	12.1	21.3
1984	14.7	12.1	21.2
1985	15.3	13.0	21.6
1986	15.5	13.3	21.6
1987	15.4	13.2	22.5
1988	15.8	13.4	21.7

[a]Calculated for all patients treated during reference year, life-table method with censoring at end of year (HCFA, 1990a).

[b]One-year mortality during reference year for prevalent patients who had survived at least one year before start of the index year, life-table method (HCFA, 1990a).

[c]One-year mortality after first 90 days of ESRD for all patients by year of incidence, Kaplan-Meier method (USRDS, 1990).

SOURCES: HCFA, 1990a; USRDS, 1990.

1989a; USRDS, 1989, 1990). Unadjusted mortality analyses indicate three things: First, in the period from 1978 through 1982, mortality was stable; second, an abrupt increase in recorded mortality occurred during the 1982-83 period; and third, mortality has remained fairly stable since 1983 (Table 4-7).

The abrupt upward shift in unadjusted incident cohort mortality reported from 1982 to 1983 (Eggers, 1990; USRDS, 1989, 1990) represents a puzzle to analysts of ESRD mortality data that is unlikely to be fully resolved. The increase is partly due to a sharp increase during 1983 in reported new patients in two high-risk groups—the elderly and the Medicare disabled (those who had qualified for disability *before* kidney failure). It also appears to reflect an artifact of the data reporting system. Evidence supporting this view includes recent analyses by Eggers (P.W. Eggers, HCFA, unpublished data, 1990) showing that a large number of cases, most of whom were elderly, were reported to HCFA on July 1, 1983, and that more incident ESRD cases were recorded in the HCFA PMMIS data set for 1983 than reported by the facilities, a virtual impossibility.

In addition to mortality for the total population, most of these unadjusted incident patient cohort analyses usually present data grouped by patient characteristics such as age, gender, race, and/or primary diagnosis. Mortality for the subgroups usually differs from the total unadjusted mortality.

It is also clear that mortality of new ESRD patients is considerably higher than mortality of those continuing treatment (e.g., those who have already survived for at least one year on treatment) or of the total patient population (gross mortality) (Table 4-7). For example, unadjusted incident cohort mortality for 1988 was 21.7 percent (USRDS, 1990), whereas it was 13.4 percent for one-year survivors. Mortality rates are generally highest during the period immediately after initiation of ESRD treatment, largely because of earlier death of more vulnerable patients.

Adjusted Mortality

Although mortality rates of a patient population may change over time, the risk of death for particular groups of patients does not necessarily follow the same trend. Gross mortality for ESRD patients has increased over time, largely because of an increased proportion of higher risk patients, but there is no a priori reason to believe that the risk of death, for example, of a white male patient, age 45, with no major comorbid conditions, increased between 1978 and 1988.

In order to assess whether the risk of death has changed over time, mortality data must be adjusted for changes in the patient population. For ESRD patients, mortality risk differs by age, race, gender, primary diagnosis, time since diagnosis of renal failure, and comorbid conditions. Various statistical methods, including a Cox proportional hazards model, Poisson regression, and subgroup analysis, can be used to adjust or control for these variables so that populations with different distribution of these variables can be more appropriately compared. HCFA data permit adjustment for age, gender, race, primary diagnosis, and time-related covariates such as year of treatment and time since renal failure. They do not permit adjustment for comorbid conditions and severity of illness, although these factors have important effects on mortality.

ESRD mortality rates for annual incident patient cohorts, when adjusted for age, race, gender, and primary diagnosis, were stable during the 1980s (Eggers, 1990; USRDS, 1990) as shown in Table 4-8. Mortality for prevalent (all) ESRD patients, adjusted for age, was stable or improving.

Subgroup Mortality

Mortality data grouped by patient characteristics generally indicate the following patterns (Table 4-9). Mortality increases with age, males have slightly higher mortality than females, and whites have higher mortality than blacks. By the major primary disease leading to ESRD, diabetes has

TABLE 4-8 Mortality for Medicare End-Stage Renal Disease (ESRD) Patients (ever entitled) Adjusted for Age, Race, Gender, and Primary Diagnosis, 1978-88 Patient Cohorts

Year	Adjusted Mortality (%)	
	Incident Cohorts[a]	Prevalent Cohorts[b]
1978	21.0	13.8
1979	20.3	13.5
1980	20.1	13.9
1981	20.9	14.2
1982	20.7	13.2
1983	21.7	13.2
1984	21.6	12.0
1985	21.6	13.8
1986	21.1	13.7
1987	21.5	13.6
1988	20.6	13.7

[a]One-year adjusted mortality calculated from day 91 to 1 year + 90 days for patients, by year of incidence of ESRD. Adjustment is by years of age (1-19, 20-44, 45-64, 65-74, 75 plus), race, gender, and primary diagnosis, Kaplan-Meier method (USRDS, 1990).

[b]One-year mortality calculated for patients who had survived at least 1 year before start of the index year. Adjustment is by 5-year age groups, life-table method (HCFA, 1990a).

the highest mortality, hypertension is next, and glomerulonephritis and polycystic disease have the lowest mortality. Mortality rates for transplant patients are lower than those for dialysis patients. The extent to which these differences reflect patient selection is not known.

In spite of the general stability in adjusted mortality, changes have occurred for different subgroups of the ESRD population between 1978 and 1988. There has been general improvement in survival of younger patients and diabetic patients on all modalities of treatment (USRDS, 1990, Tables E.69-E.89). In older patients, race- and diagnosis-adjusted survival is generally steady except for a step increase between 1982 and 1983. Mortality rates, especially in older patients, vary considerably depending on the method of analysis. For example, using age groups with 10-year spans shows a larger trend toward increased mortality than using groups with a span of 5 years or less. This is because age is less adequately controlled as the span increases.

By treatment, there has been improvement in survival for transplant patients of all ages. For example, one-year survival percentages for cadaveric transplant patients in the age groups 0-19, 20-44, and 45-64 increased from 72 to 78, 87 to 94, and 68 to 89, respectively, between 1978 and 1988

TABLE 4-9 One-Year Mortality (percent) for All End-Stage Renal Disease (ESRD) Patients, at Year of Incidence, by Age, Gender, Race, and Primary Diagnosis, 1978-88

	Year										
	1978	1979	1980	1981	1982	1983	1984	1985	1986	1987	1988
AGE GROUP (years)											
0-19[a]	6.8	5.8	5.4	4.0	4.9	3.9	4.8	5.2	4.0	4.1	4.6
20-44	12.9	10.7	11.0	10.0	8.9	9.6	9.5	9.3	8.7	9.5	8.4
45-64	18.7	18.5	17.3	18.4	18.2	19.1	19.6	19.0	18.3	18.0	17.5
65-74	25.5	24.8	27.6	27.8	27.5	29.8	29.0	30.6	29.8	29.6	28.5
75 and older	37.2	35.6	34.2	38.6	38.1	41.1	37.5	38.2	38.3	41.7	39.2
GENDER											
Female	18.4	17.3	15.6	17.9	17.6	18.4	17.9	18.9	18.4	18.2	17.3
Male	22.4	21.7	21.9	22.4	22.0	23.3	23.3	22.9	22.3	22.0	22.0
RACE											
Black	20.2	20.1	19.8	20.5	19.8	20.9	20.4	20.8	19.5	19.3	19.3
Nonblack	21.7	20.7	20.4	21.2	21.5	22.4	22.5	22.3	22.3	21.8	21.8
PRIMARY DIAGNOSIS											
Diabetes	28.5	27.2	27.5	28.9	29.6	28.7	27.1	29.5	27.6	24.8	24.8
Hypertension	17.9	16.9	18.2	18.5	18.9	20.1	21.0	19.3	19.9	20.5	20.5
Kidney diseases	14.4	12.3	13.0	14.0	14.1	14.3	13.9	14.8	14.6	14.9	14.9
Other	22.9	23.4	22.3	21.5	20.3	24.4	24.4	25.2	22.8	21.7	21.7
TOTAL	21.0	20.3	20.1	20.9	20.7	21.7	21.6	21.6	21.1	20.6	20.6

NOTE: Mortality calculated from day 91 to 1 year + 90 days.

[a]Because of possible data errors for pediatric patients (ages 0-19 years), unadjusted mortality has been used for this group. Because measured differences in incidence patterns for the pediatric population have been very small, the use of unadjusted in place of adjusted data should not have a meaningful effect.

SOURCE: USRDS, 1990, Tables E-52 and E-53.

(USRDS, 1990). Dialysis patient survival, however, does not show consistent time trends (Table 4-10), partly because of greater variability among patient age groups. In addition, it is difficult to interpret dialysis mortality because it is influenced by the outward flow of healthier patients to transplantation.

Nevertheless, by age, adjusted by gender, race, and primary diagnosis, there appears to be improved survival among dialysis patients under 45 years old and steady survival for those between ages 45 and 64. Over age 65, there is greater variability in the data; however, a trend toward higher mortality is evident in Table 4-10 for both the 65-74 and the over 75 age groups.

State and Regional Mortality Data

State and regional data, although they often differ from national data, offer insight into the experience of various patient groups. Wolfe and coworkers (1990) reported mortality outcomes for 2,754 dialysis patients using data from the Michigan Kidney Registry for patients between the ages of 20 and 60. Using a Cox regression model, they found a 6 percent per year increase in mortality between annual incident patient cohorts starting center hemodialysis (CH) treatment between 1980 and 1987. (They defined treatment as the modality of dialysis at six months after the onset of ESRD, without regard to whether patients changed to another modality after six months.) This represents a 50 percent increase in the mortality of new patient cohorts during the study years. (Time-dependent covariates, such as treatment year and time since renal failure, were not included in the study; see Wolfe, Appendix D.)

Wolfe and colleagues suggest several possible factors contributing to the observed trend: acceptance of sicker patients for ESRD therapy; selection of healthier patients to treatment modes other than CH, leaving sicker patients on CH (increased proportions of patients were treated with transplantation and peritoneal dialysis during the period of this study); and a degradation of quality of CH therapy. The investigators conclude: "If these trends continue, or if the most recent results are maintained, then future studies must confront the increase in mortality rates among center hemodialysis patients and determine its cause" (Wolfe et al., 1990, p. 439). This report differs sharply from the national pattern for the same period and it should be followed up with studies designed to disentangle patient characteristics and treatment modality effects on mortality.

Collins and associates (1990) analyzed the mortality experience of 2,985 hemodialysis patients treated within the Regional Kidney Disease Program in Minnesota. A comparison of the 1976-82 and 1983-87 periods showed that the proportion of patients starting hemodialysis with no major risk

TABLE 4-10 One-Year Mortality (percent) for Dialysis Patients at Year of Incidence by Age, Gender, Race, and Primary Diagnosis, 1978-88

	Year										
	1978	1979	1980	1981	1982	1983	1984	1985	1986	1987	1988
	AGE GROUP (years)										
0-19a	15.8	14.4	11.7	10.0	11.3	9.4	9.7	9.6	6.3	6.4	6.4
20-44	21.1	19.8	19.5	17.3	16.9	16.6	14.9	13.9	12.2	12.2	9.9
45-64	21.0	20.7	19.2	20.8	20.2	21.1	21.6	20.9	20.1	19.1	18.4
65-74	24.9	25.5	24.8	27.7	27.8	27.5	29.8	29.1	30.6	29.8	29.7
75 and older	37.2	35.6	34.2	38.6	38.1	40.1	37.5	38.2	38.3	41.7	39.2
	GENDER										
Female	22.7	22.6	22.3	22.7	21.8	23.0	22.1	22.2	20.8	21.7	19.8
Male	25.3	24.5	23.7	24.5	24.6	25.4	25.2	24.8	24.1	22.7	22.7
	RACE										
Black	20.1	19.8	17.4	19.5	19.6	20.1	19.5	20.1	19.2	17.6	17.6
Nonblack	26.0	25.3	25.3	25.6	24.9	26.3	25.8	27.2	24.2	22.9	22.9
	PRIMARY DIAGNOSIS										
Diabetes	31.9	32.7	31.6	33.1	32.9	32.1	30.1	32.4	30.3	25.8	25.8
Hypertension	20.5	20.0	20.8	20.8	21.1	22.3	22.6	20.6	21.2	21.0	21.0
Kidney diseases	17.2	15.2	15.4	16.7	16.4	16.7	15.7	16.4	15.9	15.5	15.5
Other	25.6	26.1	24.9	23.7	22.4	26.2	26.2	27.1	24.2	22.5	22.5
TOTAL	24.1	23.5	23.0	23.7	23.4	24.3	23.8	23.7	22.6	21.4	21.4

NOTE: Mortality calculated from day 91 to 1 year + 90 days.

aBecause of possible data errors for pediatric patients (ages 0-19 years), unadjusted mortality has been used for this group. Because measured differences in incidence patterns for the pediatric population have been very small, the use of unadjusted in place of adjusted data should not have a meaningful effect.

SOURCE: USRDS, 1990, Tables E-68 and E-69.

factors (atherosclerotic heart disease, cerebrovascular disease, peripheral vascular disease, chronic obstructive lung disease, and nonskin malignancies) decreased from 41 percent to 28 percent. Those with two or more such risk factors increased from 59 percent to 72 percent: diabetics increased from 29 percent to 43 percent; and the percentage of patients over age 75 nearly doubled. Between 1982-84 and 1985-88, the average annual *unadjusted* mortality rate for all dialysis patients (hemodialysis and peritoneal dialysis) increased from 16.7 percent to 25.6 percent, a 55 percent increase.

In spite of increased comorbidities, mortality among diabetics remained stable up to age 75 but increased among older patients. Mortality decreased among nondiabetic patients with no major comorbidities in these years; nondiabetic patients with increased numbers of major risk factors had increased mortality. Thus, higher comorbidity correlated with increased mortality. The investigators conclude that "the increase in the annual gross mortality rate is highly predicted based on the change in the diabetic population and the increase in single and multiple comorbid conditions in the nondiabetic population" (Collins et al., 1990, p. 422).

These regional studies show increased mortality rates among some groups of dialysis patients and point out the importance of controlling for comorbidities in the analysis of mortality. At present, however, HCFA data do not include these comorbidities.

Cross-National Mortality Data

There are usually two major objectives of international comparisons of mortality rates. (See Wolfe, Appendix D.) The first is to document the existence of differences in mortality rates or to evaluate the relative risk of mortality between countries. The second is to identify the reasons for such differences, if they exist. Using the data currently available from different national registries, it is difficult to arrive at a definitive answer to the first objective, and it is impossible to arrive at an answer to the second.

It has been reported that the mortality of U.S. dialysis patients is higher than in many other countries. The measure most commonly used is gross mortality, which has major limitations as described above. Held and co-workers (1990), however, reported that the mortality of U.S. dialysis patients is much higher even after age adjustment. They compared 5-year survival (the inverse of mortality) of new ESRD patients accepted for treatment in the U.S. Medicare program (150,862 patients), the European Dialysis and Transplant Association (EDTA) countries (124,796 patients for 1982-87), and Japan (66,244 patients for 1983-87). The patients over age 65 represented 37, 24, and 30 percent of the patients for the United States, EDTA, and Japan, respectively; the percentages diabetic were 27, 10, and 19, respectively).

Compared to the U.S. experience, survival rates, adjusted for age and diabetes as a primary diagnosis, were higher in the EDTA for all ages above 25 and in Japan for all ages above 15. Five-year survival rates for the ESRD populations, adjusted to the U.S. population age structure, are shown in Table 4-11. The authors suggest that the differences in mortality may be due to one or more of the following: patient selection rates (the U.S. accepts more patients per million for renal replacement treatment); the completeness and representativeness of the different registries; patient compliance; and the adequacy of treatment.

Kjellstrand and associates (1990) reported important factors that influenced mortality rates in U.S. and Swedish dialysis centers. Data included 2,004 cases from the Regional Kidney Disease Program at Hennepin County Medical Center in Minneapolis and 274 patients at the Karolinska Hospital in Stockholm, Sweden. Focusing on 10 comorbid conditions (arteriosclerotic heart disease, chronic heart insufficiency, peripheral vascular disease, cerebral stroke, pulmonary disease, gastrointestinal disease, cirrhosis, malignancy, hypertensive cardiomegaly, and presence of infection), the investigators found that the number of patients without complications remained stable in both centers between the early 1970s and the mid-1980s. Almost all the increase in the number of patients was among patients over age 50 with complications. Survival analyses stratified by patient comorbid conditions showed little difference between the U.S. and the Swedish experiences.

In an analysis of survival in five European areas (Benelux; British Isles—UK and Ireland; Nordic—Denmark, Norway, Sweden, and Finland; Latin—Italy, Spain and France; and Germany and Austria) and the United States, Kjellstrand and associates (1990) reported that over 90 percent of differences in cumulative survival rates among younger dialysis patients correlated with acceptance and transplantation rates. The analysis reported 4-year cumulative survival in dialysis patients aged 15-44 years. This analysis points to effects of comorbid conditions, acceptance rates, and transplantation rates on survival rates in national populations.

Wolfe (Appendix D) has identified several limitations that apply to international comparisons of mortality rates: (1) data are not collected and reported in a consistent way; (2) the level of mortality observed in a national registry is strongly related to the criteria for patient acceptance for treatment; (3) patient-specific data are not available in a unified data base on which analyses can be performed, resulting in the comparison of dissimilar data; (4) etiologies and comorbidities are not adequately reported; (5) age adjustment tends not to fully adjust for age differences—if patients are older in one nation, then they will tend to be older within each age category as well; (6) cross-national differences in withdrawal from treatment and in the reporting of withdrawal may also be relevant since withdrawal is a major cause of death among elderly U.S. patients.

In spite of these limitations, international comparisons provide important information and hypotheses for further analysis which may lead to improve-

TABLE 4-11   Five-Year Survival of Dialysis Patients
by Country and Diagnosis of Diabetes

Country	% Nondiabetic	% Diabetic
United States[a]	45	26
Europe, 1982-87[b]	55	31
United States[a]	44	26
Japan, 1983-87[c]	60	40

[a]Years and age groupings differ for the age-adjusted comparisons
with EDTA and Japan. Therefore, U.S. data are calculated twice to
match European and Japanese data.

[b]Europe consists of the countries of the European Dialysis and
Transplant Association. Age ranges for Europe are 0-14, 15-24, 25-
34, 35-44, 45-54, 55-64, 65-74, and 75-84 years.

[c]Age ranges for Japan are 0-14, 15-29, 30-44, 45-59, 60-74, and
75-89 years.

SOURCE: Held et al., 1990.

ments in provision of treatment to ESRD patients. It is important to evaluate more precisely which subgroups (both by patient and by treatment characteristics) of ESRD patients have higher, similar, or lower mortality rates than in other countries. Is quite possible that a lower overall mortality rate is achievable in the United States and that international comparisons may contribute to attaining this goal.

PROJECTIONS TO THE YEAR 2000[6]

In 1984, Eggers and coworkers (1984) suggested that the Medicare ESRD population was unlikely to level off in the near future. They projected that program enrollment would rise to 94,400 by 1990, 117,200 by 2000, and 162,100 by 2030. By 1988, however, the total Medicare enrollment had already increased to more than 133,900 people. The primary reason for Eggers and coworkers' underestimation was an unanticipated increase in the incidence of ESRD patients.

Eggers, at the request of the IOM ESRD study, prepared an estimate of the Medicare ESRD patient population for the year 2000 for this study, updating previous projections (Eggers, 1989) by incorporating new information on incidence and mortality for dialysis as well as transplant patients. His model, based on current eligibility criteria, generates low, middle, and high projections of the ESRD patient population for December 31, 2000, as presented in Table 4-12.

The middle projection anticipates that over 240,000 ESRD patients will be receiving treatment on December 31, 2000. This scenario estimates that

TABLE 4-12   Medicare End-Stage Renal Disease (ESRD) Population
Projections, Year 2000

	Estimates		
Category	Low	Middle	High
Incidence of ESRD patients	47,949	56,877	68,472
Transplant patients[a,b]	24,915	14,445	8,237
Cadaver donors	20,186	11,653	6,594
Living donors	4,729	2,792	1,643
Dialysis patients[c]	122,953	182,037	231,401
Functioning graft patients[c]	86,993	59,414	42,927
Patients leaving Medicare	5,256	3,566	2,562
Deaths[a]	34,164	43,357	49,351
Total patients[c]	209,946	241,452	274,328

[a]During calendar year 2000.

[b]Under existing statutory authority, transplant recipients are limited to 3 years of Medicare
eligibility. Increased rates of transplantation, therefore, reduce the projected Medicare patient
population, creating the counterintuitive results shown in the table.

[c]End of calendar year 2000.

SOURCE: Paul W. Eggers, HCFA, unpublished data, 1990.

almost 57,000 new patients will enter the program during the year 2000, an
increase of 57 percent from 1988. The low scenario projects that almost
210,000 patients will be undergoing treatment at the end of the year 2000,
the high scenario nearly 275,000 patients.

The model is sensitive to underlying assumptions, particularly incidence
rates. The projection based on the highest incidence rate results in almost
65,000 more ESRD patients than that using the lowest rate. Changes in the
number of transplants performed do not influence the projections of total
patient population very much but do affect the distribution by mode of therapy.
Failure to increase transplants above the current levels will lead to a decline in
the percentage of all ESRD prevalent patients with a functioning graft.

Although these projections are unlikely to predict the future of the Medicare ESRD enrollment with precision, they provide a reasonable estimate of
future enrollment based on current treatment and outcome trends. Even the
low scenario indicates that historical growth of the ESRD population will
continue well into the next century, as shown in Figure 4-3.

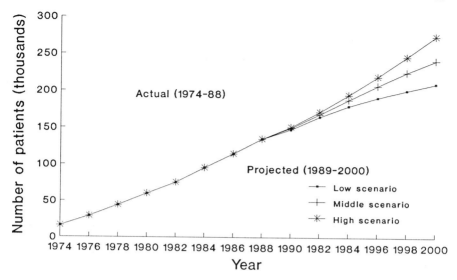

FIGURE 4-3   Number of ESRD Patients, Actual and Projected, 1974-2000
NOTE: As of December 31.
SOURCE: Paul E. Eggers, HCFA, unpublished data, 1990.

NOTES

1. Data for primary diagnosis are quite incomplete before 1982.
2. Diagnostic categories lack clarity, precision, and uniform application, especially for the diagnosis of hypertension.
3. Age adjustment largely compensates for the increased gross mortality observed in 1982 and 1983 because of a large reported increase in elderly ESRD patients in these years.
4. In their analysis of dialysis mortality, Hull and Parker (1990) used the total number of patients who died during the year as the numerator and the average of the prevalent populations on the first and last days of the year as the denominator.
5. Gross mortality may have been increasing since the inception of the Medicare ESRD program, with the increase of older patients and patients with chronic diseases such as diabetes. These trends in patient incidence, which drive up gross mortality, have continued to the present. Because of the limits of HCFA data, we report the trend quantitatively only since 1978.
6. This section is based upon projections by P.W. Eggers of HCFA prepared for this study.

REFERENCES

Acchiardo SR, Moore LW, Latour PA. 1983. Malnutrition as the main factor in morbidity and mortality of hemodialysis patients. Kidney Int 24(Suppl 16):S99-S203.
Blagg CR, Wahl PW, Lamers JY. 1983. Treatment of chronic renal failure at the Northwest Kidney Center, Seattle, from 1960 to 1982. ASAIO J 6:170-175.
Collins AJ, Hanson G, Umen A, Kjellstrand C, Keshaviah P. 1990. Changing risk factor demographics in end-stage renal disease patients entering hemodialysis and the impact on long-term mortality. Am J Kidney Dis 15:422-432.

Committee on Chronic Kidney Disease. 1967. Report of the Committee on Chronic Kidney Disease to U.S. Bureau of the Budget.

Degoulet P, Legrain M, Reach I. 1982. Mortality risk factors in patients treated by chronic hemodialysis: Report of the Daiphane Collaborative Study. Nephron 31:103-110.

Disney APS. 1990. Dialysis treatment in Australia, 1982 to 1988. Am J Kidney Dis 15:402-409.

Eggers, PW. 1989. Projections for the end-stage renal disease population to the year 2000. Proceedings of the 1989 Public Health Conference on Records and Statistics. U.S. Department of Health and Human Services, DHHS Publ. No. PHS 90-1214. November, pp. 121-126.

Eggers PW. 1990. Mortality rates among dialysis patients in Medicare's End-Stage Renal Disease Program. Am J Kidney Dis 15:414-421.

Eggers PW, Connerton R, McMullan M. 1984. The Medicare experience with end-stage renal disease: Trends in incidence, prevalence, and survival. Health Care Financing Rev 5:69-88.

Evans RW, Blagg CR, Bryan FA, Jr. 1981. Implications for health care policy: A social and demographic profile of hemodialysis patients in the United States. JAMA 245:487-491.

HCFA (Health Care Financing Administration). 1986. Health Care Financing Research Report: End-Stage Renal Disease, 1984. Baltimore, Md.

HCFA. 1987. Health Care Financing Research Report: End-Stage Renal Disease, 1985. Baltimore, Md.

HCFA. 1988. Health Care Financing Research Report: End-Stage Renal Disease, 1986. Baltimore, Md.

HCFA. 1989. Health Care Financing Research Report: End-Stage Renal Disease, 1987. Baltimore, Md.

HCFA. 1990a. ESRD Program Management and Medical Information System. March update. Baltimore, Md.

HCFA. 1990b. ESRD Program Management and Medical Information System. August update. Baltimore, Md.

Held PJ, Brunner MD, Odaka MD, Garcia BS, Port FK, Gaylin DS. 1990. Five-year survival for end-stage renal disease patients in the United States, Europe, and Japan, 1982 to 1987. Am J Kidney Dis 15:451-457.

Hull AR, Parker TF. 1990. Introduction and summary: Proceedings from the Morbidity, Mortality, and Prescription of Dialysis Symposium (Dallas, Tex., Sept. 15-17, 1989). Am J Kidney Dis 15:375-383.

Kjellstrand CM, Hylander B, Collins AC. 1990. Mortality on dialysis—On the influence of early start, patient characteristics, and transplantation and acceptance rates. Am J Kid Dis 15:483-490.

Lowie EG, Lew NL. 1990. Death risk in hemodialysis patients: the predictive value of commonly measured variables and an evaluation of death rate differences between facilities. Am J Kidney Dis 15:458-482.

Parker T, Laird NM, Lowrie EG. 1983. Comparison of the study groups. The National Cooperative Dialysis Study. A description of morbidity, mortality and patient withdrawal. Kidney Int 23(Suppl 13):S42-S49.

Shapiro FL, Umen A. 1983. Risk factors in hemodialysis patient survival. ASAIO J 6:176-184.

USRDS (U.S. Renal Data System). 1989. Annual Data Report. National Institute of Diabetes and Digestive and Kidney Diseases, Baltimore, Md.

USRDS. 1990. Annual Data Report. National Institute of Diabetes and Digestive and Kidney Diseases, Bethesda, Md.

Wolfe RA, Port FK, Hawthorne MV, Guire KE. 1990. Comparison of survival among dialytic therapies of choice: In-center hemodialysis versus continuous ambulatory peritoneal dialysis at home. Am J Kidney Dis 15:433-440.

5

The ESRD Patient Population: Special Groups

Several segments of the ESRD population deserve special consideration: pediatric, elderly, diabetic, hypertensive, and minority patients. In all but the pediatric group, renal failure risk is higher than that among the general population.

PEDIATRIC PATIENTS

Pediatric ESRD patients, ranging in age from birth to 20 years, are special patients with very special needs. Their physical and emotional growth relative to their age is often delayed as a consequence of their chronic illness. Indeed, the primary difference between the child and the adult ESRD patient lies in the child's needs to grow and develop, both physically and mentally, and in how these needs interact with treatment.

In this section, the incidence, prevalence, and survival of pediatric ESRD patients from 1978 to 1987 are described. Also discussed are morbidity, prevention of ESRD, access to treatment, and the special needs and problems of the pediatric patients, their families, and their providers.

The absolute numbers of incident and prevalent pediatric ESRD patients for 1978 and 1987 are shown in Table 5-1. During this period, the incidence of treated ESRD among infants and preschool children under age 5 years tripled, from 37 to 120; children in the 5- to 9-year age group increased 36 percent, from 81 to 110 patients; and incidence among older children was steady during this period (P.W. Eggers, S. Alexander, and J.E. Lewy, unpublished data, 1990).

As in the adult population, ESRD incidence is greater among males than among females; in particular, it is almost twofold higher among male infants. In contrast to the adult population, black children and white children

TABLE 5-1   Incidence and Prevalence of Pediatric End-Stage Renal Disease (ESRD) Patients, 1978 and 1987

	Age Group (years)					
	0-1	1-4	5-9	10-14	15-19	All
Incidence						
1978	12	25	81	208	428	754
1987	52	68	110	194	470	894
Increase (%)	333	172	36	-5	9	19
Prevalence						
1978	a	43	195	546	1,348	2,132
1987	a	262	536	930	2,203	3,931
Increase (%)	a	446	175	70	63	84

aExcluded because of small numbers.

SOURCE: P.W. Eggers (Health Care Financing Administration), S.R. Alexander (Southwestern Medical Center, University of Texas, Dallas), and J.E. Lewy (Tulane University School of Medicine, New Orleans, Louisiana), unpublished data, 1990.

have similar incidence rates until their early teens, when incidence rates among blacks begin to exceed those among whites. By ages 16 to 18 years, rates among blacks are about twice those among whites.

The increasing incidence in younger age groups combined with improved survival resulted in nearly a twofold increase in prevalence of pediatric patients between 1978 and 1987 (Table 5-1). In 1988, there were 833 new pediatric patients in the Medicare ESRD program, or 2.3 percent of all new patients; prevalence was 4,069, or 2.8 percent of all patients.

Many quality-of-life factors are unique to pediatric patients. These include growth retardation, delayed pubertal development, transfusion-dependent anemia, bone and neurologic abnormalities, as well as psychosocial and educational problems. The burdens common to all ESRD patients are often greater for pediatric patients.

The increased incidence and survival of infants and preschool children with ESRD leads to increased comorbidities and treatment problems in the older pediatric population. Major physical problems, such as bone deformities and inhibited growth, are more severe in infants and young children than in those who acquire ESRD at older ages.

Transplantation is the preferred treatment for almost all children; the needs for physical growth and pubertal development are better met through transplantation than dialysis. Table 5-2 shows the change between 1978 and

1987 in the proportion of pediatric patients who had a functioning transplant during those years.

Recently, however, two factors have adversely affected the transplantation rate among children: (1) the limited number of available kidneys despite the increased number of acceptable recipients (Chapter 8); and (2) a UNOS policy in 1988 and 1989, since revised, of allocating grafts to patients on the basis of time on a transplant waiting list. Younger children are adversely affected by these factors, since growth is a critical problem and more constrained by dialysis than transplantation. Transplantation from living related donors is sometimes undertaken as a way to ensure rapid resumption of growth in these children, since the waiting time for cadaver transplants is often prolonged. The recent availability of recombinant growth hormone may alleviate the problem of growth somewhat in young dialysis patients.

Except among infants, survival rates are higher for pediatric ESRD patients than for adults. These rates have been improving progressively among children over time, especially among the younger age groups (Table 5-3).

These survival trends are true for dialysis as well as transplant patients, but average survival rates for patients with transplants are higher than for those treated with dialysis. How much of the difference is due to patient selection and timing of the treatment (for example, preemptive transplantation) versus direct advantage of the treatment is not known. Contributing to this has been an increase in graft survival over time, a factor that has been most important for the successful rehabilitation of pediatric patients. In addition, survival for transplant patients differs by source of graft: survival is greater for patients receiving kidneys from living related donors than from cadaver donors.

Many physical problems affect ESRD pediatric patients uniquely or more severely than they affect adult patients (Fine, 1990). Bone disease may limit ambulatory activities of pediatric patients, including school attendance.

TABLE 5-2 Percentage of Pediatric End-Stage Renal Disease (ESRD) Patients with Functioning Graft, 1978 and 1987

	Age Group (years)					
	0-1	1-4	5-9	10-14	15-19	All
1978	0	19	37	34	29	30
1987	7	48	62	56	54	55

NOTE: As of December 31 of the given year.

SOURCE: P.W. Eggers (Health Care Financing Administration), S.R. Alexander (Southwestern Medical Center, University of Texas, Dallas), J.E. Lewy (Tulane School of Medicine, New Orleans, Louisiana), unpublished data, 1990.

TABLE 5-3 Pediatric End-Stage Renal Disease (ESRD) Patient Survival (percent) at One Year by Year of Incidence and Age Group, 1978 and 1987

Age Group (years)	1978	1987
Under 1	a	83.9
1-4	76.0	98.5
5-9	93.8	99.1
10-14	96.7	99.0
15-19	95.5	96.5

NOTE: Includes dialysis and transplant patients who have survived the first 90 days of end-stage renal disease (ESRD) treatment. Only 9 months of time at risk are included in this period, which ends at one year after ESRD treatment initiation.

aExcluded because of small numbers.

SOURCE: USRDS, 1989, Table D-5.

Associated abnormalities resulting from disturbed calcium/phosphorus metabolism include visual abnormalities, growth delay or growth failure, poor calcification of bone, and severe overactivity of the parathyroid gland. Neurologic abnormalities may include seizures, which occur at a greater frequency in the pediatric than in the adult ESRD patient.

Of particular importance in younger children is growth retardation. Significant psychosocial problems may arise among pediatric ESRD patients as a result of their short stature. Furthermore, delayed pubertal development limits psychosocial and psychosexual development of adolescent patients with ESRD.

Psychosocial problems among adolescent transplant patients are also exacerbated by the side effects of immunosuppressive medications, such as corticosteroids and cyclosporine. A full, rounded face (Cushingoid facies), acne, and obesity may result from corticosteroid therapy. Hirsutism (excessive hair) may result from cyclosporine treatment of transplant recipients. The negative psychological reaction to these side effects may result in noncompliance with immunosuppressive drug treatment and may lead to graft failure.

Other treatments have important side effects on pediatric patients. Various antihypertensive medications may adversely influence the patient's level of activity, academic achievement, and sleep patterns. Severe anemia greatly affects the pediatric patient because of the resulting fatigue, apathy, and anorexia that negatively affect social and educational activities. This problem is now helped by the use of erythropoietin.

Surgical interventions present special problems for young patients. Multiple surgical scars resulting from repetitive peritoneal and/or vascular access, bilateral nephrectomy, and one or more renal transplants negatively affect the pediatric patient's psychosocial development and sense of well-being. Multiple hospitalizations may produce fears in the younger child and interfere with schooling of the older patient. Although many of the above problems are common to all ESRD patients, the pediatric ESRD patient must cope with the problems of growth and development as well as the challenges of ESRD treatment. The pediatric ESRD patient requires more time and attention from physicians, nurses, social workers, nutritionists, psychologists, and other health care professionals. They and their families are also very sensitive to limitations on access to treatment and financial resources.

The special needs of infants, children, and adolescents with ESRD require a multidisciplinary approach to care. This calls for the availability of specially trained pediatric nephrologists, renal nursing specialists, renal nutritionists, social workers, psychologists, and, often, special teachers or vocational rehabilitation counselors. Pediatric urologists and surgeons are also required. There is a shortage, however, of trained personnel to deal with pediatric ESRD patients (Fine, 1990).

Specialized pediatric renal failure centers are necessary for the training of the nephrologists, nutritionists, social workers, and nursing personnel. The availability of these centers is essential to provide appropriate supervision of pediatric patients and to provide consultation for children and their families and physicians who reside in rural areas that are not in close proximity to the children's centers and who must use a facility that is closer to the patient's home. Such supervision and consultation may ensure that optimal care is provided to pediatric patients regardless of their residence.

Children also confront problems related to drug therapy. They are often excluded from testing for the safety and efficacy of new pharmaceuticals. Certain drugs, therefore, either are unavailable to children or must be administered without supporting clinical trial data. Multicenter collaborative studies of new therapies are needed so that enough pediatric subjects will be available to evaluate treatment effects in that population.

The pediatric ESRD population is increasing over time, and many of their problems remain unresolved. Many preventable medical, psychosocial, and educational complications associated with ESRD in the pediatric patient are related to the patient's eligibility for Medicare coverage. The committee's recommendations that Medicare ESRD coverage be extended to all U.S. citizens, independent of Social Security status (Chapter 7), and that HCFA establish special reimbursement rates for children with ESRD (Chapter 11) are steps that will help alleviate these problems.

ELDERLY ESRD PATIENTS

Medicare was established in 1965 to provide medical care to those 65 years of age and over. At the outset, Medicare covered established medical services, and neither dialysis nor kidney transplantation was recognized as an established service. After the 1967 *Report of the Committee on Chronic Kidney Disease*, dialysis and transplantation were basically elevated from "experimental" to "established" treatments (Rettig, 1981). However, few elderly patients were dialyzed in the late 1960s because advanced age was considered a contraindication for renal replacement therapy.

In 1971, Medicare received several inquiries about dialysis coverage for the elderly but had not clarified its policies regarding ESRD. Neither patients nor physicians knew that the elderly were potentially covered by Medicare for dialysis under the 1965 statute. The 1972 kidney entitlement, however, created a Medicare benefit for those under 65. By definition, a Medicare benefit could not be made available to the nonelderly and remain unavailable to the elderly. Hence, the 1972 statute sanctioned Medicare financing for elderly ESRD patients.

The earlier orientation against treating the elderly is reflected in the fact that those over 65 years of age accounted for only 5 percent of the total enrollment in 1974 and 11 percent in 1975, but climbed to 18 percent in 1978 (Rettig and Marks, 1980). By 1988, 38 percent of incident (new) ESRD patients, or 13,866, and 27 percent of prevalent (all) patients, or 39,383, were over age 65. Thus the incidence of treated renal failure is now much higher among the elderly than among the general population. In 1988, it was nearly 500 per million population for those over age 65 compared to 147 per million for the general population (USRDS, 1990). The proportion of elderly patients among all those being treated for ESRD continues to increase, perhaps in part because decreasing general mortality from other conditions, such as cardiovascular diseases, enables more patients to reach renal failure. Projections (see Chapter 4) indicate that the elderly will account for nearly half of new Medicare ESRD patients by the year 2000.

The growth among the very old ESRD population is even more striking. Among those 85 and older, new ESRD patients increased from 65 in 1978 to 580 in 1988, for an average annual growth rate of 18 percent. Changes in incidence over time for various age groups are shown in Table 5-4.

The primary diagnoses leading to renal failure among treated elderly ESRD patients have changed over time (IOM, 1990). Diabetes and hypertension have accounted for an increasing proportion of cases. Diagnostic data are unavailable for the elderly in the early 1970s. In 1978, among new elderly ESRD patients with a specified diagnosis leading to renal failure, 16 percent were diabetic and 38 percent were hypertensive. These proportions had increased to 29 and 42 percent, respectively, by 1988 (IOM, 1990). Glomerulonephritis account for a steady 17 to 18 percent of new elderly patients.[1] Similar trends hold for prevalent patients, except that diabetic patients are a lesser percentage of the prevalent population, compared to new patients, due to their higher mortality rate.

TABLE 5-4 New End-Stage Renal Disease (ESRD) Patients in 1978 and 1988, by Age Group

Age Group (years)	1978	1988	% Increase
0-64	11,258	22,294	98
65-75	2,838	8,805	210
75-86	745	4,530	508
85 and up	54	531	883

SOURCE: USRDS, 1990.

Elderly patients generally arrive at permanent kidney failure with more comorbidity than their younger counterparts, including unstable hemodynamics, vascular disease, and impaired function. In particular, elderly diabetics exhibit the various comorbidities typical of that disease, including visual problems, neuropathy, and amputations.

Treatment modality is highly age dependent, as is shown in Figure 5-1. More young people than elderly receive transplants, the primary treatment modality for the elderly ESRD patient being hemodialysis. On December 31, 1988, elderly ESRD patients were distributed among treatment modalities in the following way: 82 percent in-center hemodialysis, 2 percent home dialysis, 9 percent peritoneal dialysis, 2 percent transplant, and 5 percent other or unknown (USRDS, 1990).

Adjusted mortality of elderly patient groups, although high, appears quite stable during the 1980s except for an increase between the 1982 and 1983 incidence cohorts (IOM, 1990; USRDS, 1990). Most of this increase is eliminated by adjusting for age and primary diagnosis, but a small increase in mortality still remains in some groups of patients after adjustment (USRDS, 1990). Most reports indicate stable adjusted mortality rates since the mid-1980s (Eggers, 1990; Sehgal et al., 1990; USRDS, 1990). A stable mortality despite an increasing proportion of very elderly and of underlying conditions such as diabetes among the elderly patients may reflect increasing physician and provider experience over time in treating a more vulnerable patient population.

The leading causes of death among elderly ESRD patients are cardiac arrest, myocardial infarction, and withdrawal from treatment. In contrast to the experience among younger ESRD patient groups, withdrawal from dialysis is common among elderly ESRD patients, accounting for over 10 percent of all deaths of ESRD patients over 65 (USRDS, 1990). Patients or their families, in concert with physicians, withdraw because they decide that the burdens of treatment and the reduced quality of life outweigh the benefits of continued survival. (See Chapter 3.)

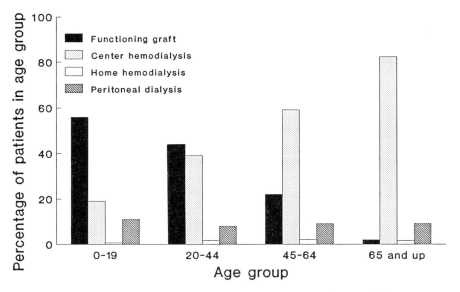

FIGURE 5-1   ESRD Patients: Treatment Modality by Age Group, 1988
NOTE: Excludes small numbers of noncenter dialysis patients.
SOURCE: USRDS, 1989.

The elderly ESRD patient population has increased in number, average age, comorbidities, and special problems in the past decade. These changes are expected to continue throughout the 1990s. The treatment needs of these patients will challenge clinicians in the years ahead to a greater extent than they have to date.

DIABETIC PATIENTS

Diabetes mellitus as a cause of ESRD has increased substantially in the past two decades. During the 1960s and early 1970s, diabetes was generally a reason for not treating ESRD patients. In the 1970s, diabetic patients were a small proportion of total ESRD patients (Table 5-5). By 1983, however, diabetic kidney disease had become the most frequent diagnosis among patients entering the Medicare ESRD program. Clinical experience in the late 1970s and the 1980s had shown that ESRD patients with a primary diagnosis of diabetes could benefit from renal replacement therapy.

Simultaneously, improvements in the treatment of diabetes have contributed to decreased mortality from cardiovascular diseases. This has led to longer life spans and increased chance of renal failure later in life. In 1988,

TABLE 5-5 Patients with Diabetic Kidney Disease as a Percentage of Total End-Stage Renal Disease (ESRD) Patients, by Age Group

Age Group (years)	1972-76[a]	1983[b]	1988[b]
1-19	0.5	0.5	0.7
20-39	5.6	14.0	18.9
40-49	4.7	13.6	21.6
50-59	6.5	15.2	24.1
60+	6.9	13.5	21.9
TOTAL	5.0	13.6	20.0

[a]Approximate, dialysis patients only.

[b]Includes dialysis as well as transplantation patients. In 1983, one-third of diagnoses were reported as missing/unknown; in 1988, one-fifth were missing/unknown. Therefore, the percentages of diabetic patients for 1983 and 1988 are higher than presented above.

SOURCES: Research Triangle Institute, 1976; HCFA, 1990.

diabetics accounted for 27 percent (or 11,034) of new ESRD patients and 20 percent (or 29,937) of prevalent patients (USRDS, 1990).

The age, gender, and racial distributions of new diabetic ESRD patients have been changing over time. Each year a greater proportion of these patients are elderly, as is true for the ESRD population as a whole. In 1982, the median age of a new diabetic ESRD patient was about 55 years, with 23 percent over age 65 and 11 percent over age 75; in 1988, the median age was 59, with 34 percent over age 65 and 18 percent over age 75.

Incidence of diabetic ESRD differs by race. Rates are higher among blacks and Native Americans than among whites, and higher among Hispanics than among non-Hispanic whites. In a study of racial disparities in Michigan, after adjustment for the higher prevalence of diabetes among blacks, the incidence of diabetic ESRD was 2.6-fold higher among blacks than among whites (Cowie et al., 1989). Incidence of diabetic patients also differs by gender. Among whites, rates are higher among men; by contrast, rates among blacks and Native Americans are higher among women (USRDS, 1990).

Incidence of ESRD differs dramatically as a function of type of diabetes. Although patients with insulin-independent diabetes mellitus (IDDM) constitute only 5 to 10 percent of all diabetics, they account for 40 percent or more of renal failure due to diabetes (Hawthorne, 1990; Rettig and Teutsch, 1990). The relative risk of renal failure appears to be 10 to 15 times greater from IDDM than from non-insulin-dependent diabetes mellitus (NIDDM).

There are racial differences in the type of diabetes leading to ESRD. In Michigan, 77 percent of black diabetic ESRD patients had NIDDM, whereas 58 percent of white diabetic ESRD patients had IDDM (Cowie et al., 1989).

Genetic factors also play a role. Familial susceptibility to diabetic nephropathy (NIDDM) has been shown among the Pima Indians (Pettitt and Saad, 1988), as well as among patients with IDDM (Seaquist et al., 1989).

Like incidence, prevalence has increased substantially since 1973, although HCFA data for primary diagnosis are highly incomplete before 1982. Between 1982 and 1988, however, there has been a threefold increase in prevalent diabetic ESRD patients, from 9,913 to 29,937 (USRDS, 1990).

Diabetic ESRD patients have higher adjusted mortality rates than the other major diagnostic groups—glomerulonephritis and hypertension. During the 1980s, however, mortality rates of diabetic ESRD patients, when controlled for age, gender, and race, decreased slightly for patients on dialysis or with transplants (USRDS, 1990) in spite of substantial increases in incident patients and, presumably, in patient complexity. This suggests that growing clinical experience with this patient segment may have reduced the risk of mortality. Most patients with diabetic ESRD die of coronary heart disease within 5 years of onset of ESRD treatment (Hawthorne, 1990).

In addition to higher mortality rates, diabetic ESRD patients have more comorbidities than the other major diagnostic groups. Major comorbidities include blindness, peripheral neuritis, and vascular disease. Hypertension is present in two out of three patients (Hawthorne, 1990). The increased severity of illness of diabetic ESRD patients leads to increased hospitalization and higher overall medical costs (Smith et al., 1989).

Knowledge of the risk factors for the development of diabetic nephropathy is critical in determining points of intervention. Major risk factors include hyperglycemia, hypertension, macrovascular disease, familial associations, race, age, and type and duration of diabetes. Some risk factors for development of ESRD in diabetics may be susceptible to intervention. In longitudinal studies, poor glucose control is a strong predictor of development of clinical diabetic nephropathy. Thus, strict glucose control may be of value in primary prevention of early diabetic nephropathy and possibly slowing or reversing early nephropathy (Hawthorne, 1990).

Hypertension is an important predictor and possible cause of diabetic nephropathy. The appearance of hypertension in a diabetic patient with previously normal blood pressure may be the first sign of renal disease (Selby et al., 1990). Blood pressure monitoring and control is indicated for all diabetic patients (Working Group on Hypertension in Diabetes, 1987). Albuminuria screening is under study as a test for the earliest phase of diabetic kidney disease; early recognition would permit institution of treatment to prevent or slow development of ESRD (Bennett, 1989; Mogensen and Christiansen, 1984; Viberti et al., 1982). In addition, some research suggests that protein restriction may slow or halt renal decline (Cohen et al., 1986; Wiseman et al., 1987). Hence, the American Diabetes Association has recommended that diabetics restrict their dietary intake of protein (American Diabetes Association, 1986).

The rapid increase of diabetics treated for renal failure underlines the urgent need to understand the etiologies of this disease process as well as potential interventions. The development of screening methods to assess renal function of diabetics and detect the early stages of diabetic nephrology should be pursued. In addition, measures to distinguish between IDDM and NIDDM as well as to classify comorbidities, including hypertension and cardiovascular diseases, should be developed and incorporated in ERSD data systems at HCFA and the USRDS.

HYPERTENSIVE PATIENTS

The incidence and prevalence of treated hypertensive ESRD has increased continually since the Medicare ESRD program was initiated. In 1974, 13.5 percent of the new patients (less than 1,000) entered the program with the diagnosis of hypertensive ESRD (Eggers et al., 1984). By 1988, 27 percent of new patients, or 9,647, carried this diagnosis; the prevalence of hypertensive patients was 21 percent, or 30,517 patients (USRDS, 1990).

Hypertension in the United States

A substantial proportion of the U.S. population has hypertension. According to the Second National Health and Nutrition Examination Survey (NHANES II), conducted during 1976-80 (NCHS, 1986), an estimated 18 percent of U.S. adults (about 25 million) had "definite hypertension," defined as a systolic blood pressure (SBP) at least 160 mmHg and/or diastolic blood pressure (DBP) at least 95 mmHg, and/or taking antihypertensive medication. Under a more liberal definition of hypertension (DBP at least 90 mmHg, SBP at least 140 mmHg, and/or medicated), hypertensives comprised nearly 30 percent of (or about 40 million) Americans.

Prevalence of hypertension increases with age; men have higher rates at younger ages, women at older ages. Blacks have higher rates than whites; the prevalence of definite hypertension for blacks and whites, by age group and gender, in the NHANES II data set is shown in Table 5-6.

Between 1960 and 1980, the prevalence of definite hypertension among black adults decreased from 33.6 to 28.6 percent; no similar decline was observed among whites (NCHS, 1986). The proportion of hypertensives taking antihypertensive medications increased from 30 to 45 percent and the proportion of those whose hypertension was controlled by medication increased from 39 to 52 percent. The prevalence of hypertension in the United States

TABLE 5-6   Percentage of U.S. Population with Definite Hypertension, 1976-80

Age Group (years)	Whites		Blacks	
	Men	Women	Men	Women
18-24	2.8	1.4	2.4	3.2
25-34	9.3	4.1	13.3	7.3
35-44	13.4	11.2	23.8	26.9
45-54	25.7	25.2	26.0	58.3
55-64	32.6	36.6	46.4	60.1
65-74	38.1	50.5	42.9	72.8

NOTE: Definite hypertension is defined as systolic blood pressure at least 160 mmHg and diastolic blood pressure at least 95 mmHg and/or taking antihypertensive medication.

SOURCE: NCHS, 1986.

has decreased as improvements in its treatment have occurred. However, a corollary, and probable consequence, of these developments is that treated hypertensive ESRD has increased strikingly.

Relationship Between Hypertension and Hypertensive ESRD

The risk of renal disease due to severe hypertension is well documented. Before the availability of effective antihypertensive drug therapy, over 90 percent of patients with accelerated and malignant hypertension died within 12 months of their initial presentation, most from uremia (Kincaid-Smith et al., 1958). The development of effective antihypertensive treatment improved survival even in patients with advanced renal insufficiency (Mroczed et al., 1969; Mamdani et al., 1974; Lee and Alderman, 1978). In people with mild to moderate hypertension, however, little information exists about the risk of renal failure and how that risk is affected by various treatments (Whelton and Klag, 1989).

Although hypertension is a cause of renal failure, renal disease also causes hypertension. Consequently, most patients with ESRD eventually develop hypertension. In new ESRD patients, it is often difficult to distinguish between hypertension as the primary cause and hypertension as a result of ESRD.

Epidemiology of ESRD Attributed to Hypertension

Physician-reported primary diagnoses, as they appear in the HCFA PMMIS, are the most comprehensive data available for evaluating hypertension-related ESRD in the United States. Although limited by the problem of inferred causality, these data strongly implicate hypertension as a primary and increasingly common cause of renal failure. Most of the following discussion is based on these data.

The age/race/gender-adjusted incidence of physician-reported ESRD due to hypertension has risen continuously over the years since the Medicare ESRD program was initiated. Although data from the 1970s concerning primary diagnoses leading to ESRD are lacking or incomplete,[2] it is clear that the numbers of patients with hypertension and diabetes who were treated for ESRD increased during the 1970s.

When the incidence of hypertensive ESRD is compared to that for glomerulonephritis, steady change is apparent. In the early years of the ESRD program, glomerulonephritis was the primary disease leading to renal failure. The ratio of new ESRD cases reported as due to hypertension compared to glomerulonephritis more than doubled between 1978 and 1988, from 0.95 to 1.93. HCFA data indicate an average annual increase in incident hypertensive ESRD patients greater than 10 percent for the period 1982-88; by contrast, the corresponding increase in new glomerulonephritis patients was less than 4 percent per year. Both the absolute numbers and the proportion of ESRD patients attributed to hypertension have increased substantially over the past two decades.

The increase of hypertensive ESRD results, in part, from decreased mortality from competing illnesses, such as coronary heart disease and stroke, attributable to improved treatment of hypertension. This allows a greater proportion of hypertensive patients to progress to renal failure.

The incidence of treated hypertensive ESRD is higher at older ages and among men than among women (USRDS, 1990). In 1988, gender- and race-adjusted incidence rates per million population for age groups 0-19, 20-44, 45-64, 65-74, and 75 and older were 0.3, 13, 70, 194, and 215, respectively. Age- and race-adjusted incidence rates per million population were 49 and 27 for males and females, respectively.

The risk of hypertensive ESRD is strikingly different for blacks compared to whites. Age-adjusted incidence is as much as eight times higher among blacks than whites, and over 20 times higher in the 25- to 44-year age group (USRDS, 1990). Table 5-7 shows age-stratified incidence of treated hypertensive ESRD per 10 million population, adjusted for gender, for blacks and whites during 1988.

The reasons for the racial disparities in hypertensive ESRD are not clear. Contributing factors may be mislabeling of hypertension as a cause of ESRD among blacks; the greater incidence, severity, and duration of hypertension among blacks; and lower rates of antihypertensive treatment among blacks (Whittle et al., 1991). Gender ratios of hypertensive ESRD patients differ between racial and ethnic groups. Among blacks, 45 percent of ESRD patients are women, whereas only 33 percent of white ESRD patients are women.

TABLE 5-7 Incidence of Treated Hypertensive End-Stage Renal Disease (ESRD) per 10 Million Population by Age Group for Blacks and Whites in 1988

Age Group[a] (years)	Whites		Blacks	
	Men	Women	Men	Women
0-19	1	4	9	9
20-44	50	32	1,060	356
45-64	433	265	3,940	2,432
67-74	1,839	955	5,864	5,485
75+	2,634	1,030	6,569	5,269
TOTAL	347	176	1,870	1,232

[a]Age adjusted.

SOURCE: USRDS, 1990.

Age- and race-adjusted survival of hypertensive ESRD patients remained stable between 1977 and 1988 for dialysis patients and improved for patients with kidney transplants (USRDS, 1990). IOM analyses of mortality, comparing new patients during 1980-82 with those during 1984-86, stratified by age and race, showed that mortality rates of younger patients decreased slightly. Rates of patients over age 55 increased slightly, largely because of higher mortality among older patients during the first year of ESRD treatment.

Intervention

Prevention and treatment of hypertension have improved substantially, but the situation is less clear with respect to prevention of hypertensive renal disease. Whelton and Klag (1989) reviewed six studies dealing with antihypertensive drug therapy and the risk of renal disease. They reported that although the majority of the trials were consistent with therapy reducing the risk of renal disease, the trials with the largest number of renal disease events failed to support the benefit of treatment.

In the Hypertension Detection and Follow-up Program (HDFP), a community-based, randomized controlled trial involving 10,940 people with high blood pressure, members of the control group received standard care by each patient's own physician whereas the treatment group received additional care for hypertension. There were 15 deaths attributed to renal disease in the treatment group and 10 in the control group after 5 years (Shulman et al., 1989). Mortality is a poor marker of treatment efficacy, however, since most treated ESRD patients die from causes other than renal disease.

The HDFP study also showed an increased risk of renal disease, defined as an elevated and increasing blood creatinine level. In those with blood pressure of 90-104 mmHg, incidence of renal disease was 16 per 1,000 patients; for those with blood pressure of 105-114 mmHg, incidence was 35 per 1,000; for those with blood pressure above 115 mmHg, incidence was 58 per 1,000. These results, although not free of confounding factors, suggest an effect of blood pressure on development of renal disease.

Klag (1990) used data from the HDFP study and from NCHS hypertension prevalence summaries to estimate the number of people expected to develop hypertensive renal disease, defined by the HDFP study, between 1990 and 1995. For the three diastolic blood pressure groups 90-104 mmHg, 105-114 mmHg, and greater than 115 mmHg, he calculated approximately 320,000, 80,000, and 47,000 new cases, respectively. According to his calculations, two-thirds of these new renal disease cases were expected in hypertensive patients with lowest blood pressure (DBP 90-104 mmHg). Klag concluded that although the risk of developing hypercreatininemia is greater at the highest levels of blood pressure, most cases of renal dysfunction will develop in those hypertensives with the mildest elevations of blood pressure. This seeming paradox occurs because the number of persons with mild diastolic hypertension is much greater than the number in the higher strata of blood pressure. Thus, therapeutic and preventive interventions directed at severe hypertensives can, at the most, prevent only a minority of renal disease cases. To substantially reduce the national burden of hypertension-related kidney disease, intervention strategies must include the large number of people with mild hypertension (Klag, 1990, pp. 22-23).

The relationship between hypertension, the decline of renal function, and the development of ESRD must be clarified for various levels of blood pressure. The effect of control of blood pressure, hyperlipidemia, and other cardiovascular disease risk factors on ESRD incidence, morbidity, and mortality also should be evaluated. In addition, high priority should be given to evaluating the causes of excess hypertensive ESRD among blacks.

MINORITY PATIENTS

Following the 1972 kidney entitlement, different patterns of treated ESRD have appeared among racial and ethnic groups (Feldman, 1990). HCFA PMMIS data are used to present the basic epidemiology, including incidence, prevalence, and survival patterns, and variability in outcomes of treatment modalities between groups.

The relative risk of developing ESRD is several times higher among blacks, Hispanics, and Native Americans than among whites, possibly because of physiologic heterogeneity of the racial and ethnic groups as well as differential access to preventive care. In 1988, nonwhite patients comprised 33 percent of incident (or 11,704) and prevalent (or 48,730) patients.

The incidence of Medicare ESRD patients of all races has increased over the years. Between 1978 and 1988, the average yearly rate of increase in incidence was 10.1 percent among blacks compared with 8.9 percent among whites. Between 1981 and 1988, the average yearly rates of increase in new Medicare ESRD patients among Native Americans and Asians/Pacific Islanders were 16.6 percent and 26.2 percent, respectively.[3] Estimated average yearly rate of increase for Hispanics, based on a sample of 9,690 Medicare patients with Hispanic surnames, was 12.7 percent (IOM, 1990).

Age- and sex-adjusted treated ESRD incidence rates are four times greater for blacks and Native Americans (404 and 109 per million population in 1988, respectively) than for whites (109 per million) (USRDS, 1990). Rates among Asians/Pacific Islanders are closest to those of whites. Hispanics in Texas have threefold higher rates than non-Hispanic whites (Pugh et al., 1988).

The age, gender, and primary disease distributions of incident patients differ considerably among races. Blacks and Native Americans, on average, experience ESRD at an earlier age than whites. Consequently, the age distributions between these groups are substantially different. The pattern for Asians/Pacific Islanders is closer to that of whites. The distribution, by age, of 1988 incident patients is shown in Figure 5-2.

By race and gender, incidence rates among white men are 1.3-1.4 times higher than among women. Incidence rates among black men are slightly

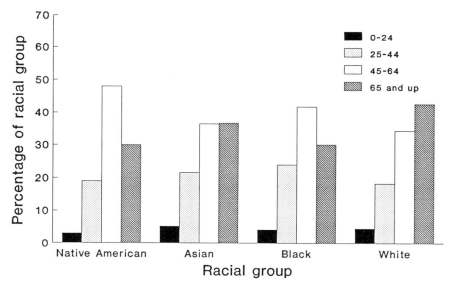

FIGURE 5-2   Age Distribution of New ESRD Patients, by Race, 1988
SOURCE: HCFA, 1990.

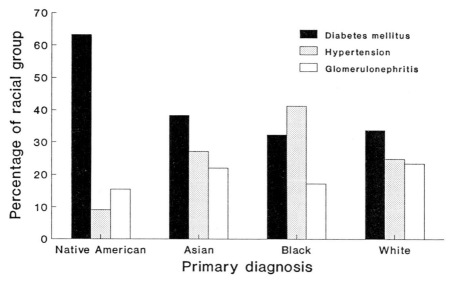

FIGURE 5-3   Distribution of Primary Diagnosis Leading to ESRD, by Race, 1986-88
SOURCE: HCFA, 1990.

higher than among women overall, but there is considerable variation by disease leading to ESRD: women have higher rates for diabetes and men have higher rates for hypertension and glomerulonephritis. Among Native Americans, Asians/Pacific Islanders, and Hispanics, men have a slightly higher risk than women (IOM, 1990; USRDS, 1990).

As shown in Figure 5-3, primary diagnosis of cause of ESRD differs considerably among races. Hypertension is the predominant diagnosis among blacks; diabetes among whites, Native Americans and Hispanics; and glomerulonephritis among Asians/Pacific Islanders.

Although Native American tribes are aggregated in the above data, they vary greatly in the incidence rates of treated ESRD across geographic and tribal boundaries.   The Navajo, the largest Native American tribe, showed age-adjusted ESRD incidence rates four times those of whites between 1976 and 1980 (Gardner et al., 1984). Diabetes accounted for 50 percent of new patients, and the incidence rate of diabetic ESRD was 9.6 times that of whites. The Pima Indians of south central Arizona have one of the world's highest incidence rates of NIDDM, with an age- and gender-adjusted rate of 27 per 1,000 population, approximately 19 times the rate among whites (Knowler et al., 1978; Rate et al., 1983). Among Pima Indians with diabetes, the incidence of ESRD has been estimated to be as high as 21,400 per million leading to a treated diabetic ESRD rate of 960 per million (Kunzelman et al., 1989). The Zuni Indians, a small, ethnically homogeneous tribe of western New Mexico, had one of the highest reported ESRD incidence rates of any Native American group (Pasinski and Pasinski, 1987); between 1978 and 1985, it averaged 11 times that reported for whites. Glomerulonephritis was identified as a cause of 40 percent of new Zuni ESRD patients between 1973 and 1983.

Although data on Hispanics are not systematically collected, Pugh and colleagues (1988) report that Mexican Americans had from 2.4 to 3.2 times higher rates of treated ESRD than non-Hispanic whites. Using data from the Texas Kidney Health Program and the 1980 U.S. census, they calculated 3-year average incidence rates of treated ESRD among Mexican Americans, blacks, and non-Hispanic whites between 1978 and 1984. Mexican Americans had 4.5 to 6.6 times the rate of diabetic ESRD among whites and 1.2 to 1.9 times the rate among blacks. Among Mexican Americans (Pugh et al., 1988) and U.S. Hispanics (IOM, 1990), diabetes is the primary diagnosis leading to ESRD. This high rate of diabetic ESRD is partly explained by the increased prevalence of diabetes mellitus: NIDDM is estimated to be about three times greater among Mexican Americans than among non-Hispanic whites (Stern et al., 1984). In addition, rates of hypertensive and glomerulonephritis-related ESRD are higher among Mexican Americans than among non-Hispanic whites.

Among blacks, rates of hypertension and hypertensive ESRD are considerably higher than among whites. In the NHANES, the age-adjusted prevalence of hypertension was 28 percent and 40 percent among black men and women, respectively, compared to 21.5 percent and 20 percent among white men and women (Rowland and Roberts, 1982). However, the prevalence of hypertension was higher among whites and blacks having an annual household income below $20,000 (NCHS, 1990). Since a greater proportion of blacks fall into the lower income groups, economic disadvantage probably contributes to this racial difference in rates of hypertension.

Once hypertension has developed, blacks have a higher risk of developing ESRD compared to whites (Shulman et al., 1989). Population-based studies have shown that hypertensive blacks have a five- to eightfold risk of developing ESRD compared to hypertensive whites (McClellan et al., 1988; USRDS, 1990). For individuals in their thirties and forties, the risk may be as much as 20 times higher among blacks than among whites (USRDS, 1990). The high risk of hypertensive ESRD among blacks suggests that blacks may have an elevated susceptibility to renal damage due to hypertension.

Both diabetes and diabetes-related ESRD are also more common among blacks than among whites. Age-adjusted estimates of the prevalence of diabetes mellitus showed a 36 percent higher rate among blacks than among whites during 1985-87 (NCHS, 1987).

Age-adjusted 1988 ESRD incidence rates were reported to be 1,094 and

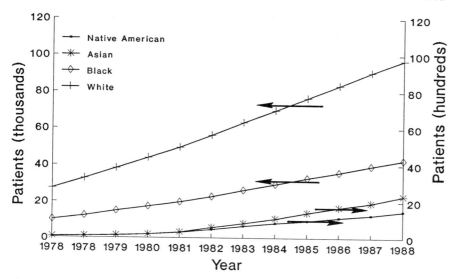

FIGURE 5-4   ESRD Patients, by Race, 1978-88
NOTE: As of December 31.
SOURCE: USRDS, 1990.

1,306 per 10 million black men and women, respectively, compared to 369 and 315 among white men and women (USRDS, 1990).

As expected from racial patterns in incidence, the prevalence rates for treated ESRD are considerably higher among blacks and Native Americans than among whites; the rates for Asians/Pacific Islanders and whites are similar. Total numbers of patients on December 31 of each year have increased for all racial groups (Figure 5-4).

The mode of treatment of ESRD patients differs by racial group. In-center hemodialysis is the principal treatment for all races, but more so for blacks than for whites. Compared to whites, the proportion of blacks with a functioning renal transplant has been consistently smaller, and this gap has grown slowly over time (see Chapter 8). Table 5-8 shows black/white differences in treatment mode for 1980, 1984, and 1988.

The 1-, 2-, and 5-year survival rates of nonwhite dialysis patients have been consistently higher than those of white patients. Table 5-9 shows these survival rates over time. Among transplant patients, black patients have lower survival than whites and other nonwhites.

Between 1981 and 1983, the overall age-adjusted mortality rate from renal failure for Native Americans was 2.6 times the corresponding rate for all Americans. Several areas within the Indian Health Service (Aberdeen, South Dakota; Tucson, Arizona; Phoenix, Arizona) experienced mortality

TABLE 5-8 End-Stage Renal Disease (ESRD) Treatment Modalities (percent) for Blacks and Whites on December 31, 1980, 1984, and 1988

	1980		1984		1988	
Modality	Blacks	Whites	Blacks	Whites	Blacks	Whites
Functioning allograft	6.5	13.4	10.0	21.5	13.8	30.3
In-center hemodialysis	77.5	64.1	74.8	55.6	73.4	50.5
Home hemodialysis	1.6	4.8	2.3	3.8	1.1	2.1
Peritoneal dialysis	1.2	2.2	5.4	8.9	6.2	9.6
Other dialysis	2.4	2.8	2.9	3.3	1.6	2.1
Unknown	10.5	12.4	4.4	6.7	3.6	5.0

NOTE: Percentages may not add to 100 because of rounding.

SOURCE: USRDS, 1990.

rates almost 5 times that of the general U.S. population (Indian Health Service, 1987). These extreme mortality rates seem to correlate best with the incidence of ESRD secondary to diabetes mellitus, recorded as high as 89 percent of incident cases in the Aberdeen area and 95 percent in the Pima tribe (Nelson et al., 1988).

The differences in survival between the races are related to the mode of

TABLE 5-9 Survival of Black Versus Other Dialysis Patients by Year of Incidence

	Survival (%)	
	Black	Other[a]
1-Year Survival		
1978	79.9	74.0
1983	79.9	73.7
1988	82.4	77.1
2-Year Survival		
1978	64.4	57.4
1983	65.0	57.0
1987	66.7	59.8
5-Year Survival		
1978	36.0	36.5
1984	31.5	30.5

NOTES: Adjusted for age, gender, and renal diagnosis. All survival rates include only patients who survived the first 90 days.
[a] P = .0001.

SOURCE: USRDS, 1990.

treatment. Overall, blacks have higher average survival than whites on dialysis and similar survival following transplantation (USRDS, 1990). However, the average survival of the transplanted kidney is poorer for blacks. Although there has been substantial improvement overall in the survival of the grafts, blacks have always lagged behind whites. This is shown in Figure 5-5 for cadaveric grafts surviving 2 years after transplantation. The result is similar for living related donor grafts for the same and longer time periods.

Although these data do not control for possible influences on allograft survival, such as HLA matching and age, gender, and race of organ donor, studies that control for these potentially confounding factors have, for the most part, shown similar shortened allograft survival in black recipients (Orial et al., 1982; Krakauer et al., 1983; USRDS, 1990). There are exceptions, including Michigan (Weller et al., 1985) and Ohio State Medical Center (Sommer et al., 1989). Other investigators (Purdue and Terasaki, 1982; Mcdonald et al., 1984) also have reported that race was not an important predictor of survival. The disparities in these results may arise in part from variations in immunosuppressive regimes, patient comorbidity, and choice of cofactors to be included in the analysis. However, considerable evidence still remains, including national data from HCFA and the USRDS, indicating that blacks reject their grafts more frequently than do whites.

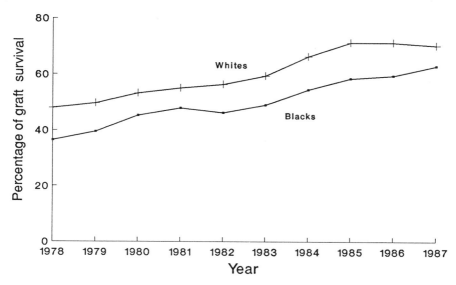

FIGURE 5-5   Two-Year Survival of Transplanted Cadaver Kidneys, by Race, 1978-88
SOURCE: USRDS, 1990.

The above data describe considerable racial and ethnic variation in incidence, treatment, and outcomes of end-stage renal failure. Although data suggest a physiologic contribution to the discrepancies in the development of ESRD among races, racial and ethnic variations in access to and utilization of preventive health care and in the implementation of renal replacement therapy are likely important contributors to these patterns. It is important that future research and policy decisions address the sociologic and economic differences in access to health care relative to outcomes in these populations.

CONCLUSION

The epidemiology of ESRD is in its early stages of development. This chapter makes clear, however, that the ESRD population is highly diverse and that its composition has changed over time. Children with ESRD have special problems that deserve explicit attention. Elderly ESRD patients are growing as a percentage of the patient population and confront providers and policy makers with an array of new challenges.

The prominence of diabetes and hypertension as causes of renal failure highlights the importance of finding ways to control and prevent these diseases and thus prevent the progression to renal failure of individuals with these diagnoses.

Finally, the striking disparities between the rates of kidney failure among minority populations and the white population underscore the need to understand the causal factors and the effective preventive interventions for individuals in these groups long before they arrive at the stage of permanent kidney failure.

The material in this and the previous chapter suggests that permanent kidney failure correlates with lower socioeconomic status (SES). However, the ESRD patient population has not been systematically studied in SES terms and existing data do not permit a direct examination of relation of SES to renal failure. Such an examination is clearly called for. The nation may pay a high price through the ESRD program for inadequate health care and the lower health status of lower socioeconomic groups.

NOTES

1. New elderly ESRD patients without a specified diagnosis were excluded from these calculations. These patients amounted to 58.5 percent of the total in 1978 but only 7.7 percent in 1988.
2. Nearly 50 percent of patient records lack primary diagnosis information through 1980.
3. Beginning in 1981, HCFA achieved relatively complete data tracking of Native Americans and Asians/Pacific Islanders treated for ESRD.

REFERENCES

American Diabetes Association. 1986. Nutritional recommendations and principles for individuals with diabetes mellitus. Diabetes Care 10:126-132.

Bennett PH. 1989. "Microalbuminuria" and diabetes: A critique: Assessment of urinary albumin excretion and its role in screening for diabetic nephropathy. Am J Kidney Dis 13:29-34.

Cohen DL, Dodds R, Viberti GC. 1986. Reduction of microalbuminuria and glomerular filtration rate by dietary protein restriction in type I (insulin-dependent) diabetic patients: An effect independent of blood glucose control and arterial pressure changes (abstract). Diabetologia 29:528a.

Cowie CC, Port FK, Wolfe RA, Savage PJ, Moll PP, Hawthorne VM. 1989. Disparities in incidence of diabetic end-stage renal disease according to race and type of diabetes. N Engl J Med 321:1074-1079.

Eggers PW. 1990. Mortality rates among dialysis patients in Medicare's End-Stage Renal Disease Program. Am J Kidney Dis 15:414-421.

Eggers PW, Connerton R, McMullan M. 1984. The Medicare experience with end-stage renal disease: Trends in incidence, prevalence, and survival. Health Care Financing Rev 5:69-88.

Feldman HI. 1990. End-stage renal disease in U.S. minority groups. Paper prepared for the Institute of Medicine ESRD Study Committee.

Fine RN. 1990. The effect of the End-Stage Renal Disease program on the pediatric patient. Paper prepared for the Institute of Medicine ESRD Study Committee.

Gardner LI, Stern MP, Hafner SM, et al. 1984. Prevalence of diabetes in Mexican-Americans: Relationship to percent of gene pool derived from Native-American sources. Diabetes 3:86-92.

Hawthorne VM. 1990. Preventing kidney disease of diabetes mellitus. Paper prepared for the Institute of Medicine ESRD Study Committee.

HCFA (Health Care Financing Administration). 1990. ESRD Program Management and Medical Information System, March update. Baltimore, Md.

Indian Health Service. 1987. Data Center Periodic Reports from Albuquerque, NM and Rockville, MD. Public Health Service, U.S. Department of Health and Human Services.

IOM (Institute of Medicine). 1990. Staff analysis of a sample of 9690 Medicare ESRD patients with Hispanic surnames.

Kincaid-Smith P, McMichael J, Murphy EA. 1958. The clinical course and pathology of hypertension with papilloedema (malignant hypertension). Q J Med 27:117-153.

Klag MJ. 1990. The patient with hypertensive end-stage renal disease. Paper prepared for the Institute of Medicine ESRD Study Committee.

Knowler WC, Bennett PH, Hamman RF, Miller M. 1978. Diabetes incidence and prevalence in Pima Indians: A 19-fold greater incidence that in Rochester, Minnesota. Am J Epidemiol 108:497-505.

Krakauer H, Spees EK, Vaughn WK, Grauman JS, Summe JP, Bailey RC. 1983. Assessment of prognostic factors and projection of outcomes in renal transplantation. Transplantation 36:378-382.

Kunzelman CL, Knowler WC, Pettitt DJ, Bennett PH. 1989. Incidence of proteinuria in type 2 diabetes mellitus in the Pima Indians. Kidney Int 35:681-687.

Lee TH, Alderman MH. 1978. Malignant hypertension: Declining mortality rate in New York City, 1958 to 1974. NY State J Med 78:1389-1391.

Mamdani BH, Lim VS, Mahurkar SD, Katz AI, Dunea G. 1974. Recovery from prolonged renal failure in patients with accelerated hypertension. N Engl J Med 291:1343-1344.

McClellan W, Elbert T, Issa A. 1988. Racial differences in the incidence of hypertensive end-stage renal disease (ESRD) are not entirely explained by differences in the prevalence of hypertension. Am J Kidney Dis 12:285-290.

Mcdonald JC, Vaughn W, Filo RS, Mendez-Picon G, Niblack G, Spees EK, Williams GM. 1981. Cadaver donor renal transplantation by Centers of the South-Eastern Organ Procurement Foundation. Ann Surg 193:1-8.

Mogensen CE, Christiansen CK. 1984. Predicting diabetic nephropathy in insulin-dependent diabetics. N Engl J Med 311:89-93.

Mroczed WJ, Davidov M, Gavrilovich L, Finnerty FA. 1969. The value of aggressive therapy in the hypertensive patient with azotremia. Circulation 15:893-904.

NCHS (National Center for Health Statistics). 1986. Blood Pressure Levels in Persons 18-74 Years of Age in 1976-80, and Trends in Blood Pressure from 1969 to 1980 in the United States. Vital & Health Statistics, Series 11, No. 234, DHHS Publ. No. (PHS) 86-1684. Public Health Service, U.S. Department of Health and Human Services, Hyattsville, Md.

NCHS. 1987. Health, United States, DHHS Publ. No. (PHS) 88-1232. Public Health Service, U.S. Department of Health and Human Services, Hyattsville, Md.

NCHS. 1990. Health of Black and White Americans, 1985-86. Vital and Health Statistics Series No. 10, No. 171, Public Health Service, U.S. Department of Health and Human Services, Hyattsville, Md. Series 10, No. 171.

Nelson RG, Newman JM, Knowler WC, et al. 1988. Incidence of end-stage renal disease in type 2 (non-insulin-dependent) diabetes mellitus in Pima Indians. Diabetologia 31:730-736.

Orial R, Le Pendu J, Chu C. 1982. Influence of the original disease, race, and center on the outcome of kidney transplantation. Transplantation 33:22.

Pasinski R, Pasinski M. 1987. End-stage renal disease among the Zuni Indians: 1973-83. Arch Intern Med 147:1093-1096.

Pettitt DJ, Saad MF. 1988. Inheritance of predisposition to renal insufficiency in diabetic men. Diabetes 37:51A.

Pugh JA, Stern MP, Haffner SM, Eifler CW, Zapata M. 1988. Excess incidence of treatment of end-stage renal disease in Mexican-Americans. Am J Epidemiol 127:135-144.

Purdue ST, Terasaki PI. 1982. Analysis of interracial variations in kidney transplant and patient survival. Transplantation 34:75-77.

Rate RG, Knowler WC, Morse HG, et al. 1983. Diabetes mellitus in Hopi and Navajo Indians. Diabetes 32:894-899.

Research Triangle Institute. 1976. The National Dialysis Registry. Development of a Medical Registry of Patients on Chronic Dialysis, Final Report, August. Research Triangle Park, North Carolina.

Rettig BS, Teutsch SM. 1990. The incidence of end-stage renal disease in type I and type II diabetes mellitus. Diabetic Nephrol 3:26-27.

Rettig RA. 1981. Formal analysis, policy formulation, and end-stage renal disease, case study #1. In: Background Paper #2: Case Studies of Medical Technologies; The Implications of Cost-Effectiveness Analysis of Medical Technology, Washington, D.C.: Office of Technology Assessment, U.S. Congress.

Rettig RA, Marks EL. 1980. Implementing the End-Stage Renal Disease Program of Medicare. Rept R-2505-HCFA/HEW. The RAND Corporation, Santa Monica, California.

Rowland M, Roberts J. 1982. Blood pressure levels and hypertension in persons ages 6-74 years: United States, 1976-1980. Advance Data, Vol. 84. Washington, D.C.: National Center for Health Statistics.

Seaquist ER, Goetz FC, Rich S, Barbosa J. 1989. Familial clustering of diabetic kidney disease. N Engl J Med 320:1161-1165.

Sehgal A, Rennie D, Showstack J, Amend W, Lo B. 1990. Chronic end-stage renal disease in the elderly. Paper prepared for the Institute of Medicine ESRD Study Committee.

Selby JV, FitzSimmons SC, Newman JM, Katz PP, Sepe S, Showstack J. 1990. The natural history and epidemiology of diabetic nephropathy: Implications for prevention and control. JAMA 263:1954-1960.

Shulman NB, Ford CE, Hall WD, et al. 1989. Prognostic value of serum creatinine and effect of treatment of hypertension on renal function: Results from the Hypertension Detection and Follow-up Program. Hypertension 13(Suppl. I):I80-I93.

Smith DG, Harlan LC, Hawthorne VM. 1989. The charges for ESRD treatment of diabetics. J Clin Epidemiol 42:111-118.

Sommer BG, Sing DE, Ferguson RM. 1989. The influence of recipient race on renal allograft survival: A single institution analysis. Trans Proc 21:3929-3930.

Stern MP, Rosenthal M, Haffner SM, et al. 1984. Sex differences in the effects of sociocultural status on diabetes and cardiovascular risk factors in Mexican Americans: the San Antonio Heart Study. Am J Epidemiol 120:834-851.

USRDS (U.S. Renal Data System). 1989. Annual Data Report. National Institute of Diabetes and Digestive and Kidney Diseases. Bethesda, Md.

USRDS. 1990. Annual Data Report. National Institute of Diabetes and Digestive and Kidney Diseases. Bethesda, Md.

Viberti GC, Hill RD, Jarrett RJ, et al. 1982. Microalbuminuria as a predictor of clinical nephropathy in insulin-dependent diabetes mellitus. Lancet 1:1430-1432.

Weller JM, Wu SCH, Ferguson CW, et al. 1985. End-stage renal disease in Michigan: incidence, underlying causes, prevalence, and modalities of treatment. Am J Nephrol 5:84.

Whelton PK, Klag JH. 1989. Hypertension as a risk factor for renal disease: Review of clinical and epidemiological evidence. Hypertension 13(Suppl. I):I19-I27.

Whittle JC, Whelton PK, Seidler AJ, Klag MJ. 1991. Does racial variation in risk factors explain black-white differences in the incidence of hypertensive end-stage renal disease? Arch Intern Med (in press).

Wiseman MJ, Bogneth E, Dodds R, Keen H, Viberti GC. 1987. Changes in renal function in response to protein restricted diet in type I diabetes. Diabetologia 30:154-159.

Working Group on Hypertension in Diabetes. 1987. Statement on hypertension in diabetes mellitus. Arch Intern Med 147:830-842, 1160-1162.

6

Structure of the Provider Community

Providers[1] of outpatient dialysis treatment now represent the vast majority of the renal treatment provider community, and thus they are the primary focus of this chapter. Transplant centers, organ procurement agencies, and pediatric facilities are also discussed in order to provide information about the complete spectrum of renal treatment providers.

Structural change in the provider community is analyzed in terms of:

• overall growth in treatment capacity, especially in relation to the increase in patient population;
• growth of hospital-based versus independent facilities;
• growth of for-profit versus not-for-profit facilities; and
• growth of large versus small facilities.

The policy implications of these structural changes for access, patient choice, and quality of care are then briefly discussed with the committee's statements and recommendations.

The analyses in this chapter are based mainly on the data from HCFA's annual facility survey. All dialysis and transplant units are required to respond to the survey, and the information collected ranges from provider characteristics, such as size and ownership, to volume and type of treatments provided. Medicare as well as non-Medicare patients are included in the statistics, so the data may not agree completely with other HCFA data bases, which generally contain only Medicare beneficiary data.

Information about providers is generally well defined. HCFA distinguishes the following types of facilities by ownership: individual for-profit; partnership for-profit; corporation not-for-profit, individual not-for-profit; partnership not-for-profit; corporation not-for-profit; state government; county government; municipal government; Veterans Administration; and other federal government. This analysis groups all facilities into two categories—for-profit and not-for-profit. Current information on the chain ownership of dialysis units is limited. Although such information was included in the annual facility survey report before 1986, it was omitted thereafter.[2] HFCA facility ownership data do not indicate chain affiliation.

OVERVIEW

During the 1980s, major changes occurred in the structure of the renal treatment provider community:

• From 1980 to 1988, the total U.S. dialysis patient population increased from 52,364 to 105,958, an average annual growth of 9.2 percent.
• The total number of Medicare-certified renal dialysis treatment providers grew from 1,004 in 1980 to 1,740 in 1988, with independent facilities contributing to over 90 percent of this growth.
• In 1988, approximately 62 percent of all renal dialysis facilities were independent units, compared to about 40 percent in 1980. These units were generally larger than hospital-based units. By 1988, they accounted for almost 70 percent of the total number of dialysis stations,[3] up from 50 percent in 1980.
• The number of for-profit renal dialysis facilities almost tripled from 342 in 1980 to 912 in 1988, an average annual growth rate of 13 percent; not-for-profit facilities grew at a rate of only 2.8 percent annually over the same period.
• Growth rates were slightly higher for larger dialysis facilities. From 1980 to 1988, small facilities (1 to 9 stations) decreased from 44 percent to 38 percent of all facilities, medium-size units (10 to 20 stations) increased from less than 41 percent to more than 47 percent, and large units (20+ stations) increased from 12 percent to 14 percent.
• In 1980, the largest group of dialysis providers consisted of small, not-for-profit, hospital-based units. By 1988, medium-size, for-profit, independent facilities made up the largest group.
• The number of renal transplant centers grew from 151 units in 1980 to 219 units in 1989; the number of kidney transplants grew from 4,697 in 1980 to 8,976 in 1986 and since then has leveled off at around 9,000. Patients on transplant waiting lists, however, increased steadily from 5,072 in 1980 to 14,669 in 1989.
• Since 1987, following the National Organ Transplant Act of 1986, multiple organ procurement organizations (OPOs) in a single statistical metropolitan area (SMA) have been consolidated. As a result, there were only 70 OPOs [20 of which were hospital-based (HOPOs) and 50 of which were independent (IOPOs)] in 1990 compared to 115 in 1986.

• In addition to these documented changes, rural dialysis facilities have received some attention in recent years. The definition of rural units, however, is not well developed, and historical data do not exist for these units. In general, it appears that rural dialysis facilities are smaller, have fewer patients, and thus are less able to realize the efficiencies generated by volume.

• Currently, 18 facilities are dedicated solely to pediatric ESRD patients. All are hospital-based units located in children's hospitals, and they tend to be smaller than other facilities. The total number of pediatric facilities has not increased over the years in spite of an increasing number of pediatric ESRD patients.

Outpatient Dialysis Facilities

Since the ESRD program began in 1973, the total number of Medicare-certified renal treatment providers has grown from 606 to 1,819 in 1988, primarily in dialysis facilities. From 1980 to 1988, such facilities grew from 1,004 units to 1,740, an average annual growth rate of 7.1 percent (Table 6-1).

The number of approved dialysis stations also has increased steadily since 1976. In 1976, there were 7,093 stations; this number increased to 12,216 in 1980 and to 22,803 by 1988. From 1980 to 1988, the average annual growth rate in stations was approximately 8 percent (Table 6-1). During this same period, the total U.S. dialysis population increased from

TABLE 6-1 Growth of Outpatient Dialysis Providers, 1980-88

Year	No. of Units	No. of Stations	No. of Patients	No. of Treatments[a]
1980	1,004	12,216	52,364	5,672,277
1981	1,124	13,510	58,924	6,443,624
1982	1,155	14,270	65,765	7,072,072
1983	1,217	15,216	71,987	7,675,641
1984	1,307	17,138	78,483	8,463,376
1985	1,392	18,226	84,797	9,246,027
1986	1,507	19,799	90,886	10,137,701
1987	1,618	21,380	98,432	10,798,202
1988	1,740	22,803	105,958	11,866,112
Average annual growth (%)	7.1	8.1	9.2	9.7

[a]Outpatient hemodialysis (including training) treatments only.

SOURCE: HCFA, 1980-88.

TABLE 6-2   Definitions of Dialysis Unit Size, Demand, Capacity, and Utilization

---

Dialysis facility size = number of stations:
    Small, 1-9
    Medium, 10-20
    Large, 20+
Demand:
    Unit demand = Actual hemodialysis treatments per year
    System demand = Actual treatments per year (all units)
Capacity:
    Station capacity = (2 treatments per day) x (6 days per week) x (52 weeks per year)
      = 624 treatments per year
    Unit capacity = (624 treatments per year) x (number of stations in the unit)
    System capacity = (624 treatments per year) x (total number of stations in the provider community)
Utilization:
    Actual treatments per year per unit capacity

52,364 to 105,958, an average annual growth rate of 9.2 percent,[4] and the number of outpatient hemodialysis treatments grew correspondingly at 9.7 percent annually (Table 6-1). Thus, total capacity of all renal treatment providers, measured by the aggregate number of hemodialysis stations, grew somewhat slower than the patient population and the number of dialysis treatments provided between 1980 and 1988.

The optimal level of facility utilization has never been clearly defined, and justifiable geographic variations may exist. If the number of dialysis stations is used as the measure of capacity, unit capacity can then be defined as the number of stations in a dialysis facility that operate two patient treatment shifts a day for 6 days a week.[5] This is equivalent to 624 treatments per station per year when a facility is running at full capacity (Table 6-2). If utilization or demand is measured in terms of hemodialysis treatments administered per station, then the treatment/station ratio can serve as a proxy indication of utilization rate; i.e., when the facility's average treatment/station ratio is 624 treatments per station per year, it can be regarded as operating at full capacity. These measures, though imperfect, are commonly used by the renal treatment community (REN Corporation, 1989; Community Psychiatric Centers, 1989).

In the past decade, the more rapid increase in patient treatments compared to treatment capacity has resulted in a higher use of treatment at the program level. The number of hemodialysis treatments per station per year increased 12 percent, from 464 in 1980 to 520 treatments per station per year in 1988.[6] On the other hand, there are substantial variations among states in the utilization rate of dialysis facilities. These variations may be due partly to state certificate-of-need or other regulatory constraints on capacity (see Chapter 7).

Kidney Transplant Centers

There were 167 renal transplant centers when the Medicare ESRD program was established in 1973. Each year the number decreased slightly until the early 1980s when the trend reversed, and the number of renal transplant centers grew at 4.2 percent annually from 151 in 1980 to 219 in 1989.

On the basis of 1988 facility survey data, 55 percent of transplant centers perform 11 to 49 procedures annually. Fewer than 10 percent perform more than 100 procedures during any given year, but the largest centers perform more than 200 procedures per year. About 15 percent of the centers perform fewer than 10 procedures per year. The median transplant center size, as measured by the number of procedures performed, increased from 24 procedures in 1980 to 32 procedures in 1988.

An effective transplantation program depends on the donation of organs and a system to procure and distribute the donated organs. The first programs to increase the procurement and distribution of cadaver kidneys began in 1968 in Boston and Los Angeles; several other centers were established in 1969. The Medicare ESRD program made federal funds available for kidney procurement and distribution through the reimbursement system, beginning in 1973. In 1986, about 115 OPOs were operating across the country (Task Force on Organ Transplantation, 1986). Although these agencies were initially established to procure kidneys, they now also procure and distribute other organs, including hearts and livers.

Two types of organizations procure organs: IOPOs and HOPOs. In 1986, nearly one-half of the 115 organ procurement agencies were IOPOs—private, not-for-profit organizations created solely for the purpose of procuring organs. IOPOs usually supply organs to several transplant centers and serve more than half of the nation's hospitals. A HOPO is affiliated with a single transplant center at a given hospital and obtains organs primarily for that center. All organs procured, whether obtained by IOPOs or HOPOs, are offered first to local transplant centers, then regionally and nationally if no local recipients are identified.[7]

IOPOs generally obtain more organs and serve more hospitals than do HOPOs. However, the size and effectiveness of OPOs varies widely (Prottas, 1985). Some OPOs procure less than 10 organs a year; others obtain more than 300 organs a year. Since 1987, following the Omnibus Budget Reconciliation Act of 1986, multiple OPOs in a single SMA have been consolidated. As a result, there were only 70 OPOs (20 HOPOs and 50 IOPOs) in 1990, compared to 115 in 1986.

Pretransplant laboratory costs account for about 20 percent of all Medicare expenditures for kidney acquisition and must not be overlooked. Questions regarding the practices of tissue typing laboratories have been raised in recent years. A report from the DHHS Office of Inspector General (OIG, 1987) indicates that, in some areas of the country, there is widespread variation in pretransplant testing procedures, including duplication of testing. In many areas, renal transplant centers have agreed to use a single laboratory for all pretransplant testings. In other areas, however, individual renal transplant centers continue to operate their own laboratories.

Pediatric Facilities

Children with ESRD have special needs. Only a small number of renal treatment providers dedicate themselves exclusively to children. Currently, there are 18 Medicare-approved pediatric ESRD facilities, most of which were developed after 1973. All are connected with children's hospitals, and most also have pediatric transplantation units.[8]

Compared to the adult renal treatment facilities, pediatric units tend to be smaller. HCFA's 1987 facility survey, for example, shows that the median pediatric facility has only 4 dialysis stations and the largest pediatric unit has 10 stations. The number of patients in each facility ranged from 2 to 53, with an average of 16 patients. In 1987, only 289 patients—fewer than 10 percent of the total pediatric ESRD population—were being treated in these 18 pediatric units. The remaining children with ESRD receive their treatments from facilities that predominantly treat adults.

There is general agreement that the treatment of choice for children with ESRD is transplantation. However, although patients who receive their care from pediatric facilities have more direct access to pediatric transplant units, they have a lower rate of transplantation than the general pediatric ESRD patients. On the basis of a survey conducted by the National Association of Children's Hospitals and Related Institutions (1987), only 46 percent of pediatric ESRD patients treated in the children's hospitals had been transplanted, compared to nearly 65 percent of pediatric patients who are treated elsewhere. The reasons for this difference are not clear. Patients treated in pediatric facilities are generally younger than other pediatric ESRD patients, and this may be one reason for the lower transplantation rate. Second, the proportion of black children treated in pediatric facilities is higher than in the adult facilities, and black patients receive transplants at lower rates than do whites.

The number of pediatric ESRD patients is increasing (see Chapter 5), but the number of renal pediatric facilities is not. Hence, access to appropriate care for these children is becoming more difficult (see Chapter 7). Most pediatric ESRD patients are treated in adult-oriented renal treatment facilities that treat limited numbers of children. Thus, access to specialized care provided by pediatric nephrologists is needed for these patients.

CHANGING STRUCTURE OF THE OUTPATIENT DIALYSIS COMMUNITY

HCFA defines dialysis facilities as units (hospital-based or independent) approved to furnish outpatient maintenance dialysis services to ESRD patients. Outpatient dialysis providers can be categorized along three dimensions: hospital-based or independent; for-profit or not-for-profit; and size as measured by number of stations.

Hospital-Based Versus Independent Providers[9]

Hospital-Based Providers

The growth of hospital-based outpatient dialysis facilities can be examined in terms of increases in the numbers of facilities, dialysis stations, and patients, and their "market share" relative to that of independent facilities.

Outpatient Dialysis Facilities   The number of hospital-based dialysis facilities increased slightly from 600 in 1980 to 661 in 1988, a growth rate of 1.2 percent annually.   By 1988, only 38 percent of dialysis facilities were hospital-based, a significant decrease from almost 60 percent in 1980 (Table 6-3).   Over 97 percent of hospital dialysis facilities are not-for-profit, and this has not changed between 1980 and 1988.

Dialysis Stations   The total number of stations in hospital-based facilities has not grown rapidly.   There were 6,105 dialysis stations in hospital-based facilities in 1980, increasing to 7,285 in 1988, an average annual growth rate of 2.2 percent (Table 6-3).   These hospital-based stations accounted for half of the total number of dialysis stations in 1980, but only one-third in 1988.   The average-size hospital-based dialysis unit grew slightly from just under 10 stations in 1980 to 10.3 stations in 1988.

Patients   In 1980, 26,537 patients received their outpatient dialysis treatments in hospital-based facilities. This number increased to 38,657 by 1988 for an average annual growth of 4.8 percent. The ESRD "patient share" of hospital-based facilities, however, declined dramatically from over 50 percent in 1980 to less than 37 percent in 1988 (Table 6-3).

Although hospital-based facilities grew slowly in treatment capacity, their number of patients grew faster and, consequently, the average utilization rate increased.   The median (50th percentile) hospital-based dialysis facility had 31 patients in 1988 compared to 17 patients in 1980.   An analysis

TABLE 6-3 Outpatient Dialysis Providers, Independent Versus Hospital-Based, 1980-88

	Independent			Hospital-Based		
Year	No. of Units	No. of Stations	No. of Patients	No. of Units	No. of Stations	No. of Patients
1980	404	6,111	25,827	600	6,105	26,537
1981	296	7,082	30,112	628	6,428	28,812
1982	522	7,701	34,215	633	6,569	31,550
1983	610	8,837	40,163	607	6,379	31,824
1984	686	10,509	45,082	621	6,629	33,401
1985	763	11,486	49,817	629	6,740	34,980
1986	869	12,835	54,902	638	6,964	35,984
1987	961	14,089	60,815	657	7,291	37,617
1988	1,079	15,518	67,301	661	7,285	38,657
Average annual growth (%)	13.1	12.4	12.7	1.2	2.2	4.8
Total share (%):						
1980	40.2	50.0	49.3	59.8	50.0	50.7
1988	62.0	68.1	63.5	38.0	32.0	36.5

SOURCE: HCFA, 1980-88.

based on USRDS data shows that about 18 percent of the hospital-based facilities had more than 100 patients in 1988, compared to only 8.5 percent in 1980 (USRDS, 1989).

Independent Providers

The growth of independent outpatient dialysis facilities can be examined in a manner similar to that used for hospital-based providers.

Outpatient Dialysis Facilities The number of independent outpatient dialysis facilities grew much more rapidly than the number of hospital-based units (Figure 6-1), increasing from 404 units in 1980 to 1,079 units in 1988, an average annual growth rate of 13.1 percent (Table 6-3). By the end of 1988, about 62 percent of all dialysis facilities were independent, compared to approximately 40 percent in 1980. During this time, the independent facilities accounted for 92 percent of the increase in all outpatient dialysis facilities. Unlike their hospital-based counterparts, independent dialysis facilities are predominantly for-profit. From 1980 to 1988, for-profit facilities accounted for over 80 percent of the total independent facilities, and for 84 percent of the 675 new independent units established during this period.

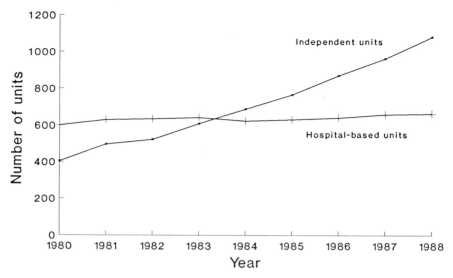

FIGURE 6-1   Outpatient Dialysis Units, 1980-88: Independent Versus Hospital-Based
SOURCE: HCFA, 1980-88.

Dialysis Stations   The total number of stations in independent facilities also grew significantly from 6,111 dialysis stations in 1980 to 15,518 stations in 1988, at an average annual growth rate of 12.4 percent (Table 6-3 and Figure 6-2).   By 1988, dialysis stations in independent facilities accounted for over 68 percent of all dialysis stations, up by 50 percent from 1980.

Patients   Independent facilities provided maintenance dialysis to 25,827 patients in 1980.   This increased to 67,301 patients by 1988, an average annual increase of 12.7 percent.   The proportion of patients in independent facilities increased from just under 50 percent in 1980 to over 63 percent in 1988 (Table 6-3).

The number of patients treated by the median independent for-profit dialysis facility was 48 patients in 1988 compared to 49 patients in 1980 (USRDS, 1989).   The median independent not-for-profit dialysis facility had 56 patients in 1988, down from 65 patients in 1980.   By contrast, the median hospital-based unit increased from 17 patients in 1980 to 31 patients in 1988.

Utilization of dialysis stations is lower in independent units compared to hospital-based units.   Independent facilities accounted for over 68 percent of total national dialysis stations but treated slightly less than 64 percent of the patients in 1988.   The *average* size of an independent facility decreased slightly from 14.6 stations in 1980 to 14.1 stations in 1988, whereas the

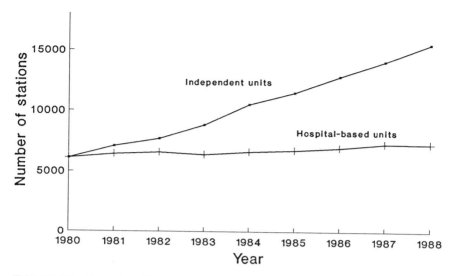

FIGURE 6-2   Outpatient Hemodialysis Stations, 1980-88: Independent Versus Hospital-Based Units
SOURCE: HCFA, 1980-88.

number of facilities grew significantly. Since the growth in the number of independent facilities and stations was comparable to the increase in demand for patient treatments from 1980 to 1988, on a national level the independent facilities experienced no significant utilization rate increase.[10]

Not-For-Profit Versus For-Profit Providers[11]

In 1988, about 52 percent of all outpatient dialysis facilities were proprietary (Table 6-4), a substantial increase from 34 percent in 1980. Since there are only 18 hospital-based for-profit facilities, almost all growth of the proprietary sector was accounted for by independent facilities (Table 6-5). Not-for-profit renal treatment facilities are mainly hospital-based, although the number of independent not-for-profit facilities increased during the 1980s.

Not-For-Profit Providers

Examination of not-for-profit outpatient dialysis facilities in terms of the increases of numbers of facilities, dialysis stations, and patients shows that their market share relative to that of for-profit facilities has declined over the past decade.

Outpatient Dialysis Facilities   Not-for-profit renal treatment facilities grew relatively slowly during the 1980s from 662 units in 1980 to 828 units in

TABLE 6-4   Outpatient Dialysis Providers, For-Profit Versus Not-For-Profit, 1980-88

	For-Profit			Not-For-Profit		
Year	No. of Units	No. of Stations	No. of Patients	No. of Units	No. of Stations	No. of Patients
1980	342	4,986	20,317	662	7,230	32,047
1981	413	5,758	23,835	711	7,752	35,089
1982	429	6,221	26,940	726	8,049	38,825
1983	495	7,028	30,911	722	8,188	41,076
1984	554	8,376	34,675	753	8,762	43,808
1985	622	9,187	38,458	770	9,039	46,339
1986	722	10,507	43,361	785	9,292	47,525
1987	803	11,718	48,846	815	9,662	49,586
1988	912	13,077	54,528	828	9,726	51,430
Average annual growth (%)	13.0	12.8	13.1	2.8	3.8	6.1
Total share (%):						
1980	34.1	40.8	38.8	65.9	59.2	61.2
1988	52.4	57.4	51.5	47.6	42.7	48.5

SOURCE: HCFA, 1980-88.

1988, for an average annual growth rate of 2.8 percent. By 1988, not-for-profit facilities represented less than half of all dialysis facilities, a significant decrease from nearly two-thirds in 1980 (Table 6-4).

Although hospital-based facilities still made up about 78 percent of the not-for-profit sector in 1988, that was down from 88 percent in 1980. Independent not-for-profit facilities grew at a faster pace, from 79 units in 1980 to 185 units in 1988, an average annual growth rate of 11.2 percent (Table 6-5).

Dialysis Stations   The total number of stations in not-for-profit facilities grew slowly from 7,230 in 1980 to 9,726 in 1988, an average annual growth rate of 3.8 percent. The not-for-profit facilities accounted for almost 60 percent of total stations in 1980, but declined to less than 43 percent in 1988 (Table 6-4). Hospital-based facilities provided about 74 percent of the stations in the not-for-profit sector in 1988, down from 83 percent in 1980.

Patients   Outpatient treatments in not-for-profit facilities were provided to 32,047 patients in 1980, which increased an average of 6 percent annually to 51,430 patients in 1988. However, the proportion of patients under

TABLE 6-5 Outpatient Dialysis Providers, by Profit Status and Type of Facility, 1980-88

| | For-Profit | | | | | | Not-For-Profit | | | | | |
| | Independent | | | Hospital-Based | | | Independent | | | Hospital-Based | | |
Year	No. of Units	No. of Stations	No. of Patients	No. of Units	No. of Stations	No. of Patients	No. of Units	No. of Stations	No. of Patients	No. of Units	No. of Stations	No. of Patients
1980	325	4,846	19,782	17	140	535	79	1,265	6,045	583	5,965	26,002
1981	397	5,621	23,341	16	137	494	99	1,461	6,771	612	6,291	28,318
1982	416	6,102	26,482	13	119	458	106	1,599	7,733	620	6,450	31,092
1983	482	6,950	30,560	13	78	351	128	1,887	9,603	594	6,301	31,473
1984	538	8,265	34,272	16	111	403	148	2,244	10,810	605	6,518	32,998
1985	605	9,073	38,120	17	114	338	158	2,413	11,697	612	6,626	34,642
1986	704	10,385	42,984	18	122	377	165	2,450	11,918	620	6,842	35,607
1987	786	11,594	48,478	17	124	368	175	2,495	12,337	640	7,152	37,249
1988	894	12,944	54,105	18	133	423	185	2,574	13,196	643	7,152	38,234
Average annual growth (%)	13.5	13.1	13.4	0.7	-0.6	2.9	11.2	9.3	10.3	1.2	2.3	4.9
Total share (%):												
1980	32.4	29.7	37.8	1.7	1.1	1.0	7.9	10.4	11.5	58.1	8.8	49.7
1988	51.45	56.8	51.1	1.0	0.6	0.4	0.6	11.3	12.5	37.0	31.4	36.1

SOURCE: HCFA, 1980-88.

care by the not-for-profit sector declined steadily from 61 percent in 1980 to less than 49 percent in 1988 (Table 6-4).

Although the increase in average facility size was small—from 10.6 to 11.2 stations between 1980 and 1988—the overall utilization rate for the not-for-profit sector still increased significantly from 4.4 patients per station in 1980 to 5.3 patients per station in 1988. The not-for-profit sector accounted for 42.7 percent of the treatment capacity in 1988 but 48.5 percent of the total patient population.

For-Profit Providers

For-profit providers have been a major source of growth in outpatient dialysis since 1980 with increases in the numbers of facilities, dialysis stations, and patients receiving treatment.

Outpatient Dialysis Facilities For-profit units accounted for about 34 percent of all renal dialysis facilities in 1980 but more than 52 percent by 1988 (Figure 6-3), increasing from 325 to 894 at an average annual growth rate of 13.5 percent (Table 6-5). Proprietary dialysis facilities are predominantly independent units and included only 18 hospital-based units in 1988, up from 17 in 1980 (Table 6-5).

Dialysis Stations The total number of stations in for-profit facilities grew from 4,986 stations in 1980 to 13,077 stations in 1988, an average annual growth rate of 12.8 percent. The share of for-profit dialysis stations increased from 41 percent in 1980 to over 57 percent in 1988 (Table 6-4 and Figure 6-4).

Patients For-profit dialysis facilities provided maintenance dialysis to 20,317 patients in 1980 and to 54,528 patients by 1988, for an average annual increase of 13.1 percent (Table 6-4). The "patient share" treated by the for-profit sector increased from under 39 percent in 1980 to over 51 percent in 1988.

From 1980 to 1988, for-profit facilities and stations grew at a rate comparable to their patient load. Average facility size decreased slightly from 14.2 stations in 1980 to 14.0 stations in 1988. Consequently, the national patient/station ratio increased only slightly from 4.1 patients per station in 1980 to 4.2 patients per station in 1988.

Size of Outpatient Dialysis Facilities[12]

In general, the size of dialysis facilities, as measured by the number of stations in each unit, increased slightly during the 1980s. Small facilities (1-9 stations) grew at an average rate of only 4.9 percent annually, whereas medium-size (10-20 stations) and large (over 20 stations) facilities increased

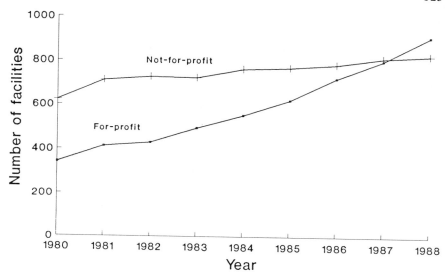

FIGURE 6-3   Outpatient Hemodialysis Units, 1980-88: For-Profit Versus Not-For-Profit
SOURCE: HCFA, 1980-88.

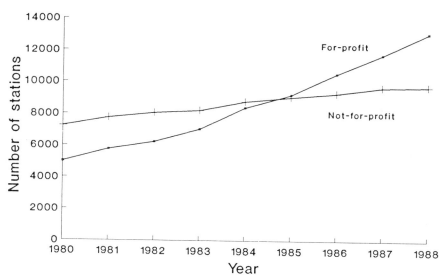

FIGURE 6-4   Outpatient Hemodialysis Stations, 1980-88: For-Profit Versus Not-For-Profit Units
SOURCE: HCFA, 1980-88.

almost twice as fast at an average annual rate of nearly 9 percent from 1980 to 1988. The number of small facilities grew from 456 units in 1980 to 666 units in 1988, whereas the number of medium-size and large facilities nearly doubled during the same period from 419 units to 824 units and from 129 units to 250 units, respectively (Table 6-6 and Figure 6-5).

In 1980, over 45 percent of all facilities were small, 42 percent were medium-size, and 13 percent were large. By 1988, however, that distribution had changed to 38 percent, 47 percent, and 14 percent, respectively (Table 6-6).

A shift toward larger facilities is also evident in the relative shares of "treatment capacity." From 1980 to 1988, small facilities changed from accounting for over 22 percent of all dialysis stations to only about 18 percent; medium-size facilities increased from less than 48 percent of stations to over 50 percent; and large facilities increased from 30 percent of stations to 31 percent (Table 6-6).

Most hospital-based facilities remain small; they made up the second largest number of facilities in 1988 (Table 6-7). However, the medium-size and large facilities accounted for the growth of hospital-based renal treatment facilities during the 1980s. Although independent facilities are predominantly medium or large in size, they increased during the 1980s in all three size categories.

The growth of medium-size and large independent facilities is most evident in the for-profit sector. Medium-size for-profit independent facilities increased from 173 in 1980 to 490 by 1988, making them the single largest sector and accounting for over 28 percent of the number of facilities (Table 6-7) and almost 30 percent of the stations (Table 6-8). Additionally, the medium-size and large for-profit independent facilities together represented over 50 percent of the total dialysis stations in the entire provider community in 1988.

The largest renal treatment provider group in 1980 was small not-for-profit hospital-based facilities. By 1988, medium-size for-profit independent facilities made up the largest provider group. This is the most telling summary of structural changes in the renal treatment provider community. It is plausible that the growth of facility size has been stimulated by an effort to realize economies of scale. Other factors that are likely to have affected both facility size and the number of facilities are the changes in the availability of nursing staff and in the timing of patient treatment shifts. In the earlier years of the ESRD program, some units operated 24 hours a day, with four or five patient shifts. Over the past 10 to 15 years, physicians, nurses, and patients increasingly have rejected treatment at night. Consequently, either larger units or more units were needed to accommodate a reduction in the number of shifts and an increasing patient population.

TABLE 6-6 Outpatient Dialysis Providers, by Facility Size, 1980-88

Year	Small (1-9 stations)			Medium (10-20 stations)			Large (20+ stations)		
	No. of Units	No. of Stations	No. of Patients	No. of Units	No. of Stations	No. of Patients	No. of Units	No. of Stations	No. of Patients
1980	456	2,697	10,799	419	5,823	24,648	129	3,696	16,475
1981	527	3,146	12,904	454	6,304	27,320	143	4,060	18,480
1982	512	3,093	13,351	488	6,764	30,788	155	4,413	20,770
1983	545	3,366	14,822	508	7,134	33,089	164	4,716	22,426
1984	525	3,237	13,967	584	8,229	36,896	198	5,672	27,424
1985	556	3,406	15,427	627	8,838	40,073	209	5,982	28,959
1986	593	3,659	16,357	690	9,692	43,684	223	6,448	30,277
1987	630	3,953	17,448	751	10,579	48,368	237	6,848	32,182
1988	666	4,205	18,866	824	11,509	52,235	250	7,089	34,195
Average annual growth (%)	4.9	5.7	7.2	8.8	8.9	9.8	8.6	8.5	9.6
Total share (%):									
1980	45.4	22.1	20.6	41.7	47.7	47.1	12.8	30.3	31.5
1988	38.2	18.4	17.8	47.4	50.5	49.3	14.4	31.1	32.3

SOURCE: HCFA, 1980-88.

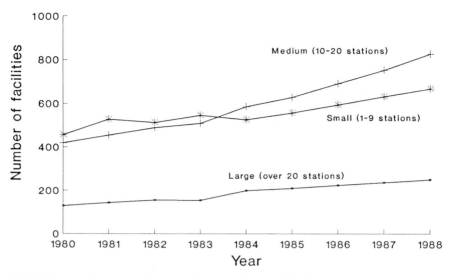

FIGURE 6-5   Outpatient Dialysis Units, by Size, 1980-88
SOURCE: HCFA, 1980-88.

Facility Ownership

Facility ownership has long been of great concern in the health care sector. The past decade's growth of outpatient dialysis chains, defined by HCFA as two or more units under the same ownership, thus deserves attention. However, information about the chain affiliations of dialysis units is limited. A question on such affiliation was originally included in HCFA's annual facility survey, but many facilities, especially for-profit ones, did not indicate whether they were affiliated with a chain. After 1985, the question was removed. The following discussion is based, in part, on the information provided by Dialysis Management, Incorporated (D.L. Vlchek, Dialysis Management Incorporated, personal communication, October 10, 1989) which has not been independently validated.

As previously noted, independent dialysis facilities, especially the for-profit ones, have grown far more rapidly than hospital-based units during the past decade. This growth of proprietary independent facilities has been accompanied by an increase of multiunit "chains." The project staff estimate that by 1988 more than half of all 912 for-profit renal dialysis facilities were affiliated with a chain.

National Medical Care (NMC) is by far the largest for-profit chain. On the basis of the most recent data that were available to the study committee, almost 20 percent of all U.S. dialysis patients receive their regular maintenance dialysis treatments in one of the 300+ NMC-owned facilities. NMC

TABLE 6-7 Outpatient Dialysis Providers, by Type of Facility, Profit Status, and Size, 1980-88

	Independent						Hospital-Based					
	For-Profit			Not-For-Profit			For-Profit			Not-For-Profit		
Year	Small	Medium	Large	Small	Medium	Large	Small	Medium	Large	Small	Medium	Large
1980	87	173	65	18	43	18	13	3	1	338	200	45
1981	132	192	73	31	48	20	12	3	1	352	211	49
1982	120	215	81	35	46	25	9	3	1	348	224	48
1983	156	237	89	46	55	27	12	1	0	331	215	48
1984	135	293	110	47	66	35	13	3	0	330	222	53
1985	164	322	119	45	77	36	14	3	0	333	225	54
1986	195	380	129	50	81	34	14	3	0	334	226	60
1987	220	425	141	55	85	35	14	3	0	341	238	61
1988	250	490	155	61	90	34	14	4	0	341	241	61
Average annual growth (%)	14.1	13.9	11.5	16.5	9.7	8.3	0.9	3.7	-100	0.1	2.4	3.9
Total share (%):												
1980	8.7	17.2	6.5	1.8	4.3	1.8	1.3	0.3	0.1	33.7	19.9	4.5
1988	4.4	28.2	8.9	3.5	5.2	2.0	0.8	0.2	0.0	19.6	13.9	3.5

NOTE: Small = 1-9 stations; medium = 10-20 stations; large = 20+ stations.
SOURCE: HCFA, 1980-88.

TABLE 6-8 Hemodialysis Stations, by Type of Facility, Profit Status, and Size, 1980-88

| | Independent | | | | | | Hospital-Based | | | | | |
| | For-Profit | | | Not-for-Profit | | | For-Profit | | | Not-For-Profit | | |
Year	Small	Medium	Large	Small	Medium	Large	Small	Medium	Large	Small	Medium	Large
1980	555	2,415	1,876	114	666	485	76	43	21	1,952	2,699	1,314
1981	840	2,689	2,092	196	733	532	73	43	21	2,037	2,839	1,415
1982	785	2,979	2,338	217	711	671	55	43	21	2,036	3,031	1,383
1983	1,071	3,334	2,545	290	847	750	66	12	0	1,939	2,941	1,421
1984	940	4,182	3,143	290	979	975	66	45	0	1,960	3,079	1,587
1985	1,109	4,583	3,381	268	1,131	1,041	69	45	0	1,960	3,079	1,587
1986	1,334	5,385	3,666	293	1,181	976	75	47	0	1,957	3,079	1,806
1987	1,504	6,038	4,052	329	1,200	966	84	40	0	2,036	3,301	1,830
1988	1,714	6,828	4,402	369	1,275	930	82	51	0	2,040	3,355	1,757
Average annual growth	15.1	13.9	11.3	15.8	8.5	8.5	1.0	2.2	-100	0.5	2.8	3.7
Total share (%):												
1980	4.5	19.8	15.4	0.9	5.5	4.0	0.6	0.4	0.2	16.0	22.1	10.8
1988	7.5	29.9	19.3	1.6	5.6	4.1	0.4	0.2	0.0	9.0	14.7	7.7

NOTE: Small = 1-9 stations; medium = 10-20 stations; large = 20+ stations.
SOURCE: HCFA, 1980-88.

also provides dialysis supplies in the product market through its Dialysis Products Division, as well as laboratory services to over 30 percent of the dialysis market. Because NMC is a wholly owned subsidiary of W.R. Grace, Inc., the publicly available information reported to the Securities and Exchange Commission is quite limited.

In addition to NMC, there are four other major chains: Community Psychiatric Centers (which recently separated its dialysis division and formed a new publicly traded common stock company, Vivra Incorporated), Laguna Hills, California; Dialysis Clinics, Incorporated (DCI), Nashville, Tennessee; National Medical Enterprises—Medical Ambulatory Care (MAC), Tacoma, Washington; and REN Corporation-USA, Nashville, Tennessee. Of these, DCI is the only not-for-profit chain. The size of these chains varies from approximately 18 facilities (REN Corporation) to 85 facilities (Vivra). Together, these four chains owned nearly 200 facilities and provided services to about 10,000 patients in 1989. Vivra and REN, in 1989, became the first publicly traded all-dialysis service corporations.

Additionally, there are a number of smaller chains, including Greenfield Health Systems Corporation, Detroit, Michigan; Renal Treatment Centers Corporation, Philadelphia, Pennsylvania; Satellite Dialysis, San Francisco, California; Northwest Kidney Center, Seattle, Washington; Salick Health Care, Los Angeles, California; Kidney Care, Jackson, Mississippi; Clinishare, Los Angeles, California; Neomedica Dialysis Centers, Inc., Chicago, Illinois; Home Intensive Care, N. Miami Beach, Florida; Hemodialysis, Inc., Los Angeles, California; West Suburban Kidney Centers, Chicago, Illinois; Health Systems Management, southeastern United States; New West Dialysis, Sacramento, California; Tidewater Nephrology Associates, Norfolk, Virginia; Regional Kidney Disease Program, Minneapolis, Minnesota; and American Outpatient Services Corporation, Los Angeles, California. These chains together serve an estimated 8,000 to 10,000 dialysis patients. Allowing for some other small chains not accounted for, we estimate that in 1989 nearly 50,000 out of a total of 116,000 dialysis patients received their dialysis treatments in chain-affiliated facilities.

HCFA's current renal data systems do not identify ownership except as for-profit or not-for-profit, and as individual, corporate, or public institutions. Individual units, however, may be owned by one or more nephrologists, or by nonnephrologists (physicians as well as nonphysicians), or jointly by nephrologists and nonnephrologists. The possibility of conflicts of interest over physician ownership of dialysis units cannot be examined with current data.

A market exists for buying and selling renal dialysis facilities. A few hospitals and the large proprietary chains are the major buyers, whereas physician owners and hospitals are usually the sellers. Purchasing terms are usually based on potential revenue, i.e., number of regular patients in the facilities (Dialysis Management Inc. 1990. Perspectives on the renal care provider community—1989. Golden Colorado, unpublished data). Prices range from $10,000 to $40,000 per patient. During 1988-89, one hospital in Ohio bought a unit with 50 patients for $2.3 million, i.e., $46,000 per patient. The average purchase price in 1988, however, was estimated at $18,000 to $20,000 per patient. Prices apparently fell in 1989 to an estimated range of $15,000 to $18,000 per patient; changes in federal income tax law, quite independent of ESRD, significantly slowed corporate acquisitions. In states without CON regulations, the prices tend to be lower.

Proprietary health care facilities grew rapidly in the American health care system in the past decade. Consequently, concerns have been raised about the effect of profit-seeking on medical decision making (Gray, 1986). In the ESRD program, it is unclear whether the quality of care is affected by facility ownership or chain affiliation. The multiunit chains presumably realize economies of scale and generate higher profit margins on the firm level than do sole-owner units. However, some studies have suggested that competition in local markets may reduce facilities' profits by driving them to provide more amenities to patients (Held and Pauly, 1983). Objective and credible information about the profitability of renal dialysis chains is still quite limited, as is the relation between ownership and quality of care.

CONCLUSIONS

Renal dialysis facilities have increased substantially in number since the ESRD program started in 1973. This increase has paralleled the growth of the patient population, although certain geographic areas still lack adequate treatment capacity to meet increasing demand. In addition, other factors may influence growth in the number of facilities. Facilities seeking to protect their existing patient base (or local market share) from competitors may open additional units conveniently located for their patients.[13] Growth in the number of units also may respond to a desire for independence from a corporate organization or from a hospital by physicians. *In light of the increased demand for treatment, the committee finds that the rate of growth in outpatient treatment capacity is reasonable.*

The quality-of-care implications of the changing composition of the dialysis provider community need careful monitoring. The continued expansion of dialysis capacity, especially in the independent for-profit sector, cannot in itself be taken as evidence that reimbursement is adequate to provide quality care. Only an integrated assessment of cost and quality would permit such judgments to be made. However, as discussed in Chapters 11 and 12, neither the federal government nor providers have monitored quality systematically or developed adequate tools for its assessment.

The quality implications of the shift toward for-profit and physician ownership merit careful assessment. The committee is aware of no evidence that the shift from hospital-based to independent and from not-for-profit to for-profit dialysis facilities has resulted in problems in access or quality. The lack of systematic efforts to assess quality, as indicated above, preclude the development of such evidence at this time. *The commitee recommends, however, that ownership changes be monitored closely over time and that means be developed to assess their implications for access and quality.*

NOTES

1. In this chapter, the term "provider" refers to treatment facilities, not physicians, unless otherwise noted.

2. HCFA defines a chain as two or more facilities under the same ownership.

3. A dialysis station consists of a dialysis machine, a chair or a bed, and the associated floor space required to dialyze a single patient.

4. About 80 percent of all dialysis patients are treated as in-center hemodialysis patients; the remaining 20 percent are primarily home dialysis patients, most of whom receive peritoneal dialysis.

5. Treatments here refer to outpatient hemodialysis only. Peritoneal dialysis treatments are excluded from the statistics to better capture the relationship between number of hemodialysis treatments and number of dialysis stations, and thus to estimate utilization more precisely.

6. Average treatment/station ratios provided here are national, not facility-specific, figures.

7. The primary exception to this practice is the rule that a six-antigen match between an organ and a prospective donor must be shared.

8. See Chapter 5 for a discussion of pediatric ESRD patients. According to the prevalent patient count, there were 3,989 patients under age 20 in 1987.

9. The distinction between hospital-based and independent outpatient dialysis providers is based on HCFA's categorization of renal treatment facilities. Currently, HCFA distinguishes between hospital-based and independent (sometimes called freestanding) units by ownership, not by operational characteristics. Major differences exist, however, among "hospital-based" facilities in terms of their operation and patient population: Some are physically located within a hospital and dialyze mainly inpatients and a very limited number of outpatients; many, however, are not physically located within a hospital, care mainly for outpatients, and do not differ operationally from independent units.

10. Data on utilization, measured by the number of treatments per station per year, were not readily available for the period from 1980 to 1988. The number of patients per station per year is used as a rough equivalent here. The patient/station ratio for independent facilities was 4.3 patients per station in 1988, a slight increase from 4.2 in 1980.

11. The discussion here refers to dialysis facilities only. Physician ownership should not be confused with the for-profit or not-for-profit status of such facilities. Nephrologists who serve as medical directors or attending physicians at for-profit facilities do not necessarily own them.

12. The size of a dialysis facility is defined here by the number of stations: a small facility has 1 to 9 stations; a medium-size facility has 10 to 20 stations; and a large facility has more than 20 stations.

13. This point was suggested by Dr. David D. Zinn, Medical Director of Northeast Alabama Kidney Clinic, Inc., personal communication, May 17, 1990.

REFERENCES

Community Psychiatric Centers. 1989. Proxy Statement, July 12. Laguna Hills, Calif.

Gray BN., ed. 1986. For-Profit Enterprise in Health Care. Institute of Medicine. Washington, D.C.: National Academy Press.

HCFA (Health Care Financing Administration). 1980-88. Annual Facility Surveys. Baltimore, Md.

Held PJ, Pauly MV. 1983. Competition and efficiency in the End-Stage Renal Disease program. J Health Econ 2:95-118.

IHPP (Intergovernmental Health Policy Project). 1989. Certificate of Need (CON) Regulation of ESRD Service: Findings of a 50-State Survey. Report prepared for the Institute of Medicine. George Washington University, Washington, D.C.

National Association of Children's Hospitals and Related Institutions. 1987. Pediatric Patient Profile. Unpublished data.

OIG (Office of the Inspector General, U.S. Department of Health and Human Services). 1987. Organ acquisition costs: An overview. Washington, D.C., September.

Prottas J. 1985. The structure and effectiveness of the U.S. organ procurement system. Inquiry 22:366.

REN Corporation-USA. 1989. Prospectus, November 28. Nashville, Tenn.

Task Force on Organ Transplantation. 1986. Organ Transplantation: Issues and Answers. Washington, D.C.: U.S. Department of Health and Human Services, pp. 214-216.

USRDS (U.S. Renal Data System). 1989. USRDS 1989 Annual Data Report. National Institute of Diabetes and Digestive and Kidney Diseases, Bethesda, Md., August.

PART III
Access

Access to health care arises as a policy question because some individuals lack appropriate health care services. Access deals with limits to care, primarily financial barriers to care, especially the resources that enable individuals to purchase care. Medicare and Medicaid were enacted in 1965 to remove financial barriers to health care for the elderly and the poor. In 1972, Medicare was expanded to include those disabled, eligible for cash Social Security benefits, after a two-year period.

The Social Security Amendments of 1972 also established an entitlement to Medicare for most Americans individuals with permanent kidney failure. Medicare coverage meant that dialysis and kidney transplantation services would be covered as well as other medical services covered under the Medicare program. Despite this virtually universal coverage, a variety of access issues have arisen over the history of the program.

Congress, in the Omnibus Budget Reconciliation Act of 1987, asked the IOM to examine access for two groups of individuals with kidney failure—those eligible for Medicare benefits and those not eligible for such benefits. Chapter 7 addresses the problems of both groups. Chapter 8 deals with limits of access to kidney transplantation that may stem from the limited period of Medicare eligibility after transplantation and from restrictions on payment for immunosuppressive drugs. This chapter also considers the issue of equitable allocation of donated organs but places greatest emphasis on the problems created by the shortage of kidneys suitable for transplantation.

7

Access Problems of ESRD Patients

The high costs of dialysis and transplantation severely limited the access of most Americans to care for ESRD before 1973. Section 2991 of the Social Security Amendments of 1972 effectively resolved access problems stemming from financial considerations. That statute defined eligibility for ESRD beneficiaries in the following language:

(e) Notwithstanding the foregoing provisions of this section, every individual who—

(1) has not attained the age of 65;

(2)(A) is fully or currently insured (as terms are defined in section 214 of this Act), or (B) is entitled to monthly insurance benefits under title II of this Act, or (C) is the spouse or dependent child (as defined in regulations) of an individual who is fully or currently insured, or (D) is the spouse or dependent child (as defined in regulations) of an individual entitled to monthly insurance benefits under title II of this Act; and

(3) is medically determined to have chronic renal disease and who requires hemodialysis or renal transplantation for such disease; shall be deemed to be disabled for purposes of coverage under parts A and B of Medicare subject to the deductible, premium, and co-payment provisions of title XVIII.[1]

The 1972 amendment created a "near-universal" entitlement to Medicare coverage of ESRD treatment for most Americans. It did not, however, create an entitlement for all.[2] Consequently, one question that Congress asked in its OBRA 1987 charge dealt with access problems of ESRD patients who are not eligible for Medicare coverage. The congressional charge also asked that the study consider access problems of Medicare-covered ESRD beneficiaries. Both are considered below, with a focus on dialysis patients. (Chapter 8 deals with access problems of kidney transplant patients.) This chapter also deals with access limitations that flow from state laws and regulations, especially certificate-of-need (CON).

ESRD PATIENTS NOT ELIGIBLE FOR MEDICARE

Congress, in 1978, directed the Secretary of Health, Education, and Welfare

to conduct a study of the number of patients with ESRD who are not eligible for benefits with respect to such disease under this title, and of the economic impact of such non-eligibility of such individuals. Such study shall include consideration of mechanisms whereby governmental and other health plans might be instituted or modified to permit the purchase of actuarially sound coverage for the costs of ESRD. [Public Law No. 95-292, § 181(f)(6).]

HCFA responded belatedly in 1984 (HCFA, 1984). The report, using 1981 data, estimated that of the 55,000 ESRD patients in the United States who received dialysis treatments from Medicare-certified dialysis facilities, about 8,500 were not then entitled to Medicare benefits. Half of these unentitled patients were awaiting entitlement to the Medicare program and approval was expected: For these individuals, Blue Cross and other private insurers were the major sources of support for 50 percent, whereas Medicaid was the primary payment source for another 27 percent.

However, more than 4,000 of the 8,500 patients were reported as not eligible for Medicare benefits. The reasons are not entirely clear. Either they had not established fully or currently insured status under Social Security, or they had not filed an application for benefits. For 70 percent of these ESRD patients, public programs—the Veterans Administration, state Medicaid, and state kidney programs—constituted the major sources of support. The ESRD facilities surveyed for this study identified bad debts and delays in payment from non-Medicare sources as the two financial problems associated with unentitled patients. This was particularly true among self-pay patients—citizens as well as noncitizens—who lacked any public or private health insurance.

HCFA estimated that the cost of covering these unentitled ESRD patients who were not eligible for Medicare benefits would be $170 million for FY 1984 and $290 million for FY 1988. Since many unentitled ESRD patients were being supported wholly or partly by other federal programs, HCFA concluded that extending Medicare coverage to them would simply transfer responsibility from one federal source to another and recommended against legislation to do so.

The prevailing view, expressed by HCFA's 1984 report and accepted by many others, is that access limitations to ESRD treatment have been relatively minor. In addition to stability in the percentage of reported noneligibles and the existence of other government programs to finance ESRD treatment, other factors supporting this view include the continuing growth of the patient population and the existence of an aggressive medical specialty that is dedicated to treating patients.

Who Are the Reported Noneligibles?

Although aliens not legally residing in the United States may present themselves for treatment as ESRD patients, and may represent a significant proportion of the noneligibles, as a practical matter they are seldom eligible for either Medicare or state Medicaid coverage. Citizenship or resident alien status is effectively a requirement for Medicare and Medicaid eligibility for ESRD treatment.[3]

Eligibility for Medicare coverage for ESRD is a function of Social Security insured status, which results from active labor force participation. Workers are eligible for Social Security benefits if they have established fully or currently insured status, measured by quarters of coverage, and meet other criteria (age 62 for some, age 65 for others, disabled, blind) that entitle them to receive benefit payments. Workers are fully insured for themselves and their families if they have a minimum of 6 quarters of covered employment; after 40 quarters of coverage, a person is fully insured for life. They are currently insured if they have 6 quarters of covered employment in the past 3 years. In 1989, covered earnings of $470 were required to earn one quarter of coverage.

Since 1981, there have been two major expansions of Medicare coverage. The Tax Equity and Fiscal Responsibility Act of 1982 (Public Law 97-248) extended Medicare coverage to federal government employees. The Social Security Amendments of 1983 (Public Law 98-21) made coverage mandatory for all new state and local government employees; voluntary participation had been available to such individuals since 1950.

Individuals with a diagnosis of ESRD who are not eligible for Medicare ESRD coverage either do not qualify for fully or currently insured status under Social Security or have not filed an application for Social Security coverage. This includes those with no work experience, or employed in jobs not covered by Social Security, or employed in covered occupations but who have not applied, and who are neither the spouse nor dependent child of an eligible person.

What individuals or groups of individuals are at risk of lacking Medicare ESRD coverage because they are not covered under Social Security? Data to answer this question are not collected currently by HCFA. Practically speaking, the ineligibles include some federal, state, and local government employees; domestic, farm, and all other workers in covered occupations who have not applied for coverage; and those who have never worked, such as young, unmarried, nonworking mothers and their children. People in most of these categories are disproportionately concentrated among the poor and minorities.

Magnitude of the Problem

The total number of dialysis patients increased from 52,364 in 1980 to 90,886 in 1986; during this time, the reported noneligible patients accounted for 6 to 7 percent (Table 7-1). In the 3 years from 1987 to 1989, however, that percentage increased to 7.2, 7.3, and 7.5 percent. Although the percentages were stable until recently, the absolute numbers of noneligible ESRD patients more than doubled from 3,697 in 1980 to 8,722 in 1989. The implications of this growth are examined below.

Geographic Variations

Although the national percentage of reported noneligibles has been stable, HCFA ESRD data show marked variation by state. In Table 7-2, these data are summarized for selected states, and several different patterns emerge. In the first pattern, some states have been consistently high over time and more recently have abruptly dropped to a very low percentage of non-Medicare patients. In Arkansas, for example, the reported noneligibles declined from 20.1 percent in 1980 to 12.5 percent in 1986 and then fell

TABLE 7-1 Medicare Eligibility Status of Dialysis Patients, 1980-89

Year	Total Dialysis Patients[a]	Medicare-Eligible Patients		Non-Medicare Patients	
		Number of Enrollees	Applications Pending	Number	% of Total Patients
1980	52,364	44,827	3,840	3,697	7.1
1981	58,924	51,359	3,768	3,797	6.4
1982	65,765	57,784	3,998	3,983	6.1
1983	71,987	63,624	3,945	4,418	6.1
1984	78,483	69,258	4,227	4,998	6.4
1985	84,797	74,169	4,965	5,663	6.7
1986	90,886	79,739	5,076	6,071	6.7
1987	98,432	85,774	5,587	7,071	7.2
1988	105,958	91,820	6,371	7,767	7.3
1989	116,169	100,857	6,590	8,722	7.5

[a]As of December 31 of the calendar year.

SOURCE: HCFA, 1980-89.

TABLE 7-2   Percentage of Non-Medicare Patients Among Total Dialysis Patients, by State and Year, 1980-89

State	1980	1981	1982	1983	1984	1985	1986	1987	1988	1989
Arizona	16.2	16.1	16.2	14.8	12.3	13.7	12.2	12.8	15.2	15.1
Arkansas	20.1	15.0	14.1	13.1	12.2	12.4	12.5	3.5	4.8	4.6
California	7.8	7.2	7.6	7.6	8.0	8.4	8.5	10.1	10.9	11.0
Illinois	5.5	5.6	5.5	5.3	6.3	8.0	9.2	7.0	8.5	9.7
Iowa	12.6	11.9	12.2	11.2	2.4	10.2	0.9	3.1	4.2	2.6
Maryland	6.0	6.1	7.4	7.3	9.2	6.5	6.7	11.3	9.3	8.7
New Mexico	24.9	21.7	17.9	13.9	12.2	12.0	10.1	8.9	14.6	12.3
New York	7.9	7.5	6.6	6.8	7.5	7.8	8.4	9.0	10.2	9.8
Puerto Rico	12.8	7.7	8.7	7.0	7.4	8.3	6.3	10.0	9.2	7.7
Virginia	11.8	9.8	8.2	7.9	7.4	8.0	9.0	7.8	8.3	8.0
Washington, D.C.	29.1	27.5	15.9	17.4	16.3	20.6	15.5	26.4	17.4	17.6
All states	7.1	6.4	6.1	6.1	6.4	6.7	6.7	7.2	7.3	7.5

NOTE: As of December 31 of the calendar year.

SOURCE: HCFA, 1980-89.

precipitously to 4.6 percent in 1989. The recent drop may be due to the fact that patients treated at the Little Rock Veterans Hospital were counted as Medicare-eligible after the hospital obtained Medicare certification in 1986-87, although this does not explain the entire historical pattern (C.W. Roach, ESRD Network 13, personal communication, December 13, 1989).

A second pattern involves a stable rate suddenly increasing. For example, from 1980 through 1984, Illinois hovered around 6 percent for reported noneligibles, but from 1985 onward, it fluctuated between 7 and 10 percent. The reported noneligibles for Maryland were stable in the 6 to 7 percent range until 1983, increased briefly to 9.2 percent in 1984, returned to the lower level, then increased again to 11.3 percent in 1987, and have remained above 8 percent since then.

A third pattern involves percentages consistently higher than the national level over time. This is dramatically shown in the cases of Arizona and New Mexico. In 1988, Arizona had 222 noneligible ESRD patients (15 percent). Of these, 42 percent were whites, 29 percent Native Americans, and 22 percent Hispanics; one-quarter were covered under the Department of Veterans Affairs (DVA); three-quarters had "other" coverage. In New Mexico, for the same year, 71 patients (13 percent) were reported not eligible. Of these, 43 percent were Native Americans, 32 percent Hispanics, and 20 percent whites; more than one-quarter had no insurance; two-thirds had "other" insurance (S.K. Stiles, Intermountain End-Stage Renal Disease Network, Inc., personal communication, December 21, 1989). Furthermore, the data strongly suggest that the reported noneligibles are concentrated among ethnic minorities. What is not known is the adequacy of coverage from non-Medicare sources or the financial effects of ESRD on other insurers such as state Medicaid, the DVA, and the Indian Health Service (IHS).

An examination of the percentage of reported noneligibles in 20 major U.S. cities relative to their states' percentages showed that some, but not all, had markedly greater concentrations of reported noneligibles than did their home states (Table 7-3). This was true for Boston, Chicago, Detroit, Los Angeles, Miami, New York City, Newark, and Philadelphia. In addition, Washington, D.C., fluctuated between a high of 29.1 percent and a low of 15.5 percent of reported noneligibles, a significant proportion of whom had Medicaid coverage only. These data suggest that proportionately more noneligible patients are found among urban residents, as well as among ethnic minorities.

Existing data on reported noneligibles do not include the extent and adequacy of other sources of support. Thus, they do not permit direct examination of the effects of noneligible status on access to or denial of treatment, nor do they allow comparison of the Medicare benefit package to non-Medicare coverage. Most important, they do not permit examination of the effect of eligibility status on patient outcomes.

Payment Sources

Potential sources of financial support available to noneligible ESRD patients are personal resources, private health insurance, or public programs. Personal wealth and private insurance may cover a few, but public programs must provide the support for most patients. The latter include state Medicaid programs, state kidney disease programs, the IHS, and the DVA.

State Medicaid Programs

A survey of ESRD-related expenditures by state Medicaid programs, state general assistance (welfare-medical) programs, and state kidney programs performed by the Intergovernmental Health Policy Project generated responses from 47 states and the District of Columbia (IHPP, 1989a).[4] It showed that state Medicaid programs have very inadequate data on ESRD patients and expenditures. Only 23 states could provide Medicaid expenditure data for FY 1988, the most recent fiscal year; for fiscal years 1983 through 1987, the numbers reporting such data were 6, 8, 9, 14, and 18, respectively. Those 23 states reported $68 million in expenditures in 1988 but indicated that this underestimated true expenditures.[5]

State Medicaid programs serve two ESRD patient groups. Copayments are made for those Medicare-entitled patients who are also eligible for Medicaid (dual eligibles). In addition, treatment for individuals who lack any

TABLE 7-3 Percentage of Non-Medicare Patients Among Total Dialysis Patients, by City Versus State, and Year, 1980-87

City and State	1980	1981	1982	1983	1984	1985	1986	1987
Boston	8.7	8.2	8.2	7.6	7.3	7.3	12.9	10.1
Massachusetts	5.7	5.8	5.8	6.3	6.7	5.7	8.7	8.0
Chicago	10.6	9.8	8.9	8.4	9.4	11.8	15.8	10.6
Illinois	6.5	5.6	5.5	5.3	6.3	8.0	9.2	7.0
Cleveland	5.7	4.6	3.8	4.1	3.0	9.5	9.5	8.6
Ohio	4.8	5.1	5.1	5.2	5.4	7.1	5.6	5.6
Dallas	7.5	5.0	5.4	7.2	8.0	9.6	10.0	9.0
Texas	7.0	6.0	5.2	5.8	5.6	6.4	5.9	5.9
Detroit	8.5	8.2	11.2	8.3	11.2	8.2	8.0	7.9
Michigan	6.2	6.4	6.5	7.0	8.2	7.5	7.7	6.7
Indianapolis	13.2	12.6	10.8	3.1	4.7	0.8	4.1	2.4
Indiana	7.1	6.2	5.7	1.9	2.7	1.1	2.4	3.1
Los Angeles	11.8	11.9	10.5	9.5	13.6	13.5	15.9	14.3
California	7.8	7.2	7.6	7.6	8.0	8.4	8.5	10.1
Miami	9.0	12.0	12.6	12.1	11.8	9.8	9.9	10.0
Florida	4.5	4.8	5.2	5.4	5.4	5.3	5.9	4.9
New York City	11.5	10.9	8.2	9.2	10.8	12.5	11.5	11.8
New York	7.9	7.5	6.6	6.8	7.5	7.8	8.4	9.0
Newark	6.1	5.7	7.0	10.5	7.8	8.4	17.4	7.1
New Jersey	4.8	3.9	4.0	4.8	5.6	5.2	6.0	8.5
Philadelphia	8.2	6.5	6.6	7.1	7.8	8.2	8.1	9.1
Pennsylvania	6.6	5.1	5.4	5.4	5.7	6.2	4.8	5.8
Phoenix	13.8	8.6	12.9	8.9	7.9	10.2	10.1	10.6
Arizona	16.2	16.1	16.2	14.8	12.3	13.7	12.2	12.8
Washington, D.C.	29.1	27.5	15.9	17.4	16.3	20.6	15.5	26.4

NOTE: As of December 31 of the calendar year.

SOURCE: HCFA, 1980-87.

Medicare coverage is paid for. Although state Medicaid ESRD expenditures for dual eligibles and reported noneligibles are undoubtedly substantial, neither a direct count nor a good estimate exists.

A follow-up survey of 10 states—California, Florida, Illinois, Louisiana, Maryland, Massachusetts, Michigan, New York, Pennsylvania, and Texas— addressed the extent of Medicaid coverage of ESRD services and related medications for those with Medicaid coverage only (not eligible for Medicare) and for the dual eligibles (Laudicina, 1990). The services examined included outpatient hemodialysis; in-center peritoneal dialysis; inpatient hemodialysis; kidney transplant surgery; blood transfusions; transportation; home hemodialysis; intermittent peritoneal dialysis; continuous cycling peritoneal dialysis; continuous ambulatory peritoneal dialysis; dialysis equipment, supplies, and dialysis support services; self-dialysis training; and paid aides to assist at home. Seven of the 10 states examined provide Medicaid coverage for nearly all of the 15 benefits surveyed.

Eight of the 10 surveyed state Medicaid programs reimburse for outpatient dialysis treatment at payment levels ranging from $110 to $150 per session. Illinois, Maryland, and Massachusetts pay the equivalent of the Medicare composite rate under their Medicaid programs. In contrast, Florida pays only for dialysis in a hospital-based center and sets an annual payment cap of $1,000 per Medicaid ESRD patient! Louisiana reimburses hospital-based centers up to 72 percent of billed charges. Texas Medicaid does not pay for home and routine hemodialysis. State Medicaid agencies generally pay the same for center-based and home dialysis, except New York, which pays lower rates for home dialysis, and Pennsylvania, which sets a lower rate for home dialysis but makes an additional payment for dialysis equipment rental.

With regard to Medicaid reimbursement policy for dual eligibles (Medicare and Medicaid), six states pay providers for the Medicare Part B deductibles and 20 percent coinsurance. Four other states—California, Michigan, New York, and Pennsylvania—reimburse Medicare Part B coinsurance and deductibles for dual eligibles for facility and home dialysis, not to exceed the Medicare-approved amount. Texas indicated that coverage of ESRD services constituted a financial burden, a result of the growth in recent years of the overall Medicaid case load and an assessment that all chronic care expenditures are expensive.

The survey also investigated reimbursement for medications in the following categories: antihypertensives, anemia treatment, calcium/phosphorus metabolism control, multivitamin compounds, and kidney transplant immunosuppressives. Although state Medicaid programs routinely reimburse the drug costs for Medicaid-eligible patients, various restrictions exist. Florida does not yet provide erythropoietin (EPO) for its Medicaid recipients; California will not honor more than three prescriptions for antihypertensive drugs within a 75-day period. Maryland limits payment for EPO to no more than $400 per prescription and attempts to get Medicare to cover the cost of Imuran and cyclosporine for Medicaid recipients who have received transplants within the year; Texas limits coverage of EPO to no more than three injections per week and will not pay for more than three prescriptions per month for drugs intended for home use (e.g., antihypertensives, calcium/phosphorus metabolism controllers, multivitamin compounds, and cyclosporine). Medicaid agencies in most states do not reimburse separately for all ESRD-related drugs, although some drugs are included in the dialysis facility's rate (e.g., heparin, protamine, saline, pressor drugs, glucose, and antihypertensives).

Since the inception of the Medicaid program in 1965, states have been allowed to "buy into" a private health insurance program for Medicaid recipients, provided this option is exercised on a statewide basis. California, New York, Minnesota, and Washington have chosen this option. The option is not based on patient diagnosis, so there is no way of knowing how many ESRD patients benefit from it. New York Medicaid officials believe that it is sometimes cost-effective for the state to pay for private insurance premiums in lieu of caring for a Medicaid-eligible individual under the Medicaid rate structure. However, it is estimated that only a minority of Medicaid-eligibles have their health costs reimbursed in this manner.

State Kidney Programs

Twenty states administer kidney programs independent of their state Medicaid programs. Nineteen of these programs support a variety of ESRD-related services, from direct patient financial support to public education for organ donation; Michigan's program is basically a data registry (IHPP, 1989a). In Table 7-4, state kidney programs and their services are listed.

Patterns of state kidney disease program expenditures, shown in Table 7-5 are mixed. The Texas Kidney Health Care Program (which is different from the Texas Medicaid program) is unique in offering comprehensive financial assistance in all areas of patient care: transportation, medication, transplant workup procedures, dental care, and transplant follow-up care. It expanded in the early 1980s, experienced a major cut during FY 1986, and has been stable at just under $10 million. Given the budget pressures that many state governments face at the present time, it is probably not realistic to expect that these state kidney programs will increase their financial support for noneligible ESRD patients or that more states will add such programs.[6]

Other ESRD Programs

The IHS is responsible for providing comprehensive medical care to Native Americans living on reservations. IHS health care benefits vary

TABLE 7-4 Services of State Kidney Programs

State	Medicare Copay	Dialysis and Related Treatment	Prescription Drugs	Transportation	Transplants	Transplant Medications	Related Hospital Services
Delaware	X	X	X[a]	X		X	
Georgia	X	X					
Hawaii	X	X	X		X	X	X
Illinois	X	X				X	
Indiana	X	X				X	
Iowa	X	X	X	X	X	X	X
Maryland	X	X	X		X	X	X
Missouri	X	X	X	X	X	X	
Montana	X	X	X		X	X	X
Nebraska	X	X	X		X	X	X
New Jersey			[a]				
New York	X	X[b]	X				
North Carolina		X	X[a]			X	
Pennsylvania	X	X	X	X	X	X	
South Dakota	X	X	X	X	X	X	
Tennessee	X	X	X[a]		X	X	X
Texas		X	X	X		X	
Washington	X	X	X	X	X	X	
Wyoming	X	X	X	X		X	
TOTAL 19	16	18	16	8	10	16	6

[a]Includes over-the-counter medications.
[b]Program provides services to home dialysis patients only.

SOURCE: IHPP, 1989a.

TABLE 7-5 Trends in State Kidney Program Expenditures[a]

State	Fiscal Year						
	1984	1985	1986	1987	1988	1989	1990
Delaware		178,200[b]	178,200	174,034	185,719		
Georgia		600,000	500,000	400,000	400,000		
Hawaii		311,170[b]	424,726[b]	377,827	436,134	453,639	
Illinois	1,500,000	1,500,000	1,500,000	1,500,000	1,500,000	1,500,000	1,500,000
Indiana		397,653	425,725	371,388	442,606	432,783	
Iowa		838,000	504,000	768,000	904,000	764,000	
Maryland	2,710,442	3,794,853	2,833,278	3,626,369	4,127,305		
Montana		125,000	125,000	125,000	125,000		
Nebraska	669,098	486,384	729,309	726,918	543,629	833,000	
New Jersey		438,000	438,000	438,000	438,000	434,000	
New York	4,775,000	3,057,000					
North Carolina	1,800,000	1,800,000	1,800,000	1,800,000	1,800,000		
Pennsylvania	8,852,000	8,987,000	8,987,000	7,986,000	6,640,000		
South Dakota	238,479	242,949	245,517	240,346	186,184	209,372	
Tennessee	1,000,000	1,000,000	1,000,000	1,247,300			
Texas	11,913,586	15,549,022	9,548,438	9,969,953	9,973,442	9,985,739	
Washington	2,208,371[c]	2,960,000[c]					
Wyoming			412,000[b]	412,000[b]	412,000[b]	412,000[b]	

[a]Data reflect information provided by the programs, but some programs had limited expenditure data available.
[b]Budget.
[c]Amount reflects a 2-year appropriation.

SOURCE: IHPP, 1989a.

from year to year and from area to area, based on area-determined priorities and the annual congressional appropriation to IHS. IHS does not maintain its own dialysis facilities, but units managed by private contractors have been established within several IHS hospitals. In recent years, ESRD costs not covered by Medicare or other third parties have placed an increasing burden on the IHS budget.

The DVA provides dialysis treatment for slightly fewer than 3,000 veterans in DVA hospitals and satellite hospital programs.[7] Although the distribution of DVA patients between those eligible and not eligible for Medicare coverage is unknown, it is believed that most DVA ESRD patients are eligible. They apparently choose DVA treatment to avoid Medicare deductible and copayment liabilities. Thirteen DVA dialysis units are also certified by Medicare for reimbursement of treatment for a small number of non-DVA Medicare ESRD patients.

The number of DVA centers has declined slightly in recent years, but the number of DVA center dialysis patients remained stable at about 3,300 patients from 1982 through 1985, and then declined to 2,553 in 1989; the number of patients in satellite facilities ranged from 302 to 375 for the years 1982 through 1988. DVA ESRD expenditures grew from $105 million in 1980 to $151 million in 1986, then declined to $122 million in 1989 (Table 7-6). A DVA dialysis program that is shrinking in numbers of patients and expenditures could not absorb the growing number of Medicare noneligible ESRD patients, even if veterans' eligibility were not a problem.

State Medicaid programs, then, constitute the first line of financial support for ESRD patients who lack Medicare coverage. The extent and adequacy of state Medicaid ESRD benefits compared to Medicare coverage are not known in detail. It is known that states exercise discretion regarding Medicaid eligibility criteria and covered services and that the resulting variability severely limits access to treatment financing for ESRD patients in some states. (It is also known that state Medicaid programs are under budgetary constraints of varying severity and are subjected to an increasing number of mandated benefits.) The 19 state kidney programs vary substantially in funding and provide relatively modest financial support to ESRD patients not eligible for Medicare. The IHS faces a number of budgetary priorities that can be adversely affected by ESRD expenditures. The DVA resources for ESRD are shrinking, as is the number of DVA ESRD patients.

Conclusions and Recommendations

The available evidence on ESRD patients who are reported as not eligible for Medicare coverage points to the following conclusions. First, little is known about these patients, and their demographic characteristics, health status, and socioeconomic profiles should be examined carefully.

TABLE 7-6 Department of Veterans Affairs (DVA) Expenditures for Dialysis Patients, 1980-89

	1980	1981	1982	1983	1984	1985	1986	1987	1988	1989
Total DVA expenditures (millions of dollars)	104.9	107.9	114.3	120.4	132.7	148.4	150.8	143.4	129.1	121.7
Total patients	3,131	3,171	3,330	3,327	3,337	3,327	3,195	3,157	3,132	2,878
Center patients	2,879	2,887	3,011	3,008	3,030	3,025	2,893	2,818	2,757	2,553
Satellite patients	252	284	319	319	347	302	302	339	375	325

NOTE: As of December 31 of the calendar year.

SOURCE: Neil Otchin, Department of Veterans Affairs, personal communication, June 1990.

Second, the proportion of ESRD patients reported as not eligible for Medicare coverage, having been stable for some time, may now be increasing and varies substantially by state and city. Third, the absolute number of reported noneligibles has more than doubled in the past decade. Fourth, several major sources for financing the ESRD care of reported noneligibles, such as the DVA, the IHS, and state kidney programs, are stable or shrinking. State Medicaid programs have thus become the payer of last resort for reported noneligible ESRD patients. Although quite adequate in some states, Medicaid coverage for ESRD in other states is virtually nonexistent. Furthermore, Medicaid programs vary in coverage and eligibility according to state discretion.

The committee believes that there is no justifiable basis for a "near-universal" Medicare ESRD benefit that falls short of a benefit for all citizens and resident aliens. Limiting Medicare eligibility for ESRD treatment to those who are fully or currently insured under Social Security or entitled to monthly benefits puts some excluded individuals at risk of death from ESRD. The U.S. government, therefore, having assumed the responsibility as principal payer for ESRD treatment for over 90 percent of the country's population, should extend that coverage to all citizens and resident aliens. An estimate of the additional expenditures required to finance this recommendation is found as an appendix to this chapter. (Undocumented aliens are generally not eligible for Medicare benefits under existing statutory authority; the committee does not recommend any change in this area.[3])

A large share of Medicare ESRD benefits is paid through the Part B Supplemental Medical Insurance (SMI) Trust Fund. However, the SMI Trust Fund is financed by a combination of beneficiary premiums and general revenues, unlike the Part A Hospital Insurance Trust Fund, which is financed by a portion of the Social Security payroll tax. It is doubly ironic, then, that current eligibility criteria for ESRD treatment exclude some Americans from coverage on the basis of their tie to Social Security, even though much of the benefit is financed from the income tax, a broader tax than the payroll tax.

> **The committee recommends, as a matter of equitable treatment of all individuals with ESRD, that Congress modify the criteria for Medicare eligibility for ESRD patients and extend the entitlement to all citizens and resident aliens.[8]**

MEDICARE-ELIGIBLE ESRD PATIENTS

ESRD patients who are eligible for Medicare benefits also confront some problems of access to care. This section examines the specific access problems of pediatric and elderly ESRD patients, and general barriers to information, insurance, rehabilitation services, transportation, and preventive services.

Pediatric Patients

Access to care is particularly important for the pediatric ESRD patient because early diagnosis and treatment so strongly affect prognosis and outcome. Current Medicare entitlement criteria do not apply to the treatment of children with progressive irreversible renal insufficiency until they reach the ESRD stage. Consequently, many pediatric patients enter the Medicare ESRD program suffering from potentially avoidable clinical consequences of severe chronic renal failure. Quality of life is adversely affected, and the treatment of these problems is often difficult and inadequate. Early access to adequate care before renal failure could limit the nutrition-related and growth problems including defective bone formation experienced by ESRD pediatric patients. Such interventions also would be cost-effective.

Compared to the entire ESRD population, the pediatric ESRD population is less likely to be covered by Medicare. The North American Pediatric Renal Transplant Cooperative Study (Alexander et al., 1990) found that 13 percent of 754 transplant patients under age 18 were not Medicare-eligible, a rate much higher than the reported national rate of 6 to 7 percent for all ages. Four groups of pediatric patients who are not currently eligible for Medicare entitlement include (1) children of young, usually unwed, mothers receiving public assistance; (2) children of nonworking single parents (usually not working because of family responsibilities) who do not participate in the Social Security system; (3) children of nonqualifying intact families; and (4) children of undocumented aliens who are permanently residing in the United States. The effects of a lack of Medicare coverage on access to needed care are not known. Coverage through non-Medicare sources is often inadequate, however, and the expenses for this younger population are generally higher than for the general ESRD population because of the greater complexity of their care.

Preventing adverse outcomes in children is strongly related to the early treatment of chronic renal failure before ESRD is reached, which can delay or prevent progression to ESRD. If a child reaches ESRD, then transplantation is the best treatment. The European Dialysis and Transplant Association (EDTA) evaluated young adults who entered renal replacement therapy as children (Rizzoni, 1989). The data indicated that most disabilities (motor, auditory, and visual) were present at the start of treatment for ESRD, and that treatment resulted in only limited improvement in these disabilities. The EDTA report concluded that the maximum effort should be made to prevent or minimize the development of the disabilities in the period between the initial diagnosis of renal failure and before the initiation of treatment for ESRD.

Many treatment requirements of children can be met only by specially trained personnel, including board-certified pediatric nephrologists, specially trained nurses, nutritionists, social workers, psychologists, and, often, teachers. Such personnel are required to provide essential care, improve quality of life and compliance with treatment, and provide crisis intervention and educational and vocational training for the disadvantaged pediatric patients.

Family income significantly affects the quality of life of the pediatric ESRD patient. The financial demands of caring for a pediatric ESRD patient may place a heavy burden on financially disadvantaged families, as in providing the nutritional prescription required for optimal care or meeting transportation expenses. Thus, in many ways, ESRD in the pediatric population places additional burdens on patients, their families, and caregivers compared to the general ESRD population.

Elderly Patients

In the initial year of the Medicare ESRD program, only 5 percent of prevalent ESRD patients were over age 65 (Rettig, 1980). This proportion has grown over the years to nearly 40 percent of the incident ESRD population and over 25 percent of the prevalent population.

Elderly patients are treated mainly by dialysis; although kidney transplants were once extremely uncommon among the elderly, they have increased in recent years. However, the proportion of elderly patients receiving transplants remains far smaller than for younger patients: of the 17,891 kidney transplants performed in 1988 and 1989, only 2.1 percent (or 371) were in people 65 or older (UNOS, 1990); of all patients with functioning kidneys, only 2.6 percent were over age 65 (IOM, 1990).[9] Given limited availability of kidneys and a growing demand for transplantation, it is unlikely that transplantation will become a major treatment modality for the elderly.

Barriers to Access

Information

The Medicare conditions of participation (42 CFR Part 405, Subpart U, 2138) require ESRD treatment facilities to inform patients of their rights and responsibilities, their medical condition, the available services, the unit's policy toward dialyzer reuse, their treatment options, and their suitability for transplantation and home dialysis. The effective provision of information to patients remains, however, a matter of concern to many.

Patients attach a high priority to information about their disease, health status, and treatment, as the focus groups reflected in Chapter 2. Although they need this information soon after the initial diagnosis of ESRD, this is not always an optimal time to receive information. Patient receptivity to information may be affected by their physiological, emotional, and health status during this period. Patients also differ in their information-seeking behavior, with some being more active than others.

Physicians and other health professionals differ in their ability and inclination to communicate with their patients. Many routinely provide information to patients about their disease and treatment options. Moreover, they do so with awareness of the effect of health status on receptivity and of personality on information seeking. Not all providers do equally well in communicating to patients. However, respect for patients should lead all physicians and caregivers to place a high value on conveying information to patients about their health status and treatment options. Although peer education is very useful to new ESRD patients, they rely heavily on their physicians to educate them and their families.

Information about transplantation is a recurring concern of many patients. Some patients actively ask about transplantation, but many do not. Newmann and colleagues (1989) conducted a study of 300 dialysis patients and their information-seeking behavior. Most patients, they found, had discussed transplantation with their nephrologist, but few understood the procedure, and less than one-third had direct contact with someone from a transplant center. Black patients felt less competent than whites to decide about transplantation and were less inclined to talk to their nephrologist about the procedure; they seldom had access to a transplant surgeon.

Here again, physician behavior differs. Some physicians actively inform patients about transplantation, some refer patients to transplant physicians and surgeons for evaluation, and some shield patients from such information. Since dialysis patients have fewer independent sources of information about transplantation, nephrologists can easily encourage or dampen their interest by subtle interpersonal communication. Thus, nephrologists must take the initiative and responsibility to inform their patients.

Although existing regulations appear adequate, implementing procedures may be needed in some situations for referring ESRD patients to transplant centers for assessment. The Health Standards and Quality Bureau of HCFA is actually addressing the referral issue as part of its quality assurance efforts (discussed in Chapter 12). Nephrology training programs, fellowship programs, and continuing education programs can often be strengthened regarding kidney transplantation.

Transplant centers can also provide better follow-up information on transplant patients to referring nephrologists and dialysis units, thus increasing patient referrals. This might include working with dialysis unit staff to teach patients about transplantation on an ongoing basis. Training programs with an emphasis on patient education for dialysis nurses, technicians, and social workers could also be useful in this respect.

The committee recommends that the provision of information and education programs about choices among the various treatment modalities, including transplantation, be provided to all patients at all ESRD facilities. The presence of effective patient education should be documented and recognized as a necessary service by reimbursement policy.

Insurance

Little information exists on the availability of insurance to ESRD patients. Hawthorne and co-workers (1991) surveyed Michigan ESRD patients regarding the effects of insurance coverage on access to care. Ninety-four percent qualified for Medicare coverage and nearly 80 percent had some additional insurance, either public or private. These ESRD patients did not differ in Medicare coverage by age or gender, but 95 percent of white patients had such coverage compared to 90 percent of black patients.

Regarding other (non-Medicare) insurance coverage, there were no gender-related differences, but only 62 percent of blacks had such insurance compared to 87 percent of whites. Younger patients were less likely than older patients to have other insurance: 72 percent of those 19 to 40 years had other insurance, compared to 84 percent of those 41 to 60 years as well as those 61 to 90 years. Self-reported medical and physician expenses that were not covered by Medicare or other insurance, such as prescription and nonprescription drugs, outpatient charges, and doctor bills, ranged from zero to $36,000 per year, with an average of $1,072; almost 15 percent reported no out-of-pocket expenses.

In a single-center study, 55 percent of the patients who began ESRD treatment in Dialysis Clinic, Inc.-Cincinnati from 1976 through 1989 lacked private health insurance. Of these, 41 percent were black women. The relative risk of death of patients without private insurance, controlled for other factors, was 50 percent higher than for those with such insurance. That study, performed under contract with the IOM, is the only known analysis that links private insurance coverage to patient outcomes of any kind (Pollack and Pesce, 1990).

The issue of the extent and type of insurance coverage of ESRD patients deserves further attention. Analyses of coverage are needed in terms of Medicare only, Medicare plus private insurance, Medicare and Medicaid, and Medicaid only. The questions that need to be addressed are the effects of insurance on access to treatment modality and on patient outcomes. Particular attention needs to be given to those having the least adequate insurance coverage.

Medicare as Secondary Payer In OBRA 1981, Congress made Medicare the secondary payer in the first year of eligibility of an ESRD patient who is covered by an employee group health plan. In the first year, then, the health plan is the primary payer and Medicare assumes copayment liabilities. Medicare regulations were issued several years later, and facility implementation of the provision with non-Medicare third-party payers has occurred subsequently.

The DHHS Office of Inspector General, in a December 1987 report, recommended that the 12-month limit on the Medicare-as-secondary-payer provision for ESRD patients be removed entirely in the interest of consistency with other secondary-payer provisions of Medicare and for cost-saving purposes (OIG, 1987). The cost savings were to be realized by cost shifting from Medicare to the private sector. HCFA, in a September 1987 response to the draft report, basically rejected the proposal.

During 1989 and 1990, several provider organizations advocated extending the secondary-payer provision by varying lengths, the longest being 5 years. The President's budget for FY 1991, submitted to Congress in January 1990, recommended extending the secondary-payer provision for 18 months. Congress, in OBRA 1990, adopted this provision. It also directed the General Accounting Office to study the effects of this provision on patients before any further extension is considered.

Support for Medicare as secondary payer for ESRD patients derives from two basic sources. First, providers generally receive higher reimbursement from private insurers than they do from Medicare. This may be due in part to the limited ability of such insurers to track expenditures for such patients within their claims processing systems or, as providers argue, because they are more reasonable payers than Medicare.

The committee discussed the implications of extending the secondary-payer provision. Its first concern was that a substantial extension, such as 5 years, or eliminating the time limit entirely would substantially weaken the federal government's commitment to the ESRD program and clearly erode public support. The rationale for cost shifting from Medicare to the private sector is far from clear in this context. Such a step is not likely to be in the long-term interest of patients or providers.

The committee's second concern was that at least some non-Medicare payers, as their financial burden is increased for ESRD patients, would respond by seeking ways to avoid this new, unexpected demand. The requirements of risk-based insurance drive them in this direction.

Finally, and most important, the committee is concerned that extending the secondary-payer provision would in time place ESRD patients at risk.

In particular, patients with employer-based group health insurance are likely to be the most active labor force participants, otherwise healthy individuals, and those most likely to return to work after their illness is diagnosed and their treatment begun. Two problems are likely to arise. If an ESRD patient loses employment, purchasing private insurance with a preexisting condition is likely to be prohibitive. If the employer of an ESRD patient goes "shopping" for a new insurer, as many are doing in the current insurance market (GAO, 1990), the ESRD patient is again likely to be rejected by the new insurer because of the preexisting condition. The net effect is apt to be a stripping away of private insurance as sources of primary and secondary coverage, leaving Medicare as primary and no other party as secondary.

The committee commends the Congress for directing the Comptroller General to study the effects of extending the secondary-payer provision to 18 months for ESRD patients.

The committee recommends that the focus of such a study be the effects on patient access to treatment modalities and services and on patient outcomes.

Transportation

The key service needed by dialysis patients that is not reimbursed is transportation. The distance between a patient's residence or place of work and the site of treatment, the available means of transportation, the average travel time, and the financial resources to meet the travel and patient time costs are important issues to patients. Rural patients, for example, may have more difficulty in reaching a treatment facility than their urban counterparts, and poor, urban patients may have fewer transportation resources than do suburban patients. Little is known, however, about access limits imposed by the costs and availability of transportation.

For a dialysis patient needing treatment three times a week, having to travel long distances can be very troublesome. Among the St. Louis focus-group participants were individuals who traveled almost 100 miles from rural areas into the city for care. Alternatives for rural patients may include home dialysis or moving closer to caregivers. These options may be economically infeasible or medically inappropriate. No literature exists on this subject.

In 1990, Congress considered legislation to provide a special entitlement for dialysis patients with severe mobility problems and whose illness was such that traveling to a treatment facility endangered their lives. Separately, HCFA analyzed high ambulance users among ESRD beneficiaries on the assumption that patients lacking mobility constitute the ambulance-using group of ESRD patients. Transportation costs, although reimbursed by HCFA for ambulance use in some cases, are also borne by state Medicaid agencies in a larger number of cases. OBRA 1990 called for a 3-year demonstration of staff-assisted home dialysis for patients with severe mobility problems.

Rehabilitation Services

The publicly financed Medicare and Medicaid programs cover the elderly, the disabled, and the poor, all of whom are weakly tied to the labor force. As a consequence, Medicare policy is not geared to returning individuals to work, and HCFA has few statutory, organizational, or financial resources to help individuals do so. In fact, in the 1972 statute, ESRD patients are "deemed to be disabled" for purposes of Medicare coverage. Many ESRD patients, once they establish their eligibility for Medicare benefits, apply for Social Security disability status. Eligibility for disability benefits provides monthly income. In early 1990, about one-half of Medicare ESRD beneficiaries between the ages of 18 and 64 were also classified as disabled for purposes of receiving Social Security benefits. Social Security monthly disability benefits, not subject to income tax, often replace income from prior employment. Consequently, problems associated with reentering the labor force lead many patients to regard Social Security disability benefits as their first line of economic support.

Efforts to address the problems of rehabilitation encounter several obstacles. First, ESRD patients are not always able to return to their prior employment, especially to physically demanding jobs. Second, employers are not always receptive to having ESRD patients as employees, for reasons of both dependability and effect on insurance premiums. Third, federal regulations governing the Social Security disability programs provide disincentives to patients' return to work. Finally, Medicare does not finance rehabilitation other than through payment for outpatient treatment, and social services (discussed in Chapter 10) have been decreasing over time.

Rehabilitation services are no more available for kidney transplant recipients than for dialysis patients. Such patients, however, are more likely to be employed. Evans and co-workers (1990) surveyed patients between 30 and 44 months after their transplant. Of those with a functioning primary graft, 44 percent were working either full- or part-time; of patients who had received a second transplant, 44 percent were working; only 18 percent of the patients on dialysis had a job. Age, gender, primary diagnosis, and education of transplant recipients all have an effect on their ability to return to work. Younger transplant recipients are twice as likely to be working than those older than 60; men are 1.5 times more likely to be employed than women; nondiabetics are 1.5 times as likely to have a job as diabetics; and college graduates are nearly twice as likely to be working as those with less education.

Rehabilitation services for ESRD patients deserve sustained attention, especially in light of the report that EPO reduces the fatigue of dialysis patients and equips them to engage in more active pursuits, and because transplant patients should be encouraged to take advantage of their better functional status. The issue of rehabilitation also should be examined in the context of all chronic disease patients as the challenges of ESRD are apt to be encountered elsewhere.

Preventive Services

The human and economic burden of kidney failure makes it necessary to consider the access of individuals to services that may prevent ESRD. Reduced access to preventive health care has been postulated as a partial explanation for the enormous burden of ESRD among black Americans (Feldman, 1990). Implicit in this hypothesis is the notion that there exist medical regimens that may be effective in the prevention of ESRD, such as the control of hypertension and the control of hyperglycemia in diabetics. There is also some evidence for the beneficial effects of reducing dietary protein and phosphorus, and the administration of certain medications may be of some value (Feldman, 1990).

Preventive care for blacks, long documented as deficient, has steadily improved over the past decade. DHHS reported that the proportion of blacks seeing a physician annually was 18 percent less than that of whites in 1963 and that this disparity had been virtually eliminated by 1983. The differences between blacks and whites in utilization of many specific types of health care also diminished over this period. Despite these gains and their accompanying improved health outcomes, morbidity among the black population remains, on average, higher than for whites (HCFA, 1984; NCHS, 1987).

Blendon and co-workers (1989) reported on disparities in the use of health services and in health status between blacks and whites. A significantly higher proportion of blacks had not seen a physician within a one-year period. Additionally, despite evidence that serious illness is more common among blacks, their average number of physician visits was lower (3.4 per year) than that of whites (4.4 per year). Blacks with a chronic or serious illness were also more likely to have had no ambulatory physician visits during the previous year (25.1 percent versus 16.6 percent). The figures for blacks and whites with hypertension were 30 percent and 19 percent, respectively. Blacks were also less likely than whites to have any health insurance; for those blacks with coverage, it was less likely to be private insurance. These differences were reduced but still significant when adjusted for self-reported health status and income.

Shulman and co-workers (1986) investigated the economic barriers to medical care for 4,688 ambulatory patients in Georgia. Nearly one-quarter were hypertensive. Sixteen percent reported occasions on which they could not afford their medications. Blacks were substantially more likely to report this than whites, a phenomenon partially accounted for by the lower mean per-capita income of blacks and their greater prevalence of moderate-to-severe hypertension.

Although barriers to preventive health care are easy to demonstrate, their relationship to the high incidence of ESRD among minority groups is not established. Several investigators have explored socioeconomic status indicators—proxies of access to preventive medical care—and related them to the development of renal insufficiency and hypertensive ESRD. Rostand and co-workers (1989) explored the effects of income and level of education on blood pressure control in an ambulatory-care practice in which hypertensive blacks had a twofold risk of developing renal insufficiency. Neither income nor education predicted the occurrence of renal disease. These data suggest that some of the differences in risk of renal failure among blacks may be due to factors other than differences in access to antihypertensive therapy.

Another study (Whittle et al., 1991) of hypertensive ESRD patients also showed that low socioeconomic status was an independent predictor for the development of ESRD; controlling for it did not eradicate the significant influence that black race had on the occurrence of kidney failure.

Little research has been performed in the Hispanic community regarding access to preventive health care. The San Antonio Heart Study, a community-based study of 1,288 Mexican Americans and 929 whites in Texas, evaluated the prevalence and severity of hypertension among these populations. The prevalence of hypertension adjusted for body weight and socioeconomic status tended to be lower among Mexican Americans. Nonetheless, Mexican Americans had somewhat lower awareness, received treatment less frequently, and had worse control of hypertension than did whites. These findings suggest that socioeconomic barriers to preventive health care services exist in the Mexican American community.

In summary, significant barriers to the acquisition of preventive care have been identified for minority groups, especially for blacks. More research is needed, however, to elucidate the importance of control of hypertension on the development and progression of renal disease. Although barriers to preventive care are accompanied by a significantly impaired health status of the black population, a specific causal relationship between impaired access to care and the predisposition to ESRD has not been established.

STATE REGULATIONS

Some states have stringent CON regulations, and the committee has examined the implications of CON laws on ESRD patients' access to care. A major concern with the CON regulations is their effect on the treatment capacity, both at the program level and at the unit level. As defined in Chapter 6, the number of dialysis stations is the measure of capacity. Unit capacity then can be further defined as the number of hemodialysis stations in a dialysis facility that operates two patient treatment shifts a day for 6 days a week.

A survey conducted by the Intergovernmental Health Policy Project of the George Washington University (IHHP, 1989a) identified 15 states (Alabama, Connecticut, Hawaii, Illinois, Kentucky, Maine, Massachusetts, Nebraska, New Jersey, New York, North Carolina, Pennsylvania, Rhode Island, South Carolina, and Washington) and the District of Columbia as having CON regulations affecting hospital-based as well as independent dialysis providers as of June 1989.[10] The results of this survey were reviewed and confirmed by Dialysis Management, Inc., Denver, Colorado. Information on state CON programs was then combined with the 1984 and 1988 HCFA facility survey data to generate the following summary statistics.

Nationally, treatment capacity grew at an average annual rate of 8.1 percent between 1980 and 1988 whereas the number of total treatments increased 9.7 percent.[11] Station utilization increased slightly from an average of 484 treatments per station in 1984 to 517 in 1988, as Table 7-7 indicates. Utilization of the median facility shifted upward from 465 treatments per station in 1984 to 494 in 1988, a 6 percent increase. Large variations in utilization were noted among states, especially between CON states and non-CON states. In states with CON regulations, utilization increased 16 percent from an average 491 treatments per station in 1984 to 568 in 1988, whereas in states without CON programs the ratios increased only 12 percent.

Using our definition of full capacity as 624 treatments per station per year, the national average utilization rate in 1988 was 83 percent (517/624). States with CON had a utilization rate of 91 percent; states without CON had a 77 percent utilization rate. This CON-related difference in utilization appears to be widening over time: the average difference was 63 treatments per station in 1984, and 89 in 1988.

The substantial increase of the utilization rate over time in the CON states does not appear to be due solely to the growth of the patient population in those states. If anything, the patient population in CON states grew more slowly than in non-CON states between 1984 and 1988. Limited facility capacity (due to CON or other regulations) is more likely to be causing higher utilization rates in the CON states. Experience in California,

TABLE 7-7 ESRD Facility Capacity and Utilization, 1984 and 1988

	Total No. of Stations/Unit		Total No. of Patients/Unit per Year		No. of Hemodialysis Treatments/Unit per Year		Hemodialysis Treatment/Station Ratio		In-Center Patient/Station Ratio	
	1984	1988	1984	1988	1984	1988	1984	1988	1984	1988
National average	13.2	13.2	60.8	61.2	6,641	6,936	484	517	3.6	3.8
Hospital-based	10.9	11.2	55.2	60.0	5,409	6,151	490	535	3.6	3.9
Independent	15.3	14.4	65.6	62.0	7,716	7,406	478	507	3.6	3.8
National distribution										
10th percentile	5.0	5.0	12.0	13.0	1,268	1,219	204	177	1.8	1.5
25th percentile	7.0	8.0	25.0	25.0	2,894	2,860	345	319	2.6	2.5
Median	11.0	11.0	47.0	48.0	5,224	5,504	465	494	3.4	3.6
75th percentile	18.0	17.0	81.0	83.0	8,996	9,415	601	665	4.5	4.8
90th percentile	25.0	24.0	122.0	126.0	13,658	14,407	776	861	5.6	6.2
States with CON	13.6	13.2	62.4	69.5	6,860	7,771	491	568	3.7	4.2
Hospital-based	11.0	10.9	56.8	64.3	5,583	6,530	502	580	3.7	4.3
Independent	15.7	15.2	67.0	73.9	7,919	8,836	482	558	3.6	4.2
States without CON	10.8	13.3	42.0	54.6	4,782	6,335	428	479	3.2	3.5
Hospital-based	9.5	11.5	40.4	55.0	4,215	5,805	446	491	3.5	3.5
Independent	12.0	14.0	43.5	54.5	5,293	6,552	411	475	2.9	3.5
Example—CON										
Connecticut	12.1	11.5	62.9	76.3	7,278	9,224	619	885	4.6	6.2
Hospital-based	10.6	10.6	57.4	71.0	6,387	8,526	619	840	4.6	5.9
Independent	32.0	17.5	140.0	113.5	19,752	14,111	617	1203	4.4	8.5
Example—No CON										
Texas	16.9	16.1	72.8	57.8	8,527	6,979	461	417	3.3	3.1
Hospital-based	13.4	13.9	56.5	44.3	5,862	5,347	415	366	3.0	2.5
Independent	18.5	16.6	80.4	61.4	9,780	7,420	482	430	3.4	3.2

NOTES: Excluded from these data are transplant-only, backup-only, and inpatient-only facilities, as well as those reporting no treatment. The number of patients includes both home patients and in-center dialysis patients, unless otherwise noted. The number of treatments refers only to outpatient hemodialysis; peritoneal dialysis treatments and various training treatments are excluded from the statistics here.

SOURCE: HCFA Annual ESRD Facility Survey, 1984 and 1988.

Florida, Georgia, Tennessee, and Texas in the mid-1980s also supports such a hypothesis. In those states, as soon as the CON regulations for ESRD facilities were eliminated, the number of renal treatment facilities grew substantially.

Specific Limits to Access and Geographic Variations

In New England, state health code and CON requirements have tended to be stringent (IHPP, 1989b). For example, Maine requires CON review and approval before a dialysis service is established in an existing health care facility or a freestanding center, regardless of cost. Vermont requires CON review for the establishment of independent dialysis centers, but not the hospital-based dialysis facilities. The strongest regulation of dialysis services occurs in Rhode Island, Massachusetts,[12] and Connecticut. In these states, the establishment of either a freestanding or a hospital-based dialysis service requires CON review and approval regardless of cost. Any additions to existing services are also subject to review, even if only one station is added. The exception in New England is New Hampshire, in which all outpatient services are exempt from CON review.

Variations in utilization, and thus their effects on access, among geographic areas are even more evident when Connecticut or New York City is compared to Texas. In Connecticut, a state with CON and other stringent regulations on the provision of health care, there was essentially no growth in either the number of facilities or the number of dialysis stations between 1984 and 1988, whereas the number of patients and dialysis treatments increased significantly. Utilization increased almost 43 percent, from 619 to 885 treatments per station per year, during the 4-year period. The calculated statewide utilization rate was 99 percent in 1984 and 142 percent in 1988. In New York City, the utilization rate was 706 treatments per station in 1984, or 113 percent of defined "full utilization." This increased to 782 treatments per station per year in 1988, or 125 percent of "full capacity."

Texas, whose health care sector has not been highly regulated, eliminated CON in August 1985. A significant increase in dialysis facilities and stations occurred: From 1984 to 1988, facilities increased by almost 70 percent, and stations increased over 60 percent, whereas the patient population increased by only 34 percent. This led to a 10 percent decrease in utilization from 461 treatments per station in 1984 to 417 in 1988.

Hypothetically, differences in facility growth between Connecticut or New York City and Texas might be due partly to geographic differences in the cost of providing dialysis rather than to CON regulations. The experience in Texas alone, however, argues otherwise. Before Texas removed its CON regulation in August 1985, growth in dialysis facilities was very slow, from 78 units in 1983 to 81 units in 1985. After the CON regulation was

TABLE 7-8 Connecticut ESRD Patient Log

June 1989: A California dialysis patient was promoted and transferred to Connecticut by his company. He eventually turned down the promotion/transfer because he could find nowhere to dialyze in southwestern Connecticut.

June 1989: A patient from Florida wished to visit his son and grandchildren in Stamford for 2 weeks. He was unable to do so since there was no place within driving distance where he could be dialyzed.

July 1989: A 27-year-old Florida woman wished to attend a conference in New Haven but needed one transient treatment. She did not make the trip because she could not be treated.

October 1989: The parents of two automobile accident victims (one in critical condition) wanted to visit their children; the dialysis patient father needed temporary treatment; his request was eventually denied and referred to the network.

November 1989: A social worker called to state that she had a woman from Long Island, New York, who was the possible victim of domestic violence. The woman had family in Darien, Connecticut, and wanted to transfer. She was referred to the network and as of January 1990 was still looking for space.

November 1989: A 73-year-old patient in Texas with a life expectancy of about one year wanted to be near her daughter and grandchildren in Darien, Connecticut. A bed had been secured at a local nursing home pending dialysis availability. She was referred to Norwalk and a file was created in case an opening originated.

---

removed, the number of dialysis facilities increased substantially: 25 new dialysis facilities began to operate in 1986, representing a 31 percent increase from the previous year. This suggests that CON regulations also play a major role in explaining differences in facility growth across states.

Connecticut, in addition to CON, has several other requirements that may limit capacity:[13] a required nurse supervisor with no patient load for every dialysis shift; a required nurse-to-patient ratio for dialysis units; and limits on the use of technicians in freestanding dialysis units. Taken together, these requirements impose an economic cost on facilities and limit incentives to expand. The data regarding utilization suggest that access problems can arise as federal reimbursement policies intersect with the cost of state regulations.

What are the consequences of capacity limits in Connecticut? First, dialysis units are unable to accept transients or new patients because of their "full-capacity" status. This is illustrated by Table 7-8, which contains entries from a log of transfers, transients, and requests, prepared by a nurse at one dialysis facility. Second, the percentage of patients treated in Medicare-certified facilities who are not eligible for Medicare coverage, is shown in Table 7-9. Compared to the national average, Connecticut's acceptance of noneligible patients over time has consistently been one-third to one-half the national acceptance rate. This implies either that the state has fewer reported noneligibles presenting for treatment or that the absence of Medi-

TABLE 7-9 Percentage of Non-Medicare Total Dialysis Patients by State and Year, 1980-89

	1980	1981	1982	1983	1984	1985	1986	1987	1988	1989
United States	7.1	6.4	6.1	6.1	6.4	6.7	6.7	7.2	7.3	7.5
Connecticut	4.3	3.4	2.7	4.1	3.9	3.9	3.7	6.2	4.6	4.9
Difference	2.8	3.0	3.4	2.0	2.5	2.8	3.0	1.0	2.7	2.6
Connecticut/U.S.	61.0	53.0	44.0	67.0	61.0	58.0	55.0	86.0	63.0	65.0

SOURCE: HCFA, 1980-89.

care coverage discourages their acceptance under circumstances of full capacity. Third, since Connecticut is technically at capacity for in-center hemodialysis, anecdotal reports indicate that continuous ambulatory peritoneal dialysis is the only modality being offered by certain providers. Thus, for other than clinical reasons, capacity limits apparently restrict patient choice to modalities prescribed.

Implications of Regulations for Access and Quality

The data show that capacity growth is constrained and utilization increased in CON states relative to non-CON states. Who benefits from state CON regulation of dialysis units? What are the effects of higher utilization (or productivity) of dialysis units? Existing data permit only a limited response. First, CON results in no direct economic benefit to the federal government: higher utilization does not reduce Medicare expenditures nor does lower utilization increase them. Second, CON confers local monopoly benefits on approved providers, reducing competition among providers and raising barriers to entry. Moreover, the costs of legally defending local monopoly are more easily absorbed by provider chains than by single-owner units. Third, by sanctioning local provider monopoly, CON decreases patient choice of providers and eliminates competition among facilities for patients on the basis of amenities. Held and Pauly (1983) have shown that competition in ESRD program increases the amenities that dialysis patients receive. Fourth, CON regulation provides no assurance of quality and actually shields facilities from the need to compete on the basis of quality. Finally, in some states, CON has contributed to serious access problems.

The committee finds no persuasive reason for the application of state certificate-of-need regulations on dialysis treatment capacity

that is regulated mainly by the Medicare payment level. The committee strongly favors the elimination of CON as applied to dialysis facilities, but recognizes that this requires state government rather than federal government action. It recommends that HCFA review with each of the relevant states the effect of CON regulations on ESRD patient access to care in light of national data on utilization.

NOTES

1. Public Law 95-292 (June 13, 1978) amended Section 226A of the Social Security Act in the following ways: It removed reference to age 65 as a criterion of eligibility for ESRD coverage; it extended eligibility to those who would be eligible if employment, as defined by the Railroad Retirement Act of 1974, were included as employment under the Social Security Act; it substituted "is medically determined to have end stage renal disease" for "chronic renal disease and . . . requires hemodialysis or renal transplantation"; and it added a provision that an individual meeting the foregoing requirements have filed an application for benefits. The Tax Equity and Fiscal Responsibility Act of 1982 (Public Law No. 97-248), Sections 121 and 278, extended Medicare coverage, including coverage for ESRD, to federal government employees.

2. Legislation proposed in December 1971 (H.R. 12043, 92d Cong., 1st Sess.) by Representative Wilbur Mills (D-Ark.), then chairman of the House Committee on Ways and Means, called for a renal entitlement that included all citizens and resident aliens. This language was not used in Section 299(I) of the Social Security Amendments of 1972.

3. The relationship between United States citizenship and resident alien status and eligibility for Medicare and Medicaid benefits is complicated. An individual may be eligible for Medicare Part A (Hospital Insurance) benefits if he or she has established eligibility for Social Security benefits under Title II of the Social Security Act [Section 1818(a)(3) of the Social Security Act, 42 USC § 1395i-2(a)(3)]. Eligibility for Medicare Part A benefits, for those not eligible under Title II of the Social Security Act, and eligibility for Medicare Part B benefits [Section 1836(2)(B) of the Social Security Act] requires that an individual be a resident of the United States and either a citizen or an alien lawfully admitted for permanent residence who has resided in the U.S. continuously during the five years immediately before applying for benefits. Ordinarily, to qualify for state Medicaid benefits under federal law, an individual must be a citizen or national of the United States or in a satisfactory immigration status [Section 1137(d) of the Social Security Act, 42 USC § 1320b-7(d)], except for emergency care [Section 1903(v) of the Social Security Act, 42 USC § 13966b(v)].

4. The medical component of state general assistance programs provided no support for ESRD patients.

5. The Medicare-Medicaid tape-to-tape project, which has been administered variously by HCFA's Office of Research, the Office of the Actuary, and the Bureau of Data Management and Strategy (BDMS), was discussed with the HCFA Office of Research project officer as a data source. Under the Office of Research, this project included Medicaid records for 3, 4, or 5 state programs, depending on the year; under the Actuary and BDMS, it included more states. However, merging these data with Medicare data to link the records of dual-eligible and noneligible ESRD patients was judged to be a large and difficult research effort that was beyond the scope of this study.

6. In late 1990, the Maryland state kidney program became a target for elimination in that state's budget retrenchment.

7. Satellite dialysis units are typically located in small DVA hospitals that do not have a full nephrology service.
8. In December 1990, the New York State Health Department released a report of an advisory committee on ESRD in New York State. That committee recommended that "all U.S. citizens and resident aliens with ESRD should be eligible for Medicare benefits, not just those who meet the [Social Security] work history requirements" (New York State Department of Health, 1990, p. 11).
9. The percentage of patients over age 65 who currently have transplants includes those who received transplants before age 65, and thus is larger than the percentage who were over 65 when they received transplants.
10. Since the mid-1980s, several states either have eliminated their CON programs entirely or have exempted certain services from them. The analysis in the text reflects the changes that have taken place through mid-1990.
11. The IOM study used the number of stations to measure capacity and the number of hemodialysis treatments (rather than the number of patients) to measure demand.
12. Massachusetts, in late 1989 or early 1990, eliminated its Determination of Need program.
13. See State of Connecticut, Regulation of the Department of Health Services, § 19-13-D55a, for the licensure of an outpatient dialysis unit and standards for in-hospital dialysis units.

REFERENCES

Alexander SR, Arbus GS, Butt K, et al. 1990. 1989 Report of the North American Pediatric Renal Transplant Cooperative Study. Pediatr Nephrol 4:542-553.

Blendon RJ, Aiken LH, Freeman HE, Corey CR. 1989. Access to medical care for black and white Americans: A matter of continuing concern. JAMA 261:278-281.

Eggers, PW. 1989. Projections of the ESRD population to the year 2000. Proceedings of the Annual Public Health Conference on Records and Statistics. DHHS (PHS) 90-1214, Public Health Service, Washington, D.C., 121-126.

Evans RW, Manninen DL, Dugan MK, et al. 1990. The Kidney Transplant Health Insurance Study. Seattle, Wash.: Battelle Memorial Institute.

Feldman HI. 1990. End-stage renal disease in U.S. minority groups. Paper prepared for the Institute of Medicine ESRD Study Committee. Philadelphia, Pa.

GAO (General Accounting Office). 1990. Health Insurance: Cost Increases Lead to Coverage Limitations and Cost Shifting. GAO/HRD-90-68. Washington, D.C.

Hawthorne VM, Julius M, Kneisley J, Port FK, Dennisot L, Wolfe RA. 1991. Access to medical care in ESRD. Michigan Academician 23:87-97.

HCFA (Health Care Financing Administration). 1980-89. Annual ESRD Facility Surveys. Baltimore, Md.

HCFA. 1984. Report to Congress: Study of Unentitled End-Stage Renal Disease Patients. Baltimore, Md.

Held JH, Pauly MV. 1983. Competition and efficiency in the end stage renal disease program. J Health Econ 2:95-118.

IHPP (Intergovernmental Health Policy Project). 1989a. The Medicaid experience with end-stage renal disease: Findings of a national survey. Report prepared for the Institute of Medicine ESRD Study Committee. George Washington University, Washington, D.C.

IHPP. 1989b. Certificate of Need (CON) Regulation of ESRD Services: Findings of a 50-State Survey. Report prepared for the Institute of Medicine ESRD Study Committee. George Washington University, Washington, D.C.

IOM (Institute of Medicine). 1990. ESRD Staff Analysis of HCFA PIMMIS data. Washington, D.C.

Laudicina S. 1990. Medicaid coverage and payment of ESRD services. Report prepared for the Institute of Medicine ESRD Study Committee. Washington, D.C.

NCHS (National Center for Health Statistics). 1987. Health. DHHS Publ. No. (PHS)88-1232. Public Health Service, U.S. Department of Health and Human Services. Washington, D.C.

Newmann JM, Held PJ, Hutchinson T. 1989. Access to Renal Transplantation: Patients' Knowledge and Perceptions. Washington, D.C.: The Urban Institute. Washington, D.C.

New York State Department of Health. 1990. End-Stage Renal Disease in New York State: A Report of an Advisory Committee. Albany, N.Y.

OIG (Office of Inspector General, U.S. Department of Health and Human Services). 1987. Amending the Medicare Secondary Payer Provision for ESRD Beneficiaries Could Save the Medicare Program $3 Billion over the Next 5 Years. Draft report. Washington, D.C.

Pollack VE, Pesce A. 1990. Analysis of Data Related to the 1976-1989 Patient Population: Treatment Characteristics and Patient Outcomes. Report prepared for the Institute of Medicine ESRD Study Committee. Cincinnati: Dialysis Clinic, Inc.-Cincinnati.

Rettig RA, Marks EL. 1980. Implementing the End-Stage Renal Disease Program of Medicare. Rept. R-2505-HCFA/HEW, The RAND Corporation, Santa Monica, Calif.

Rizzoni G. 1989. Combined report on regular dialysis and transplantation in Europe, XIX, 1988: Renal replacement therapy in children. Presented at the XXVth Congress of the EDTA-ERA, Goteborg, Sweden, June 11-15.

Rostand SG, Brown G, Kirk KA, Rutsky FA, Dustian HP. 1989. Renal insufficiency in treated essential hypertension. N Engl J Med 320:684-688.

Shulman NB, Martinez B, Brogran D, Carr AA, Miles CG. 1986. Financial cost as an obstacle to hypertension therapy. Am J Public Health 76:1105-1108.

UNOS (United Network for Organ Sharing). 1990. Annual Report on the U.S. Scientific Registry for Organ Transplantation and the Organ Procurement and Transplantation Network, 1988 and 1989. Washington, D.C.: U.S. Department of Health and Human Services.

Whittle J, Whelton PK, Seidler AJ, Klag MJ, et al. 1991. Does racial variation in risk factors explain black-white differences in the incidence of hypertensive end-stage renal disease? Arch Intern Med (in press).

APPENDIX

Estimated Additional Program Expenditures Required for Universal Entitlement of Medicare ESRD Program, 1990-95

Year	Projected No. of Total Patients[a]	Non-eligible Patients (7.5%)	Annual Program Expenditures per Enrollee[b]	Annual Average EPO Expenditure per Treated Patient[c]	Midline Estimate of Additional Program Expenditures[d] (million of dollars)	Estimated Range of Additional Program Expenditures[e] (million of dollars)
1990	159,800	12,000	26,370	5,500	370	240-480
1991	170,100	12,800	27,161	5,665	400	270-530
1992	181,000	13,600	27,976	5,835	440	290-590
1993	192,100	14,400	28,815	6,010	480	320-640
1994	203,400	15,300	29,680	6,190	530	350-700
1995	214,600	16,100	30,570	6,376	570	380-760

NOTE: All current provisions, such as 12 months of Medicare as a second payer and a 3-year limit on eligibility of transplant patients, are assumed to remain unchanged.

[a]Based on midline projections of Eggers (1989).

[b]Estimate is based on 1987 figure with a projected 3% annual growth. Expenditures on EPO are not included.

[c]Estimate is based on 1989 HCFA interim reimbursement rate with a projected 3% annual growth. Market penetration of EPO is assumed to be 75% throughout the projection years.

[d]An estimated 45 to 50% of this estimate will actually be a transfer of funds from other federal programs, such as VA program and federal grants to state Medicaid programs.

[e]Based on a low estimate of 5% and a high estimate of 10% noneligible ESRD patients.

8

Access to Kidney Transplantation

This chapter presents an overview of kidney transplantation in the ESRD program and examines the restrictions of the Medicare entitlement for successful transplant recipients, the distribution of kidneys, and the limited supply of organs. Transplant reimbursement issues are addressed in Chapter 9.

There are a number of issues regarding kidney transplantation that the committee did not address. These include, among others, the performance of organ procurement organizations, the effects of required request on organ donation, and the scoring system for the distribution of organs. The committee focused its attention on a few issues (discussed in Chapters 7, 8, and 9) for two reasons: A large number of other organizations have many of the questions of kidney and other whole-organ transplantation under continuing study; and the rate-limiting factor in making transplantation more available to ESRD patients, as the committee believes it should be, is the shortage of suitable kidneys.

OVERVIEW

Kidney transplantation occupies a unique place in the treatment of ESRD. It is the preferred treatment for a majority of ESRD patients, there are fewer contraindications to transplantation today than ever before, and patient and graft outcomes have improved markedly in the past decade (Eggers, 1988; USRDS, 1990). The availability of donated kidneys, however, has consistently fallen short of both the estimated need and the actual demand for transplantation. Consequently, concerns over equitable distribution of donor kidneys among potential recipients have also been raised in recent years.

Kidney transplantation is the preferred treatment because, when successful, it restores a renal failure patient more nearly to a normal and satisfactory quality of life than does dialysis. It relieves the individual of continued dependence on a machine or on repeated fluid exchanges. Transplant recipients, however, face a continuing threat that the transplanted kidney will be rejected and, therefore, must take immunosuppressive drugs to prevent rejection for the duration of their functioning transplant.

From Medicare's perspective, a successful transplant is cost-effective compared to dialysis. HCFA data show that the annualized Medicare expenditure for a dialysis patient was $32,000. Patients with functioning kidney grafts require a higher first-year per-capita expenditure of $56,000, but they cost Medicare only $6,400 on average in succeeding years. Given certain assumptions about patient and graft survival rates, it has been estimated that the cumulative dialysis and transplantation costs reach a break-even point in about 3 years. From then on transplantation provides a net financial gain to Medicare (P.W. Eggers, HCFA, personal communication, 1990).

Clinically, the reasons for not transplanting an ESRD patient have diminished in the past decade. ESRD patients with diabetes are no longer viewed as poor risks. Today, a diabetic transplant patient does better than a diabetic dialysis patient, but not as well as a nondiabetic transplant patient. Age limits on kidney transplantation have also diminished in clinical importance, although dispute exists about the ethics of using a scarce donated kidney to extend the life of an older ESRD patient when dialysis treatment is available. As an empirical matter, only 193 ESRD patients 65 years of age or older received transplants in 1988 and 178 in 1989 (UNOS, 1990b). This is 2 percent of all kidney transplants, a proportion that is small and likely to remain so.

The number of kidney transplant procedures performed annually has increased from about 3,200 in 1974 to 8,889 in 1989[1] (HCFA, 1990). These data, broken down by living-donor and cadaver-donor transplants, are shown in Table 8-1. The number of living-donor transplants has been stable, just under 2,000 procedures annually, over an extended period. Cadaver-donor transplants, which grew rapidly before 1986, have leveled off at approximately 7,000.

The number of all kidney transplants grew an average of 5.5 percent per year from 1974 through 1978, then at more than 10 percent annually from 1978 to 1986. Since 1986, however, no growth has occurred, and the numbers have actually decreased slightly. The total numbers of procedures for each year of the 1986-89 period, according to HCFA data, have been 8,976, 8,892, 8,932, and 8,882, respectively. During this time, the outcomes of kidney transplantation, measured by both patient and graft (or transplanted kidney) survival, have improved for living-donor and cadaver-donor transplant recipients (USRDS, 1990). One-year patient survival[2] for living-related-donor (LRD) recipients increased from 78 percent in 1980 to 94 percent in 1988; for recipients of cadaver kidneys, the corresponding in-

TABLE 8-1 Number and Type of Kidney Transplant Procedures (Medicare and Non-Medicare), by Donor Type, 1980-89

Donor	1981	1982	1983	1984	1985	1986	1987	1988	1989
Living	1,460	1,677	1,784	1,704	1,876	1,887	1,907	1,760	1,900
Related	—	—	—	—	—	—	—	1,704	1,830
Unrelated	—	—	—	—	—	—	—	56	70
Cadaver	3,445	3,681	4,328	5,264	5,819	7,089	7,060	7,116	6,982
TOTAL	4,905	5,358	6,112	6,968	7,695	8,976	8,967	8,932	8,882

SOURCES: HCFA, 1990; P.W. Eggers, HCFA, personal communication, 1990.

TABLE 8-2   One-Year Survival of Kidney Transplant Patients 1980, 1984, and 1988

Donor	1980	1984	1988
Cadaver	78.4	87.4	91.0
Living related	78.2	91.8	94.7

NOTE: Adjusted for age, race, gender, and primary diagnosis.

SOURCE: USRDS, 1990.

crease was from 78 percent to 91 percent (Table 8-2). One-year graft survival for living-donor transplants increased from 83 percent in 1980 to 88 percent in 1988; for cadaver transplants, the improvement was from 60 percent to 77 percent (USRDS, 1990). Much of the improved graft survival is attributed to the effectiveness of cyclosporine in preventing the rejection of transplanted kidneys.

How many ESRD patients can potentially benefit from a kidney transplant? Stuart (1984) expressed the view that half the new ESRD patients in 1981 were good transplant candidates, and that improved immunosuppression might increase that figure to 75 percent. Of the over 44,000 new ESRD patients in 1988, nearly 14,000 were 65 years old or over and may be arbitrarily excluded for estimation purposes. If Stuart's assumptions are correct, perhaps 11,000 to 16,000 patients of the remaining 22,300 new ESRD patients might be suitable transplant candidates, well above the current actual number of procedures being performed.

If the estimated need exceeds the available supply, so does the actual demand for kidneys expressed by the length of patient waiting lists. The number of individuals on waiting lists doubled and then trebled in the 1980s from slightly over 5,000 in 1980 to 12,000 in 1987, nearly 14,000 in 1988, and over 16,000 by the end of 1989 (UNOS, 1990b). The 1989 end-of-year waiting list exceeded the total number of 1989 transplant procedures by almost twofold. The relationship between the growing number of wait-listed individuals and the number of transplant procedures is shown in Figure 8-1.

THE MEDICARE KIDNEY TRANSPLANT BENEFIT

Kidney transplantation is governed by two distinct bodies of statutory law. It is covered by Medicare as a treatment for ESRD pursuant to the ESRD provision of the Social Security Amendments of 1972. Medicare reimburses for organ procurement, the transplant procedure, physician fees, and one year of immunosuppressive drugs under this authority, for which HCFA is administratively responsible. In addition, the National Organ Transplant

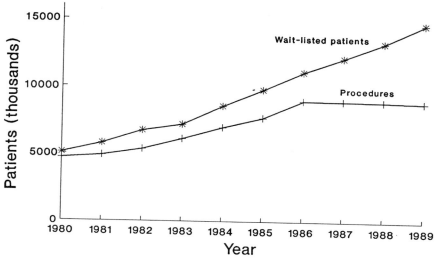

FIGURE 8-1 Kidney Transplantation Procedures and ESRD Patients on Waiting Lists, 1980-88
SOURCE: HCFA, 1980-88.

Act of 1984 (Pub. L. No. 95-292) amended the Public Health Service Act to address the acquisition and distribution of whole organs, including kidneys, through the Organ Procurement and Transplantation Network (OPTN).

The kidney transplant benefit under Medicare has two limitations that may affect access to treatment and patient outcomes. First, the 1972 statute limited the eligibility of patients with successful transplant to 12 months after the procedure, unlike the lifetime entitlement of dialysis patients. This period was extended to 36 months in 1978.

One apparent consequence of the 3-year limit on Medicare eligibility is that nearly 50 percent of the successful kidney transplant recipients who reach the 3-year posttransplant mark have established eligibility for Social Security disability benefits (P.W. Eggers, HCFA, personal communication, 1990). Although more suited to return to work than dialysis patients, they establish and maintain disability status primarily to protect their entitlement to Medicare benefits. The certainty of modest but nontaxable disability benefits reportedly acts as a disincentive to return to uncertain employment, as does employer discrimination.

The second limit on the kidney transplant benefit is that immunosuppressive drugs, which the patient must take to prevent rejection of the transplanted kidney as long as it functions, are currently reimbursed on an outpatient basis for only one year after a successful transplant. These drugs are expensive

(Showstack et al., 1990). They were not reimbursed at all until the transplant provisions of OBRA 1986 (Pub. L. No. 99-509) authorized payment for one year, mainly in response to the high cost of cyclosporine. Had the Catastrophic Health Insurance Act of 1988 been implemented, this restriction would have been removed.

In 1990, the American Society of Transplant Surgeons (ASTS, 1990), in response to a request from the Subcommittee on Health and the Environment of the House Committee on Energy and Commerce, surveyed its members to determine the effect of Medicare's limited coverage of immunosuppressive drugs on patient compliance with prescribed drug regimens and on patient outcomes. There were 107 respondents from 84 transplant centers in 36 states and the District of Columbia. Of these 37 states, 2 had programs for full coverage of immunosuppressives, 14 had partial coverage (for all patients), 3 had Medicaid coverage only (for indigent patients), and 15 had no program. Overall, respondents estimated that nearly 47 percent of patients at these 84 centers had experienced difficulty meeting the financial burdens of medication costs. The cost of drugs was regarded as a major cause of noncompliance by nearly 85 percent of the individual respondents; over 80 percent believed that extending Medicare coverage of immunosuppressives beyond the current one year would have major or significant beneficial effect. The ASTS respondents estimated that 143 kidneys had failed because of economic-related noncompliance, although the methods of estimation were not indicated. The findings of this survey, if validated, argue for the removal of this economic barrier to effective medical care.

It is not known to what extent the lack of private health insurance to pay for immunosuppressive medication after the first year deters prospective transplant recipients. Some respondents to the ASTS survey, however, indicated that the prospective financial burden of immunosuppressive drugs had led some ESRD patients to refuse a transplant. The committee also heard anecdotal reports from surgeons who stated that they could not ethically advise a patient to undergo transplantation if he or she could not pay for the medications needed to ensure its success. However, no systematic studies of this issue have been made.

It is necessary to recognize that ESRD is only controlled—not cured—by kidney transplantation. Some transplant recipients later experience failure of the transplanted kidney from a recurrence of the initial disease. All transplant patients remain at risk of rejecting the transplanted kidney throughout their lives, and the drugs they must take to prevent rejection place them at risk of various other medical problems.

Thus transplant patients face a set of predictable and very real needs for medical insurance (Evans et al., 1990). If they lose their Medicare coverage, their transplant status may be regarded as a preexisting condition by prospective insurers and prevent them from obtaining private health insurance except at very high individual rates. Transplant status may also act as a barrier to work by employers apprehensive about the dependability of the individual or their effect on the firm's health insurance premium. The limits of Medicare coverage for necessary medications may impinge on the success of the transplant or act as a disincentive to transplantation itself.

Congress, in Pub. L. No. 95-292 of 1978, the National Organ Transplant Act of 1984, certain provisions of OBRA 1986, the Health Omnibus Programs Extension of 1988, and the Transplant Amendments Act of 1990, has consistently encouraged organ transplantation for more than a decade. The committee endorses these efforts and believes that the Medicare payment system should foster transplantation rather than discourage it.

The committee recommends that Congress eliminate the three-year limit on Medicare eligibility for ESRD patients who are successful transplant recipients and authorize an entitlement equal to that of ESRD patients who are treated by dialysis.

The committee also recommends that coverage of immunosuppressive medications for kidney transplant patients be made coterminous with the period of a patient's entitlement.

The implementation of these recommendations may increase program expenditures in the short run. An estimate of that effect is found as an appendix at the end of this chapter. However, kidney transplantation is more cost-effective than dialysis as a treatment for ESRD. In the long run, the Medicare program should incur lower costs from encouraging kidney transplantation.

DISTRIBUTION OF KIDNEY TRANSPLANTS

The scarcity of organs limits the number of transplant procedures performed, however, and creates two additional access problems: how to equitably allocate a scarce supply of kidneys, and how to increase the supply of donated organs.

The legal and institutional framework for the distribution and supply of kidneys goes beyond that of the ESRD program. In the early 1980s, Congress responded to a number of highly visible cases of individuals, including very young children, who needed either a heart or a liver transplant for continued survival. It enacted the National Organ Transplant Act of 1984, which authorized the creation of the National Task Force on Organ Transplantation; grant assistance to organ procurement organizations (OPOs); establishment on a contract basis of the OPTN; and a scientific registry for organ transplantation; and it outlawed the sale of organs. Congress thus expanded the scope of federal government concern with transplantation beyond kidneys to other whole organs (especially heart and liver) and to bone marrow transplantation.

The task force recommended coverage of immunosuppressive drugs (Task Force, 1985), the implementation of the OPTN, the establishment of a national system for sharing organs, the consolidation of OPOs, a requirement that hospitals ask all prospective candidates about organ donation as a condition of participation in Medicare, and the creation of a scientific registry (Task Force, 1986). The Health Resources and Services Administration (HRSA) of the Public Health Service (PHS) currently administers the contracts for the OPTN and the scientific registry.

Before the creation of the OPTN, the distribution of donated kidneys was determined by local transplant centers and OPOs on a voluntary basis, and by sharing arrangements among centers. Regional sharing organizations developed, the largest being the Southeast Organ Procurement Foundation (SEOPF). SEOPF originally organized UNOS as a way to permit national participation in its organ-sharing activities by transplant centers across the country.

After Congress authorized the creation of the OPTN in 1984, UNOS was reconstituted separately from SEOPF. It successfully bid on the OPTN contract proposal and has operated the network since 1986. It also successfully bid on the scientific registry. The OPTN, whose rules must be proposed according to "notice and comment" procedures and be approved by the Secretary of Health and Human Services (54 Fed. Reg. 51802, December 18, 1989), establishes the policies and procedures for organ sharing and is responsible for devising and operating a system for the equitable distribution of organs.

Ideally, allocation policies ought to reflect the public consensus that donated organs are a national and a community resource that should be given to those most in need and allocated by criteria that are equitable, easily understood, and developed with broad input from all affected constituencies. Current OPTN policies on the sharing of donated organs are determined according to criteria that are first local, then regional, and finally national. This means that the determination of where a donated kidney is to be used is made by the local OPO in conjunction with the transplant centers in its area.

Mandatory national sharing of organs is required, however, under a UNOS/OPTN rule when a six-antigen match or a phenotypic identical match exists between the donor organ and the prospective recipient. The outcomes of sharing based on such matches are so favorable in such cases, but the frequency so low, that mandatory sharing is needed to ensure access to a donated kidney.

Who receives kidney transplants? Data for 1989 (UNOS, 1990b) show the following distribution by age, gender, and race of transplant recipients.

TABLE 8-3 Distribution of Kidney Transplants (percent) by Age and Type of Transplant, 1989

Age Group (years)	Living Related	Cadaver	Total
Pediatric (0-18)	16	5	7
19-45	65	58	59
46-64	19	35	31
Elderly (over 65)	0.3	2.5	2
TOTAL	100	100	100

SOURCE: UNOS, 1990b.

Pediatric patients (0-18 years) accounted for 16 percent of LRD transplants and 5 percent of cadaver transplants, or 7 percent of the total; the 19-45 age group received 65 percent of LRD transplants and 58 percent of cadaver transplants, for 59 percent of the total; the 46-64 age group received 19 percent of LRD transplants and 35 percent of cadaver transplants, for 31 percent of the total; and those 65 years of age and over accounted for 0.3 percent of LRD transplants and 2.5 percent of cadaver transplants, or 2 percent of the total (Table 8-3). Men comprised 60 percent of transplant recipients in both LRD and cadaver-donor categories. Blacks received 12 percent of the LRD transplants and 22 percent of cadaver transplants, for 20 percent of the total.

Equitable distribution of kidney transplants has emerged as an important issue, especially with publication of a report from the DHHS Office of Inspector General (OIG, 1990) that examined organ distribution practices in the United States. This analysis, based largely on UNOS data on 17,556 individuals in the United States who were awaiting or had received a first kidney transplant between October 1, 1987, and March 31, 1989, addressed the relationship between congressional and executive branch expectations[3] and actual practices. The OIG found three significant disparities in the access of individuals to cadaver kidney transplants, related to an individual's race, transplant center, and level of sensitization (reactivity to antigens).

The analysis showed that, on average, blacks waited almost twice as long as whites for their first kidney transplant, the median waiting time being 13.9 months compared to 7.6 months. The longer waiting time for blacks is not confined to a few regions, transplant centers, or procurement organizations, but is widespread. Medical considerations involving blood type, level of sensitization, and age accounted for little of the difference. The reasons for this disparity in waiting time are not known.

Second, transplant centers vary greatly in median waiting time. The time for a first kidney transplant ranged from less than 1 month at one center to

71 months at another. Among the 202 centers reviewed by the OIG, the median waiting time for 79 centers was less than 6 months for patients with low sensitization levels; 15 centers had waiting times over 18 months, however, and the other centers fell between. These wide variations existed among centers in the same OPO service area.

Finally, highly sensitized patients (i.e., highly reactive to a wide range of antigens) had considerably less access to donated organs than did others on transplant waiting lists. Their median waiting time was 32.4 months compared with 8.6 months for all others.

The causes of these observed imbalances are only partly understood. Regarding age, the original point system adopted by UNOS in 1987 for allocating organs inadvertently had a negative effect on pediatric ESRD patients by giving points for time on a waiting list; this is now being remedied. Currently, donor kidneys from individuals 10 years old or younger must be offered to prospective pediatric transplant recipients 15 years old or younger. The procuring transplant center may use such a kidney in an adult if no pediatric candidate is available. In 1989, the UNOS Board of Directors asked for an analysis of the points required to ensure that patients under age 10 would receive transplants within 1 year and that those under age 5 would receive transplants within 6 months (UNOS, 1990a).

Gender differences in transplantation rates are not well explained but may be due in part to level of sensitization. Proportionately more women are highly sensitized than men, mainly because of pregnancy, and this could affect waiting times as well as transplantation rates.

Racial differences in kidney transplantation have caused much discussion (Callender, 1989), especially as a result of the OIG's report. Given the importance of the equitable distribution of kidneys, it is worth summarizing the several facets of this complex issue: Black individuals account for 28 percent of the incident ESRD patient population, even though they represent only 12 percent of the U.S. population; their incidence of renal failure is nearly four times that of whites. Regarding kidney transplantation, black ESRD patients represent about 30 percent of those on waiting lists but wait nearly twice as long to obtain a kidney as do whites; they receive over 22 percent of cadaver transplants and 12 percent of LRD transplants (UNOS, 1990b). They donate slightly over 8 percent of cadaver donors (UNOS, 1990b). Finally, aggregate data indicate that the graft survival rate among blacks is lower than that among whites, although a number of major centers report no difference in outcomes. For 1988, one-year cadaveric graft survival (first graft only) was 78 percent among whites and 73 percent among blacks; LRD graft survival was 89 and 87 percent, respectively (USRDS, 1990).

The equity issue arises from the differences between the proportion of blacks in the ESRD population and those receiving a transplant and the longer time blacks wait for a transplant. Regarding the latter, the explanatory hypotheses include "subconscious bias" (AMA, 1990); a UNOS/OPTN organ allocation point scoring system that, until recently, favored sharing when a higher match between donor and recipient antigens existed than when fewer mismatches were present; and economic factors such as income and private health insurance.

The point scoring system warrants further explanation. In 1987, UNOS adopted a point system to determine priorities for allocating organs. This initial system emphasized both the geographic area in which a kidney was procured and the waiting time of the potential recipient. In addition, the system also emphasized human leukocyte antigen (HLA) tissue typing and matching. The immunologic characterization of individuals in terms of HLA at the A, B, and DR loci, however, has been worked out more extensively for the white population than for the black population. Since organ sharing for transplantation depends on this HLA typing system, a partial explanation for longer waiting times, as well as for actual transplant rate differences among races, is that the original UNOS point system favored more thoroughly HLA-characterized individuals, i.e., whites.

The UNOS point scoring system was modified in 1989 to give more weight to the absence of antigen mismatches. In addition, the current contract (No. 240-90-0064) between the DHHS and UNOS, as with the OPTN, calls for a monitoring effort "to identify and explain significant variations in waiting times among racial and ethnic groups" and to promote measures to eliminate such differences. Finally, the Transplant Amendments Act of 1990 called for a study by the General Accounting Office to determine "the extent to which the procurement and allocation of organs have been equitable, efficient, and effective."

In addition to the level of sensitization, the UNOS point scoring system, and race, economic factors have also been suggested as sources of disparities in access to transplantation. However, income and health insurance as economic barriers to transplantation have not yet been adequately addressed. Among the few published studies, Held and co-workers (1988) found that patients treated in predominantly white dialysis units or in units located in high-income counties are almost twice as likely to receive a transplant as patients treated in predominantly black units or those in low-income counties. The units located in the bottom-third income areas having an average annual family income of $16,000 or less in 1983 had an average transplant rate of 6.3 percent. In comparison, the rate for the top third of units by income area (average family income of $23,500) was 9.6 percent. Most important, the association of income with transplantation appears to be independent of race.

Evans and co-workers (1990) recently reported on the insurance status of patients receiving renal transplants. In a sample of 225 transplant patients, they found that 74 percent had private insurance coverage, directly or through their spouses, and 99 percent had either public or private insurance coverage. Although little is known about the adequacy of the coverage, the benefit packages for transplant recipients are consistent with those available to the general population; patients are apparently not excluded from coverage for major services such as outpatient prescription drugs.

A few patients lost private health insurance after transplantation, mostly because of job loss or change. It was unclear what percentage of those losing employment opted for policy conversion from group to individual coverage. Evans and co-workers concluded that the insurance status outlook for the vast majority of kidney transplant recipients was favorable. Not examined, however, was whether the lack of private health insurance acted as a barrier to transplantation.

A study by Dialysis Clinic, Inc.-Cincinnati (DCI-C), a dialysis unit that has a strong commitment to transplantation, compared transplantation and dialysis patients in terms of prior private health insurance (Pollack and Pesce, 1990). Of the 124 patients in the University of Cincinnati Medical Center/DCI-C system on December 31, 1975, 79 were transplant patients and 45 were dialysis patients. Only 10 percent of the transplant patients lacked private health insurance, but over half of the dialysis patients lacked such insurance. Among the 14 new patients who received transplants preemptively (i.e., were not dialyzed before receiving transplants) during the 1976-89 period, all had private health insurance. These data suggest that transplant patients are more likely to have private health insurance than are dialysis patients.

Although no national data are available on the private health insurance status of prospective transplant candidates, it is possible that the availability of private insurance affects the willingness of a prospective patient and of a transplant center to conduct the procedure. This issue, unaddressed and thus unanswered, deserves more study.

The underlying problem of equitable distribution of kidney transplants is to define equity in a way that resolves the conflict between the expected outcome of the transplant procedure and the desired social objective of nondiscrimination. Two issues require continuing attention: that social bias not exclude some individuals; and that rejection as a transplant candidate for legitimate medical factors—such as hypersensitized patients who are likely to reject the transplanted kidneys, AIDS patients, intravenous drug users—not be equated with social discrimination.

The committee believes that the differential distribution of organs by ethnic group, gender, and income should be analyzed by UNOS, HCFA, and HRSA on a continuing basis to determine the reasons for differences in kidney transplant rates and to devise remedies where appropriate.

SUPPLY OF DONOR ORGANS

The major factor limiting access to transplantation is the shortage of available kidneys. The annual rate of increase in kidney transplant procedures exceeded 10 percent from 1978 to 1986, but, as indicated earlier, no growth has occurred since 1986. Compared to this historical rate of increase, the "loss" of transplants over the 1987-89 period is approximately 5,900. Had the rate slowed to 5 percent annually, the "loss" would still be over 2,900 procedures. The effect of no growth has been substantial. During this time, the number of individuals on the UNOS-monitored kidney transplant waiting lists increased to 16,360 by the end of 1989 (UNOS, 1990a).

It has long been argued that the number of donated organs falls far short of the potential. Over the years, there have been numerous efforts to estimate the potential supply of organ donors. Among the more frequently cited studies are those of Bart et al. (1981a,b) from the Centers for Disease Control. During the 1975-79 period, Bart and his colleagues conducted two studies. The first was a pilot study in Georgia and the second a multisite study that involved organ procurement in Georgia, Kansas, and Missouri. Using criteria for ideal donors, the CDC estimated that the potential supply of kidney donors in the United States was 43 donors per million population (pmp); using more relaxed criteria of donor acceptability, the CDC estimated a potential of 116 donors pmp. Their most reasonable estimate placed the potential donor supply at 55 pmp.

A commonly cited figure, regarded as overly optimistic on the basis of recent studies, is that of 25,000 potential donors per year (AMA, 1981). A recent study of the brain death and organ donor potential for Pennsylvania estimated that the potential pool was between 38.7 and 55.2 donors pmp, depending on the stringency of criteria of organ suitability. The study estimated that, overall, 32 to 38 percent of all potential donors are realized as actual donors (Nathan et al., 1990). The Kentucky Organ Donation Agency estimated that the statewide potential was 173 for a figure of 48 donors pmp, of which 22 percent were collected in 1990 (Garrison et al., 1990). Each donor, of course, contributes two kidneys, less some loss to various factors. Actual acquisition may be one-third to one-half the potential pool, depending on the estimate of the pool.

What factors may be depressing the supply of organs? There are a number of candidate answers but few conclusive data. The factors that have been suggested include the AIDS epidemic, the advance of trauma care, and improved traffic safety. Most OPOs began rejecting potential donors who were at high risk of AIDs in 1985 and 1986, just as the number of transplants plateaued. Estimates of potential donors denied because of the risk of AIDs are 2 percent by the Tennessee OPO (L. Skelly, Tennessee Donor Services, personal communication, 1990) and 5 percent by the Delaware Valley OPO (Nathan et al., 1990).

Apparently, this results primarily from hospitals using the risk of AIDS to rule out the referral of potential donors to OPOs. Arthur Caplan (University of Minnesota, personal communication, 1990) has estimated 10 to 20 percent of potential donors are eliminated in this manner as a consequence of an expansive interpretation of risk. This range is consistent with similar estimates from San Francisco, Los Angeles, and New York City OPOs. Clearly, a careful assessment of the effects of AIDS on donation is needed.

In the matter of trauma care, 12 states had trauma centers in 1987, whereas 25 states have them today. It is believed that trauma centers save many lives, although the exact numbers are unknown (J. Morris, Vanderbilt University, personal communication, 1990). It has been estimated that advances in trauma care are able to decrease preventable deaths by about 25 percent. It is not clear, however, what effect these advances have had on organ donation.

The effect of traffic safety measures on organ donation is often mentioned but seldom analyzed. The number of traffic fatalities in the United States fell from 51,093 in 1979 to 42,589 in 1983, then increased to 47,087 in 1988; they have remained steady in the 46,000 to 47,000 range since 1986 (DOT, 1990). UNOS, however, is unable to indicate the percentage of donors who are traffic fatalities. At the margin, state and federal legislation on seat-belt use, drunken driving, minimum drinking age, and motorcycle helmet use all have reduced highway fatalities among young people, and thus may have affected the size of the potential donor pool. Air-bag use might also reduce the potential donor pool in future years.

The 55-mph speed limit is believed to have saved 2,000 to 4,000 lives per year. However, it was enacted in 1974 and any negative effects would probably have been realized long ago. If anything, the more recent authorization of a 65-mph speed limit would offset this effect. In 1987, 38 states adopted the 65-mph speed limit, and 2 states adopted it in 1988 (DOT, 1989). In the states that retained the 55-mph speed limit, fatalities remained essentially stable from 1986 to 1988.

What is known about the willingness to donate? Surveys indicate that the public's awareness of transplantation is high, but its enthusiasm for donation is lower, and individuals are more willing to donate a relative's organ than their own (Manninen and Evans, 1985; Evans and Manninen, 1988) (Table 8-4). Although public education is needed to maintain this high level of awareness, such efforts may now need to focus on promoting the discussion of transplantation by families as a way to encourage donation.

TABLE 8-4 Percentage of Responses to Organ Transplantation/Donation Surveys, 1983, 1984, and 1987

Question	Year of Public Opinion Survey		
	1983	1984	1987
Awareness of transplantation	94.0	93.0	98.7
Received information on donation	69.1	N/A	84.1
Willingness to donate own organs	50.0	45.0	49.3
Willingness to donate relative's organs	53.0	85.0	62.5
Carry organ donor card	19.2	17.02	4.6
Approached about organ donation	NA	14.0	14.9
Given consent for organ donation	NA	NA	1.7

NOTE: NA = not available.

SOURCE: Evans and Manninen, 1988.

The public's willingness to donate organs may be influenced by the newspaper and television publicity that transplantation receives. There may be a negative effect of adverse publicity, such as that about anencephalic donation or cross-species transplants (Evans and Manninen, 1988). The news value of organ transplantation may also be of limited or declining interest to newspapers and television. These dramatic procedures received substantial television coverage from 1983 through 1986, as public attention focused on the plight of a small number of individuals, often children. President Reagan made personal pleas for specific individuals, and made Air Force One available in certain notable cases. Network television programs, such as Nightline, 20-20, and the MacNeil-Lehrer Report, covered the drama of transplantation extensively (Rettig, 1989). Data developed by the IOM ESRD study staff suggest that the novelty of organ transplantation may have worn off and that the story may be less newsworthy.[4]

The attitudes of professional caregivers generally favor donation (Prottas and Batten, 1988). Recent studies, however, show substantial ignorance among neurosurgeons about brain death, a critical factor affecting organ donation which highlights the need for professional education (Youngner et al., 1989).

The hypotheses about why the supply of kidneys has not increased also include the disruptive effects of the policy interventions of the mid-1980s (Rettig, 1989; UNOS, 1990b). These interventions include the implementation of the OPTN; the requirement of a single OPO for each SMA; the requirement that individual OPOs join the OPTN network in order to be reimbursed by Medicare for organ donation costs; the requirement that hospitals establish a written policy ensuring that all prospective donors or their next-of-kin are asked about their willingness to donate organs as a condition of Medicare participation; and complex rules governing the distribution of organs that have been adopted by UNOS.

The requirement that hospitals have written protocols for asking about organ donation, although well intentioned, may have altered the character of the request for organ donation. Cadaver donation involves a complex process between the attending physicians and nurses caring for the recently deceased potential donor, the organ procurement professionals, and the family of the deceased. The initial encounter with the family is critical. It is most effective when made by professionals who show respect to the family and communicate a sensitivity that acknowledges their grief. However, if the requester is uncomfortable or lacks answers to important questions, the result is often refusal. The initial effect of required request appears to be that the process of asking for a donation became a bureaucratic requirement for all hospitals that adversely affected donation. The development of new and productive relationships among all parties is now being worked out (UNOS, 1990b).

Data show that the performance of OPOs varies substantially (UNOS, 1990b). The rate of kidney procurement ranged from 4.1 to 52.1 pmp in 1988, and from 3.7 to 58.0 pmp in 1989; the averages for these years were 30.8 and 30.3 pmp, respectively. Now, substantial attention is being directed to increasing the average rate and raising rates that are below the mean. Within the IOM committee, Held expressed the view that consolidation of multiple OPOs into a single OPO per region reduced competition and depressed the incentive to obtain organs.

OBRA 1986 required that OPOs meet performance standards prescribed by the Secretary of DHHS. The Secretary established a standard that an OPO recover 23 kidneys pmp and transplant 19 patients pmp. In 1988, however, Congress required that each OPO must "reasonably expect to procure organs from not less than fifty donors per year." This 50-donor standard provoked substantial controversy, since it was the basis of Medicare recertification. Congress, in April 1990 (Pub. L. No. 101-274), delayed the requirement until January 1, 1992; then, in OBRA 1990, it repealed the rule and again delegated authority for performance standards to the Secretary.

CONCLUSIONS AND RECOMMENDATIONS

The committee wishes to underline the urgency of increasing the organ donor supply as the central issue in making kidney transplantation available to increasing numbers of ESRD patients. However, numerous changes in the system of organ donation have been made in recent years for the purpose of increasing the supply of organs, and their results have often been disappointing. Renewed efforts to increase the supply of donated organs should be balanced, therefore, by careful design, testing, and data acquisition regarding all proposed interventions, and by extensive professional and public discussion about the social, cultural, and religious values that are involved in donation.

The committee believes that increasing the supply of donated kidneys for transplantation should receive very high priority, both from the medical community and from the federal government. It recommends that the Secretary of DHHS exercise continuing leadership on this matter. The equitable allocation of a scarce supply of organs will proceed more easily if the number to be distributed is increasing.

Many suggestions have been made about how to increase the supply of organs. Public and professional education, recommended consistently over the years, should be continued, but working assumptions should be reexamined and efforts possibly refocused, and the effects on increasing the availability of organs should be monitored closely.

The process by which the families of potential donors are asked to consider donation must be improved. This might involve requiring that hospitals refer potential donors to OPOs, instead of requiring that hospitals make requests to families of potential donors. Thus, access of skilled OPO personnel to prospective donors and their families would be increased.

Living donation should be encouraged, especially from related donors but also in appropriate cases from emotionally bonded unrelated individuals.

Efforts to increase minority donation, especially among the black community, should receive strong support. Attention also should be given to the composition of OPO staff, to ensure the selection of competent personnel skilled in the organ donation process and sensitive to the values and attitudes that different ethnic groups may have toward donation.

The families of prospective donors should not be penalized for donation. In addition to paying medical expenses for living donors, consideration should be given to paying for time off work, perhaps at the daily rate for workmen's compensation or local jury duty.

The possibilities for improving donor hospital participation in the donation process should be analyzed. The medical management of prospective donors deserves attention (Darby et al., 1989), and the associated financial costs of such management should also be analyzed. It may be appropriate to consider reimbursing donor hospitals for the workup and maintenance of prospective donors and making an allowance for professional education within the hospital.

Congress, in the Transplant Amendments Act of 1990, expanded the PHS grant program to include organizations other than OPOs. HRSA should now use this opportunity to develop a research effort focused on practical ways to increase the supply of available organs.

In the context of the above efforts, it is essential that a clear estimate of the potential national donor pool be developed against which success can be measured.

The committee recommends that the Centers for Disease Control conduct a national study of the potential donor pool, with attention to the estimated effects of AIDS, improved trauma care, traffic safety legislation, and other pertinent factors.

Two highly controversial ideas are likely to receive continuing public discussion and debate. These are consideration for donation and presumed consent. Consideration, or payment for donation, has been barred by the 1984 National Organ Transplant Act. But rewarded gifting, or a modest death benefit to the family of a donor, are ideas that have been raised and deserve thoughtful discussion (Peters, 1991).

Presumed consent, now used in several European countries, vests in the government the authority to take organs unless an individual has explicitly expressed himself to the contrary. On technical grounds, it is argued, this may facilitate the acquisition of more organs. This arrangement would alter the relationship of the state to the individual in the United States in fundamental ways, however, and the values involved should be thoroughly discussed in an open, public arena before public policy is changed.

NOTES

1. These data are based on HCFA's Annual Facility Surveys. UNOS (1990b) figures for 1987, 1988, and 1989 are slightly higher but show the same general pattern.
2. One-year survival is defined here as the survival probability from the date of the transplant procedure to one year later.
3. Strictly speaking, "expectations" are not synonymous with legislative intent as determined by an analysis of statutory law, the conference committee report, the statements of the House and Senate floor managers, and the reports of the relevant congressional committees.
4. The ESRD study staff examined newspaper coverage of organ transplantation in the *New York Times, Wall Street Journal, Washington Post, Los Angeles Times, Chicago Tribune,* and *Boston Globe,* from 1983 through 1989. News coverage was extensive in all newspapers except the *Wall Street Journal.* It was very limited before late 1982, grew in 1984 and 1985, appears to have peaked in 1986 and 1987, and declined thereafter. Most articles in

the mid-1980s dealt with heart transplantation. The *New York Times*, for example, devoted much more space to heart than to liver transplantation; the three regional papers, however, gave heart and liver transplantation approximately equal coverage from 1985 to 1987.

REFERENCES

AMA (American Medical Association, Council on Scientific Affairs). 1981. Organ donor recruitment. JAMA 246:2157-2158.

AMA (American Medical Association, Council on Ethical and Judicial Affairs). 1990. Black-white disparities in health care. JAMA 263:2345-2346.

ASTS (American Society of Transplant Surgeons). 1990. Survey on Present Status of Reimbursement for Immunosuppressive Drugs.

Bart KJ, Macon EJ, Whittier FC, Baldwin RJ, Blount JH. 1981a. Cadaveric kidneys for transplantation. Transplantation 31:379-382.

Bart KJ, Macon EJ, Humphries AL, Jr, et al. 1981b. Transplantation 31:383-387.

Callender CO. 1989. The results of transplantation in blacks: Just the tip of the iceberg. Transplantation Proc 21:3407-3410.

Darby JM, Stein K, Grenvik A, Stuart SA. 1989. Approach to management of the heartbeating "brain dead" organ donor. JAMA 261:2222-2228.

DOT (U.S. Department of Transportation). 1989. The Effects of the 65 mph Speed Limit Through 1988. Washington, D.C.

DOT. 1990. National Highway Traffic Safety Administration, Fatal Accident Reporting System.

Eggers PW. 1988. Effect of transplantation on the Medicare End-Stage Renal Disease program. N Engl J Med 318:223-229.

Evans RW, Manninen DL. 1988. U.S. public opinion concerning the procurement and distribution of donor organs. Transplantation Proc 5:781-785.

Evans RW, Manninen DL, Dugan MK, et al. 1990. The Kidney Transplant Health Insurance Study: Final Report. Seattle, Wash.: Battelle Memorial Institute.

Garrison RN, Bentley FR, Raque GH, et al. 1990. There is an answer to the organ donor shortage. Paper presented at 76th Annual Clinical Congress of the American College of Surgeons, San Francisco, October.

HCFA (Health Care Financing Administration). 1990. End Stage Renal Disease Program Quarterly Statistical Summary. August 2.

Held PJ, Pauly MV, Bovbjerg RR, Newmann J, Salvatierra O. 1988. Access to kidney transplantation: Has the United States eliminated income and racial differences? Arch Intern Med 148:2594-2600.

Kjellstrand CM. 1988. Age, sex, and race inequality in renal transplantation. Arch Int Med 148:1305-1309.

Manninen DL, Evans RW. 1985. Public attitudes and behavior regarding organ donation. JAMA 253:3111-3115.

Nathan HM, Jarrell BE, Broznik B, et al. 1990. Estimation and Characterization of the Potential Organ Donor pool in Pennsylvania: Report of the Pennsylvania Statewide Donor Study. Paper presented at the annual meeting of the American Society of Transplant Surgeons, Chicago, June.

OIG (Office of Inspector General, U.S. Department of Health and Human Services). 1990. The Distribution of Organs for Transplantation: Expectations and Practices. Washington, D.C. Draft report, August.

Peters TG. 1991. Life or death: The issue of payment in cadaveric organ donation. JAMA 265:1302-1305.

Pollack VE, Pesce A. 1990. Analysis of data related to the 1976-1989 patient population:

Treatment characteristics and patient outcomes. Report prepared for the Institute of Medicine ESRD Study Committee. Cincinnati: Dialysis Clinic, Inc.-Cincinnati.

Prottas JM, Batten HL. 1988. The health professional in organ procurement: Attitudes, reservations and their resolutions. Am J Public Health 6:642-645.

Rettig RA. 1989. The politics of organ transplantation: A parable of our time. J Health Politics Policy Law 14(1):91-227.

Showstack J, Katz P, Amend W, Salvatierra O. 1990. The association of cyclosporine with the 1-year costs of cadaver-organ kidney transplants. JAMA 264:1818-1823.

Stuart FP. 1984. Need, supply, and legal issues related to organ transplantation in the United States. Transplantation Proc 1:87-94.

Task Force on Organ Transplantation. 1985. Report to the Secretary and the Congress on Immunosuppressive Therapies. Washington, D.C.: U.S. Department of Health and Human Services.

Task Force on Organ Transplantation. 1986. Organ Transplantation: Issues and Recommendations. Washington, D.C.: U.S. Department of Health and Human Services.

UNOS (United Network for Organ Sharing). 1990a. Annual Report for 1988 and 1989. Richmond, Virginia.

UNOS. 1990b. Annual Report on the Scientific Registry for Organ Transplantation and the Organ Procurement and Transplantation Network, 1988 & 1989. Washington, D.C.: U.S. Department of Health and Human Services.

USRDS (U.S. Renal Data System). 1990. Annual Data Report. National Institute of Diabetes and Digestive and Kidney Diseases, Bethesda, Md.

Youngner SJ, Landefeld S, Coulton CJ, Juknialis BW, Leary M. 1989. "Brain death" and organ retrieval: A cross-sectional survey of knowledge and concepts among health professionals. JAMA 261:2205-2210.

APPENDIX

Estimated Additional Medicare ESRD Program Expenditures Required for Removing the 3-Year Eligibility Limit of Transplant Patients and the 1-Year Limit on Payment for Immunosuppressive Drugs, 1990-1995

Year	Removal of 3-Year Limit on Eligibility		Removal of 1-Year Limit on Payment for immunosuppressive Drugs			Estimated Total Additional Expenditures[f]
	Estimate of Former Beneficiaries[a]	Estimate of Expenditures for Former Beneficiaries[b]	Estimate of Expenditure for Former Beneficiaries[c]	Estimate of Current Beneficiaries[d]	Estimate of Expenditures of Current Beneficiaries[e]	
1990	12,000-14,000	$80-95	$60-70	25,000	$125	$265-290
1991	13,000-16,000	90-110	65-80	27,000	140	295-330
1992	14,000-18,000	100-130	70-90	29,000	150	320-370
1993	15,000-20,000	110-145	80-105	31,000	160	350-410
1994	16,000-22,000	120-160	90-120	33,000	180	390-460
1995	17,000-24,000	130-180	95-130	35,000	190	415-500

[a]These estimates are of persons with a functioning kidney transplant who, under the current 3-year eligibility limit, would have ceased to be eligible for Medicare benefits before or during the reference year. These do not include persons who would have maintained their Medicare eligibility by establishing Social Security disability status.

[b]This estimate assumes an average annual expenditure per beneficiary with a functioning kidney transplant, after the first year, of $6,800 for a 1987 base year, increased by 2 percent for each subsequent year.

[c]This estimate is based on an average annual expenditure of $5,000 per patient for immunosuppressive drugs times the number of former beneficiaries (column 1).

[d]This estimate is of current beneficiaries with a functioning kidney transplant no longer eligible for payment for immunosuppressive drugs.

[e]This estimate is based on $5,000 per year for immunosuppressive drugs times the number of current beneficiaries (column 4).

[f]This estimate is the sum of columns 2, 3, and 5. It does not include any estimates of costs saved by persons not returning to dialysis, nor of persons choosing the leave disability as a result of guaranteed medical benefits.

PART IV
Reimbursement and Quality

OBRA 1987 asked the Institute of Medicine to examine quality of care in the ESRD program and to determine how quality is affected by reimbursement. In this section, the committee offers its answers to these two questions. Chapter 9 provides background information about current reimbursement policies and the way they developed over the history of the ESRD program. Chapter 10 reviews available data (including a new study commissioned by the committee) that bear on "the effect of reimbursement on quality of treatment." The conclusions drawn from this review have implications for dialysis reimbursement policy. Reimbursement issues are discussed and recommendations are offered in Chapter 11, in the light of the committee's conclusions about the effect of reimbursement on quality.

Chapter 12 reviews the data available to answer the second question in OBRA 1987, i.e., to evaluate "quality of care . . . as measured by clinical indications, functional status of patients, and patient satisfaction." Data were found to be limited, because systematic quality assessment and assurance activities have not been implemented in the ESRD program. Therefore, Chapter 12 also discusses methods for assessing and assuring quality and suggests how they can be applied in the ESRD program.

9

Medicare ESRD Payment Policy

This chapter describes Medicare payment policy for kidney transplantation and dialysis services for ESRD beneficiaries provided by treatment facilities and physicians. Covered services for kidney transplantation include organ procurement, surgical procedure, postoperative care for three years, and immunosuppressive therapy for one year after transplantation. Dialysis services include both inpatient and outpatient treatment (whether provided in a facility or a patient's home) by either hemodialysis or peritoneal dialysis. The chapter focuses mainly on Medicare outpatient dialysis reimbursement, by far the largest part of ESRD costs, and emphasizes the facility component; inpatient dialysis treatment is addressed only briefly. ESRD patients, as Medicare beneficiaries, are entitled to *all* Medicare-covered services, not just ESRD-related services.

KIDNEY TRANSPLANT SERVICES

Medicare's payment policies for kidney transplantation are summarized below, first for the hospital component (organ acquisition and the transplant procedure) and then for the physician component (organ acquisition, the procedure, and posttransplant care).

Renal Transplant Center Reimbursement

Medicare reimburses the hospital renal transplant center (RTC) separately for kidney acquisition and the surgical procedure. Kidney acquisition costs include the surgical removal of organs from donors, living as well as cadaver; the transportation, preservation, and tissue typing of recovered organs; pretransplant costs incurred by donors, potential recipients, and recipients, including listing potential recipients on a registry (waiting list) and laboratory testing for compatibility between donor kidney and potential recipient; and public and professional education.

Medicare pays an RTC 100 percent of kidney acquisition costs on a reasonable-cost basis. The center, in turn, pays the other organizations involved in the acquisition process—organ procurement organizations (OPOs), donor hospitals, and independent laboratories.[1] At the end of the RTC hospital's fiscal year, any necessary adjustments are made on the basis of a comparison of charges with actual costs.

Payment for the transplant procedure itself is made under Diagnostic-Related Group (DRG) 302, kidney transplant surgery. This includes the surgical procedure and in-hospital preoperative care but not long-term follow-up. For hospitals reimbursed under the Prospective Payment System (PPS), the average charge for DRG 302 in FY 1988 was $38,700, with an average length of stay of 18 days (Jolene Hall, Prospective Payment Assessment Commission, personal communication, 1990).

In 1983, when the Medicare PPS for hospital inpatient services was established, HCFA considered including kidney acquisition services in DRG 302. The unique characteristics of organ procurement activities and the desirability of maintaining an adequate supply of kidneys, however, led HCFA to retain reimbursement for kidney acquisition on a reasonable-cost basis separate from the DRG. In 1987, the DHHS Office of Inspector General recommended including organ acquisition costs under DRG 302 (OIG, 1987). HCFA agreed in principle but expressed concern about the potential negative effect of such action on organ supply. The OIG, in a 1988 follow-up report, acknowledged the merit of this view but called for a demonstration project of organ acquisition under a DRG as a way to generate data on this issue (OIG, 1988).

Physician and Medication Reimbursement

Physicians are reimbursed separately for organ retrieval, transplantation-procedure-related charges, and follow-up care. In the case of retrieval of a cadaver organ, an allowance for physician payment is included in the overall Medicare payment to the RTC for acquisition, and the center pays the physician. A physician who retrieves a living-donor kidney, however, is reimbursed directly for 100 percent of the reasonable charge up to a limit of $1,250. The donor bears no out-of-pocket expense.

Procedure-related services for which physicians are reimbursed include the transplant operation, all preoperative care, and 60 days of postsurgery care, including management of immunosuppression. Physician payment for the kidney transplant procedure is based on the lesser of a maximum allowance or the amount allowed on a reasonable-charge basis. The process for updating the fee for transplant services also differs slightly from that applied to other physicians' charges.[2] The physician is reimbursed separately for the removal of a recipient's own nonfunctioning kidney(s) when that is required.

Immunosuppressive drugs administered on an outpatient basis to transplant patients are reimbursed for the first year after a transplant. Subsequently, patients pay either on an out-of-pocket basis or through their supplemental insurance. (But see the committee's recommendation in Chapter 8.)

OUTPATIENT DIALYSIS SERVICES

Medicare's payment policy is described for outpatient dialysis services, for both facility and physician reimbursement.

Facility Reimbursement

Outpatient dialysis facility reimbursement is often compared to the PPS and thus it is useful to note some similarities and important differences between the two (Table 9-1). Under the PPS and ESRD program, both the DRG payments and the dialysis Composite Rates are established prospectively. The PPS is based on a patient classification system (DRGs) which establishes per-case fixed prices for services delivered to hospitalized Medicare beneficiaries for a given diagnosis (or set of related diagnoses). The ESRD Composite Rate, on the other hand, has no patient classification system but assumes that dialysis patients are homogeneous for payment purposes and pays at a fixed per treatment rate for one service, outpatient dialysis. The Composite Rate is similar to a single DRG system. Both systems were originally based on cost reports, neither has been rebased, and only the PPS provides for an annual update of payment rates. For hospitals, Medicare payments, on average, account for approximately 35 percent of inpatient revenues. For most dialysis facilities, however, Medicare is the dominant payer. Although national data are not available, various sources indicate that Medicare accounts for between 60 and 85 percent of independent dialysis facilities' revenues (Community Psychiatric Centers, 1989; REN Corporation-USA, 1989).

Payments from non-Medicare sources result, first, from Medicare beneficiary liabilities for medical deductibles and copayments and, second, from the Medicare-as-secondary-payer (MSP) requirements of OBRA 1981 and OBRA 1990 (see Chapter 7), and are made by private health insurance, state Medicaid programs, state kidney programs, and out-of-pocket payments by beneficiaries.

Historical Overview

Medicare's payment policy for outpatient dialysis services from 1973 to 1983 reimbursed independent renal facilities on a reasonable-charge basis

TABLE 9-1 Comparison of the Inpatient Hospital Prospective Payment System (PPS) and ESRD Outpatient Dialysis Payment Policy

Features	Prospective Payment System Hospital Inpatient Reimbursement	End-Stage Renal Disease Facility Outpatient Reimbursement
Design	Prospectively set national rate Per-discharge (case) basis	Prospectively set national rate Per-treatment basis
Payment components	Standardized amount DRG weights	Composite rate No patient classification system
Original cost basis	1981 Cost reports	1977, 1978, 1979 Cost reports
Rebasing	No	No
Updating	Yearly update for change in market basket, discretionary adjustment factor, case-mix change	No update process
Payment adjustments	Differential standardized amounts Area wage index Indirect teaching Medicare case mix Disproportionate share	Dual rates for hospital-based and independent units Area wage index
Exceptions criteria	Rural referral centers Sole community hospitals	Atypical service intensity Extraordinary circumstances Isolated essential facilities Self-dialysis training costs Frequency of dialysis education costs
Exemptions	Hospitals and distinct-part units providing psychiatric, pediatric, rehabilitation, and other long-term services Capital costs Organ acquisition Certified registered nurse anesthetists	None

and hospital-based facilities on a reasonable-cost basis for both in-center and home dialysis services (Table 9-2). Under the Interim Regulations, effective July 1, 1973, reimbursement for independent as well as hospital units was limited by a screen of $138 per treatment that acted essentially as a payment ceiling (38 Fed. Reg. 17210, June 19, 1973). This screen remained in effect for 11 years (from July 1, 1973, through July 31, 1983). Home dialysis was paid for separately, and facilities managing home patients were reimbursed on a reasonable-cost basis.

Because independent units were paid the lesser of the screen or reasonable charges and only four units submitted charges less than the screen, most units were paid at the same nominal $138-per-treatment rate.[3] Hospital-based outpatient units were paid the lesser of the screen or reasonable costs. An exceptions process, however, allowed providers to obtain payment amounts in excess of the screen on the basis of actual costs. Although fewer than 10 independent units were granted exceptions, many hospital units received them during this period (48 Fed. Reg. 21255, May 11, 1983). According to HCFA, the large number of exceptions granted to hospital-based units resulted in an average payment per treatment of $159 before 1982.

Congressional hearings on the ESRD program were held in 1976, 1977, and 1978, prompted by the rapid growth of ESRD program expenditures and a concurrent decline in the proportion of patients treated by home dialysis (Rettig, 1980). On June 13, 1978, Pub. L. No. 95-292, amending the Social Security Act, was enacted with the central purpose to encourage home dialysis and transplantation.

A major provision in the law, related to outpatient dialysis facility services, called for the Secretary to establish, on a "cost-related or other economical and equitable basis," a prospective reimbursement rate for providers of dialysis services. Even though regulations were issued for various provisions of the law from 1978 onward, HCFA did not issue a Notice of Proposed Rulemaking related to outpatient dialysis facility reimbursement until 1980. These proposed rules, however, were rejected by the incoming Reagan administration in 1981.

Congress, in Section 2145 of OBRA 1981 (Pub. L. No. 97-35, August 13, 1981), again directed the Secretary to establish a prospective reimbursement system for outpatient dialysis. The 1981 legislation, however, called for a single composite weighted formula for hospital-based facilities that included home and center patients, and a similar rate for independent facilities. The implementation of this dialysis-specific prospective rate was proposed by HCFA in a Notice of Proposed Rulemaking in 1982 (47 Fed. Reg. 6556, February 12, 1982). A final rule in May 1983, effective August 1, 1983 (48 Fed. Reg. 21254, May 11, 1983), established the composite rate.

Separate rates were thus established for hospital-based and independent outpatient dialysis facilities. Payments for home dialysis and for center

TABLE 9-2 Medicare Payment for Facility Outpatient Dialysis Services

	Before 1983	1983-86	1986 to Present
Type of payment			
Hospital-based	Lesser of reasonable costs or screen	Composite rate	Composite rate
Independent	Lesser of reasonable charge or screen	Composite rate	Composite rate
Payment ceiling (screen)[a]			
Hospital-based	$138	$138	$138
Independent	$138	$138	$138
Base rate			
Hospital-based	None	$127	$125
Independent	None	$123	$121
Average rate[b]			
Hospital-based	$159	$131	$129
Independent	$138	$127	$125
Home dialysis	Reasonable-cost basis	Same rate as in-center dialysis	Same rate as in-center dialysis
Training		$20 for each self-dialysis and home dialysis training session, up to three times per week; $12 for each continuous ambulatory peritoneal dialysis training session per day, up to a maximum of 15 sessions	
Erythropoietin (EPO)[c]			$40 per EPO treatment for any dose up to 9,999 units; an additional $30 for a dose of 10,000 units or more when administered to patient in renal dialysis facilities

[a]Under the Initial Method of reimbursement, $12 was included for physician activities, resulting in a screen of $150. If the Alternate Reimbursement Method was selected, the screen was $138. Under either method, $5 of the screen accounted for laboratory testing.
[b]With wage index adjustment.
[c]Effective date of June 1, 1989.

dialysis patients were each consolidated into a single base composite rate, with the average composite rate being $131 and $127 per treatment, respectively[4] (Table 9-2). A geographic wage rate adjustment was then applied to the labor portion of the base composite rate to derive a specific composite rate for each facility. These average composite rates were down from the pre-August 1983 average rate of $159 for hospital-based units and $138 for independent units. After issuing the 1983 rule, HCFA also established more specific exceptions criteria and a more rigorous exceptions process with the intent of granting fewer exceptions than under earlier procedures.

In 1986, HCFA proposed to reduce the base composite rate on average by $6 per treatment (51 Fed. Reg. 17537, May 13, 1986). Simultaneously, it proposed to change the methodology for calculating the base rate from weighting the facility median cost per treatment by the number of facilities in each stratum (a statistical grouping of facilities that HCFA based on the number of dialysis stations in each facility) to weighting by the number of treatments in each stratum. HCFA stated that this change in methodology was supported by data that showed that 80 percent of all treatments were furnished by less than 50 percent of all renal facilities. HCFA had used this methodology when it audited a sample of facility cost reports in 1983, and the analysis showed that the Medicare costs of all renal facilities had decreased, partly because of the change in payment methodology. According to HCFA, audited data for 1986 continued to show that the Medicare costs of a dialysis treatment had not increased.

Congress, responding to this HCFA proposal in OBRA 1986, limited the reduction to $2 per treatment and froze the new rate for two fiscal years through September 30, 1988. The base composite rates were then reduced by HCFA from $127 to $125 for hospital-based facilities and from $123 to $121 for independent units, effective October 1, 1986 (Table 9-1). The basis for calculating the cost per treatment, however, reverted to the initial methodology used in 1983, i.e., weighting the facility median cost by the number of facilities in each stratum. OBRA 1986 also authorized financing of the ESRD networks by a $0.50 per treatment reduction of the facility payment.

The profile of the reimbursement rate for outpatient dialysis from 1974 through 1989 is shown in Figure 9-1 for independent units only. The rate for hospital-based outpatient units would have been higher for the period from the beginning of the program in 1973 until the introduction of the composite rate in 1983; thereafter, the rates would have been similar. The figure indicates the nominal rates and the effect of adjusting for inflation by the GNP price deflator. *On an adjusted basis, the 1989 average composite rate for independent units was less than $54 in 1974 dollars, a 61 percent reduction over this period.*

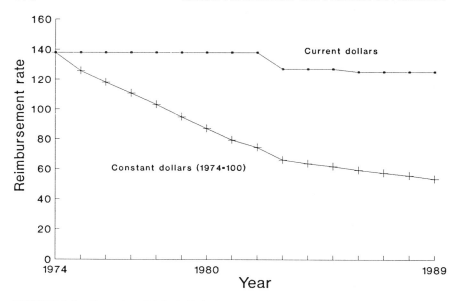

FIGURE 9-1   Outpatient Dialysis Reimbursement Rates for Independent Units, 1973-89 (current and constant dollars)
NOTES: GNP deflator used to calculate constant dollars. The same nominal rate applied to all independent units for 1973-83; after 1984, the rate is the average for all independent units.
SOURCE: HCFA

Current Policy

Current payment policy, then, includes the following elements. First, the cost base for the current composite rates remains the audited 1977-79 Medicare cost reports for a sample of 105 hospital-based and independent facilities.

Second, as has been true for the entire history of the ESRD program, no process exists to update the rates annually for inflation or other factors that influence costs. Changes in payment rates are proposed only when HCFA determines that cost report data justify rate revision. There is no adjustment for inflation. The only adjustment made to the base composite rate is the area wage index, applied annually to account for geographic differences in wages and salaries.

Third, the current rates are based on the facility median cost per treatment weighted by the number of *facilities* in each stratum, rather than weighted by the number of *treatments* in each stratum (as proposed in 1986).

Fourth, until OBRA 1990 was enacted, the existing base composite rates, for both hospital-based and independent facilities, and including both center and home patients, were those established in 1983, as reduced by $2 in

1986. In OBRA 1989, a sequester provision further reduced the composite rates by 2 percent from October 1, 1989, until March 30, 1990, and by 1.5 percent from April 1 to September 30, 1990. OBRA 1990 continued the sequester reduction through December 31, 1990; effective January 1, 1991, the application of the sequester was removed, and the composite rates were increased by $1 per treatment.

Fifth, the dual rate structure, required by statute, is reflected in base composite rates of $125 for hospital-based units and $121 for independent facilities (Table 9-2). The specific difference in rates, however, derives from a policy decision, not from a detailed analysis of the relative costs of treatment by type of facility.

Sixth, facility-specific composite rates are determined by applying the area wage index to the labor portion of the base composite rate, an adjustment performed annually.[5] Facility-specific rates are limited to a maximum of $138 per treatment, unless an exception has been obtained, and a minimum wage index of 0.9 times the labor portion of the base rate or $116 for independent units and $120 for hospital-based renal facilities. The upper limit was to prevent any excessive payment levels due to possible deficiencies in the area wage index. The lower limit on the wage index was to alleviate any adverse effect on rural facilities.

Seventh, facilities receive an additional $20 per treatment above the composite rate for self-care and home hemodialysis training. Training is limited to three sessions per week for as many sessions as needed. Facilities receive an additional $12 per treatment for each CAPD training session; these sessions are limited to one per day up to a maximum of 15 sessions. These policies are currently under review by HCFA.

An exceptions policy exists by which a facility may request a higher payment on the basis that its allowed costs exceed the composite rate.[6] One or more of the following criteria are used by HCFA to determine whether a facility's costs per treatment justify an exception: atypical service intensity (service mix), extraordinary circumstances, isolated essential facilities, self-dialysis training costs, and frequency of dialysis.[7] These criteria actually constitute a set of crude case-mix adjusters. If a facility is granted an exception based on one or more of the criteria, the composite rate for that facility is then increased. In some cases, the increased rate only applies to certain dialysis patients, such as pediatric patients or those requiring self-dialysis training. In other cases, such as isolated essential facilities, atypical service intensity, and extraordinary circumstances, the increased rate applies to all dialysis treatments performed at that facility. According to HCFA, the approval rate for exceptions is 75 percent.

No specified methodology or formula is used to calculate an exceptions adjustment to the rate. The amounts of exception increases appear somewhat arbitrary and do not derive from the criteria on which the exception was granted. For example, facilities that are granted exceptions based on the same criteria do not consistently receive the same increase above the base rate. Finally, the definitions of the criteria do not necessarily identify centers with justifiably higher costs.

Special Provisions for Home Dialysis

Medicare patients who are treated at home, whether by hemodialysis or peritoneal dialysis, may obtain their supplies and equipment either through a dialysis facility or directly from a supplier. The source of the supply determines the method of payment. If the home patient deals with a dialysis facility, Medicare pays the facility 80 percent of the composite rate, or the same as for an in-center treatment. The payment covers all necessary dialysis supplies and equipment and related support services. Payment for home dialysis under the composite rate is known as Method I. According to HCFA, about 77 percent of home patients were using Method I in March 1988, and 66 percent in June 1989.

In 1983, Medicare authorized patients to obtain supplies and equipment directly from a supplier on a reasonable-charge basis as determined by the Medicare carrier (Method II). This was done for the convenience of patients and was not required by law. Under Method II, Medicare pays 80 percent of the reasonable charge and the patient is responsible for the remaining 20 percent.

In recent years, Method II has been the subject of substantial controversy, only briefly summarized here. Home Intensive Care, Inc. (HIC), a Florida corporation, beginning in 1986, established itself as a supplier of dialysis equipment and supplies to home patients. Under Method II, HIC charged HCFA an amount for supplies and equipment equivalent to what an individual who privately contracted with a supplier would be reimbursed. The charge, approved by Florida Blue Cross and Blue Shield, was such that HIC could pay for an aide to assist the home patient without billing directly for that aide. HCFA, in February 1988, sought to limit the Method II charge to the level of the composite rate (Method I) by a directive to its Medicare carriers. In December of that year, the U.S. District Court for the District of Columbia temporarily enjoined HCFA from implementing this directive.[8]

Both the General Accounting Office (GAO) and HCFA determined that HIC charges were substantially higher than those of facilities providing home dialysis under Method I. GAO reported in October 1989 to the Senate Finance Committee that in Florida, HIC received about $2,500 per month for dialysis supplies and equipment compared to about $1,240 received by dialysis units serving home patients under the composite rate (GAO, 1989).

Faced with this cost differential, an aggressive marketing campaign by HIC, and the prospect that others would follow suit, Congress, in OBRA 1989, limited the payment for home dialysis equipment and supplies under Method II to that authorized under the composite rate (Method I). This policy reduces the incentive for an organization to establish a supply company for the purpose of receiving payment under Method II. Independently, OBRA 1989 capped payment for continuous cycling peritoneal dialysis (CCPD) provided under Method II at 130 percent of the composite rate.[9]

HIC, in December 1989, announced that it would cease to provide staff-assisted home dialysis as of February 1, 1990. Consequently, during much of 1990, HCFA, the ESRD networks, national organizations of physicians, nurses, and administrators, and individual providers sought to identify HIC patients and transfer them to the care of another provider. In addition, GAO (1990) examined various options to providing home dialysis aides. In the process, it became clear that some patients were "hardship" cases, variously described as confined to a bed or wheelchair, unable to transfer without help, lacking transportation to a dialysis unit, or having a medical condition that made such travel risky. Several legislative proposals resulted in OBRA 1990 (Section 4202) authorizing a 3-year demonstration of the cost-effectiveness and safety of staff-assisted home dialysis.

Special Provisions for Recombinant Human Erythropoietin (EPO)

EPO is the first recombinant DNA biological to be introduced into the treatment of dialysis patients. It was approved by FDA in June 1989 for use in the treatment of anemia, which affects most dialysis patients (FDA, 1989).

Effective June 1, 1989, Medicare covered EPO administered in renal dialysis facilities (HCFA, 1989). HCFA set an interim reimbursement rate that would pay dialysis facilities $40 per EPO treatment for any dose up to 9,999 units and an additional $30 for any dose of 10,000 units or more. The payment for EPO was not incorporated into the composite rate because not all patients were expected to receive it, nor were all those receiving it expected to have the same prescribed dose.

Only the product cost is recognized for EPO administered in dialysis facilities. Any additional staff time, supplies, and laboratory services required in the administration of EPO are currently absorbed by facilities in the composite rate payment. Estimates of these additional administrative costs vary.

In November 1989, HCFA extended Medicare coverage to include EPO administered in a physician's office with reimbursement on a dose-related, reasonable-charge basis. The physician can also bill Medicare for any additional supplies, such as needles and syringes, used in the administration of the biological. In some cases, staff time for administering the biological can

also be reimbursed. Home dialysis patients wishing to administer EP
themselves were not covered in 1989 and 1990 because of the statuto
prohibition against Medicare coverage of self-administered drugs.

Two reports preceded congressional action in 1990. An OTA repo
(1990) dealt with EPO payment issues. Second, a report by the DHH
Office of Inspector General (OIG, 1990) argued that the reimburseme
arrangement permitted facilities to be paid $40 per dose, but to administ
dosages lower than the amount of EPO purchased for this amount and
make money in the process.

Congress, in OBRA 1990, Section 4201(c), however, made two impo
tant changes in EPO policy. First, it authorized self-administration of EP
by home patients without medical supervision, effective July 1, 1991. Se
ond, it changed the basis for payment to $11 per 1,000 units, effecti
January 1, 1991, with the payment to be adjusted annually by the implic
price deflator of the gross national product.[10]

Physician Reimbursement

Under the original 1973 Interim Regulations, Medicare included the ph
sician payment within the payment to the treatment facility. Under thi
arrangement, Medicare allowed $12 per dialysis session for the physician
supervisory care, although this amount could be negotiated between th
physician and the unit. Physicians were paid on a fee-for-service basis f
all care provided for home dialysis patients. They could also bill Medicar
on a reasonable-charge basis for other nonsupervisory outpatient care an
for all inpatient care provided to hospitalized patients.[11]

The initial method, as it was known, generated substantial protest fror
physicians who objected to being paid as salaried employees of treatmer
units. Since no per-dialysis fee was acceptable to Medicare, an alternativ
concept of a global fee, to be paid monthly, was proposed by the nephrologist
and accepted by Medicare, pending concurrence by the American Medic
Association (AMA). The AMA, although reluctant to accept any capitatio
of physician services, was persuaded that physician services for outpatier
dialysis were similar to a standard obstetrical fee or a fee for elective service
where a set of predictable services needed for a particular condition wa
covered by a single charge.

Given AMA assent, Medicare then introduced a direct physician paymer
option, the Alternative Reimbursement Method (ARM), in July 1974 (SSA
1974). Under the ARM, renal physicians were given a monthly capitatio
payment for all routine outpatient dialysis care provided to ESRD beneficiaries
The monthly charge was based on a multiple of a brief office visit tha
assumed 20 visits for center dialysis patients and 14 for home patients. Th
lower amount for home patients reflected Medicare's judgment that thes

patients were seen less often than center patients. The ARM payment amounts varied geographically. By 1981, approximately 75 percent of all dialysis services billed by physicians were reimbursed under the ARM. Physicians assumed that the charge would be adjusted in a manner consistent with standard Medicare practice for allowable charges. The office visit code was adjusted infrequently, however; the ARM itself was modestly increased only once, in 1978.

In August 1983, regulations established a monthly capitation payment (MCP) system (48 Fed. Reg. 21254, May 11, 1983), which eliminated the initial method and replaced the ARM. The MCP system, like the ARM, pays physicians a single predetermined amount per patient per month for the outpatient dialysis services. Unlike the ARM, a physician now receives the same amount for home patients as for facility patients.

The average MCP rate for physician outpatient services was initially $184.60, with minimum and maximum limits of $144 to $220 per month. In August 1986, the MCP was reduced by more than $10, resulting in an average current rate of $173.07 per patient per month with upper and lower payment limits of $132 and $203 per month. HCFA reduced the MCP because it concluded that the amount of time necessary to treat home patients was less than that required for in-center patients (51 Fed. Reg. 9530, March 19, 1986).

The initial rate-setting payment calculation used prevailing-charge rates for visit services: a brief follow-up visit for an established patient (90040) as the unit of service multiplied to produce a rate. Visit service codes do not represent uniform or explicit services, practices vary widely, and intermediaries' rates vary correspondingly. Payment rates have been established, therefore, that differ across geographic regions. This variability also applies to the MCP payment formula: Each locality has a different MCP rate simply because payment for the brief visit varies under the reasonable-charge system of reimbursement. The MCP floor of $132 and cap of $203, however, restrict payment variation across the country.

The MCP was assumed by many nephrologists and by Medicare to cover the dialysis prescription, supervision of dialysis care, review and modification of the prescription, plus internist services for which another specialist was not required. The nephrologist was paid as the primary-care physician for the dialysis patient. The explicit reductions in the physician's monthly rate and the absence of adjustment for inflation, when coupled with the increasing age and complexity of the patient population, have raised concerns about the effects of physician payment on patient care.

The IOM staff analyzed HCFA BMAD data for 1987 for allowed charges to physicians and nonphysicians (ambulance services, medical suppliers, independent laboratories, and others). These charges totaled $866.1 million in 1987 and represent 3 percent of all Medicare Part B charges of $28.9

billion for that year; they do not include Part B charges (or payments) to facilities for outpatient dialysis.

Of the total, physician charges for ESRD beneficiaries accounted for 76 percent (or $659 million) broken down as follows: internal medicine and nephrology, 35 percent; general surgery, thoracic surgery, and anesthesia, 16 percent; and other medical specialties, 24 percent. The allocation of charges between dialysis and transplant patients and between renal and nonrenal purposes is not known. Internal medicine and nephrology are grouped together as a conservative way to estimate care provided by nephrologists. The surgical category would include charges for fistula operations (for dialysis patients), transplant procedures, as well as other nonrenal surgical procedures (for dialysis as well as transplant patients).

Although further analysis is needed, especially of changes over time, the data indicate that a significant amount of care of ESRD beneficiaries is provided by nonnephrologists. This pattern may be appropriate or it may reflect referral by nephrologists of ESRD patients to other specialists for care that they might have personally provided in the past.

These developments appear to challenge the role of the nephrologist as primary physician for the dialysis patient and may disrupt the continuity of care received by the dialysis patient. *The committee did not examine this issue to any extent but believes that it deserves further consideration in the context of a quality assurance system oriented to patient outcomes and guided by information about patient complexity.*

In OBRA 1989, Congress enacted comprehensive physician payment reform for all of Medicare, which called for a Medicare Fee Schedule (MFS) based on a resource-based relative-value scale. All Medicare-covered services paid on the basis of reasonable charges will be affected by this fee schedule, which is to be implemented effective October 1, 1991.

In 1990, HCFA announced that the MCP for dialysis physician services would not be included under the MFS. HCFA's rationale is twofold: First, from a legal standpoint, it believes that the MCP is exempt from the fee schedule because the physician payment reform act language deals with reasonable charges and the MCP does not fall under the reasonable-charge provision.[12] Second, from a practical standpoint, the MCP is set by HCFA and not calculated by carriers on the basis of reasonable charges. The 1974 visit code used as the basis for the MCP in 1983 has effectively dictated payment, although that was not intended originally.

Since the MCP is not included in the fee schedule, it is unclear how or when HCFA will update the MCP. Several possible modifications to current policy exist:

• The current formula could be retained, using visit codes as proxies and payments would be derived from the relative values for these visit codes under the fee schedule;

• The current formula could be revised, using different services for proxies of physician's outpatient dialysis services; or
• The current formula could be retained and the MCP simply updated by some process.

INPATIENT DIALYSIS SERVICES

This section briefly describes current Medicare policy for payment for inpatient dialysis treatment to the hospital and the physician.

Hospital Reimbursement

By way of background, data on ESRD program expenditures indicate that inpatient spending has grown more rapidly than outpatient spending in recent years (Table 9-3). Before 1980, payments for inpatient hospital stays consistently ranged between 25 and 28 percent of all ESRD program payments, and outpatient payments constantly claimed over 55 percent. Since the early 1980s, however, inpatient spending has claimed a larger share of program expenditures. By 1988, for example, payments for ESRD hospital stays accounted for 36 percent of Medicare ESRD payments, whereas outpatient expenditures had fallen to 40 percent of the total.

Regrettably, the literature on hospitalization of ESRD patients is very sparse. Dialysis patients are hospitalized for several purposes—initial stabilization, subsequent renal-related problems, but usually for nonrenal problems requiring inpatient care. In general, dialysis patients are not admitted as inpatients for renal purposes, but for the primary diagnosis leading to renal failure in the case of initial stabilization, or for the precipitating diagnosis in subsequent admissions. ESRD patients are chronically ill people who have a greater number of comorbid conditions (not unique to them) than non-ESRD patients. However, they are more vulnerable to these conditions because of their underlying renal failure.[13]

The hospitalization of ESRD patients under the PPS system has not been analyzed to any extent. For example, DRG 316 (renal failure without dialysis) is used for both acute renal failure and ESRD patients, although the distribution is not known. According to Medpar file data from the Prospective Payment Assessment Commission (personal communication from Jolene Hall, July 1990), there were 39,500 admissions under this DRG in 1988, the average hospital charge was $7,100, and the average length of stay was 9.35 days. However, a study of hospitalization episodes in (old) ESRD Network 8 (Nebraska and Iowa), which occurred between July 1 and December 31, 1983, showed that 7.6 percent of admissions were coded DRG 316 (Cobe Laboratories, n.d.). Similarly, in 1988, 6.9 percent of the inpatients with dialysis treatments at the Henry Ford Health Care Corporation were classi-

TABLE 9-3 Medicare ESRD Benefit Payments, by Type of Service, 1974-87 (in millions of dollars and as percent of total)

Year	Total ESRD Payments	Inpatient Payments			Outpatient Payments		
		$ Millions	% Annual Increase	% Total ESRD	$ Millions	% Annual Increase	% Total ESRD
1974	229	65	—	28.4	136	—	59.4
1975	361	99	52	27.4	205	51	56.8
1976	512	136	37	26.6	290	41	56.6
1977	641	164	21	25.6	368	27	57.4
1978	800	209	27	26.1	453	23	56.6
1979	1,011	268	28	26.5	558	23	55.2
1980	1,253	345	29	27.5	666	19	49.6
1981	1,477	436	26	29.5	733	10	49.6
1982	1,662	520	19	31.3	782	7	47.1
1983	1,898	625	20	32.9	855	9	45.0
1984	2,003	732	17	36.5	855	1	43.3
1985	2,128	822	12	38.6	867	-4	39.0
1986[a]	2,423	904	10	37.3	980	18	40.4
1987[a]	2,702	973	8	36.0	1,095	12	40.5
1988[a]	3,011	1,084	11	36.0	1,213	11	40.3

NOTE: These figures may underestimate the actual benefit payments; see note 10.
[a]Data are incomplete because of outstanding bills.
SOURCE: HCFA, ESRD Quarterly Statistical Summary.

fied as DRG 316 (David F. Shepherd, Greenfield Health Systems Corporation, personal communication, December 1990). DRG 317 (renal failure with dialysis) is practically never used; there were 1,550 discharges from PPS hospitals in 1988, with an average hospital charge of $2,675 and an average length of stay of 3.4 days. This DRG accounted for a single case at Henry Ford in that year.

Jencks and Kay (1987) examined the relationship between total Medicare charges per hospitalization and eight beneficiary characteristics to determine whether DRG-based payment resulted in misclassification of certain classes of patients. One of eight patient characteristics they used was younger ESRD beneficiaries who were less than 65 years of age when discharged. These patients accounted for 0.97 percent of discharges in the study sample (5 percent of all discharges in 1983). Their charges were 5.1 percent higher than those for other beneficiaries. Discharges were concentrated in a few DRGS: 65 percent of younger patients with ESRD fell in the 20 most frequent DRGs; no other beneficiary characteristic (nursing home residents, prior hospitalization, the poor, those over 79 years of age, those over 84 years of age; the disabled less than 65 years of age, and older disabled patients) had more than 55 percent and most had less than half in these 20 DRGs. The main purpose of this exploratory study was to examine the relationship of severity of illness to hospitalization costs, and the potential for discrimination against severely ill patients. They found, overall, that the effect was more subtle than expected.

Trude and Carter (1989) examined PPS data to determine the likelihood that patients with certain characteristics would become DRG outliers, defined as those DRG cases falling in the 5 percent of the longest stay and the 5 percent of the largest losses. They note a previous study by Guterman (1986) that found that ESRD patients were more likely to become length-of-stay outliers and cost outliers, and had higher average costs and charges. Trude and Carter found that ESRD patients not coded into DRGs 302-333 (the major diagnostic categories for kidney diseases) were a greater risk of becoming the most costly 5 percent of cases for hospitals compared to all hospitalized non-ESRD patients and to those ESRD patients assigned to DRGs 302-333.

These few studies serve to indicate how little is known about the hospitalization of ESRD patients. A careful analysis of the experience of such patients under the DRG system deserves further attention.[14] The questions that might be addressed include the following: For what medical and surgical conditions are ESRD patients most frequently hospitalized? How likely are such cases to become outliers (length-of-stay and cost)? What is the distribution of hospitalized ESRD patients within a given DRG among all outliers (days and cost), the 5 percent outlier tail, and the non-outliers? What change is occurring over time?

Physician Reimbursement

In 1973, physicians could bill Medicare on a reasonable-charge basis for all inpatient care of ESRD dialysis patients. With the introduction of the ARM in 1974, renal physicians were given the option of continuing to receive the monthly capitation payment during a patient's hospitalization or billing separately for each service on a reasonable-charge basis. Physicians selecting the latter option had their ARM payment (and later their MCP payment) for outpatient dialysis services reduced by one-thirtieth for each day a patient was hospitalized.[15]

The difference in payment between the outpatient dialysis MCP and the reasonable-charge basis for inpatient care varies with the services provided to the patient. HCFA data indicate that payments on a reasonable-charge basis are dramatically higher. Payment under the inpatient dialysis codes fall between $50 and $500 per treatment depending upon the level of the code and the area of the country. Separate charges are billed for seeing patients on nondialysis days. The average MCP payment for inpatient care, on the other hand, is $55 for an average stay of 9 days, based on a daily reduction of the average MCP of $5.77 (one-thirtieth of $173.07). HCFA believes that the majority of physicians bill on the reasonable-charge basis for inpatient dialysis visits.

Before April 1989, physicians billed for inpatient dialysis services using 18 special CPT-4 codes, which were related to the severity of the patient's condition (acute, chronic, stable, or unstable) rather than a definition of the service. It is unclear whether these codes, established by carriers after consultation with renal physicians in their areas, accorded with HCFA policy. One GAO report (1985) found that almost all of the dialysis visits were billed and paid as acute (highest) or chronic-level (lowest) visits. Furthermore, some carriers were claims based on an hourly rate for inpatient physician services provided during dialysis treatment.

This coding methodology differed significantly from how Medicare determined payments for other hospital visits. Procedure codes generally used by Medicare for surgical procedures or office and hospital visits describe the service provided unrelated to severity. According to the 1985 GAO report, the severity coding used by renal physicians for dialysis hospital visits resulted in average daily Medicare amounts that were nearly twice the average allowed other specialists for non-ESRD hospital visits. This was followed in several areas by paying only a visit charge and denying dialysis as a physician procedure.

In April 1989, after prolonged negotiations with the Renal Physicians Association which insisted that dialysis is a procedure directed and supervised by a nephrologist, HCFA instructed carriers to accept dialysis as a procedure with four new CPT codes. These codes reflect one visit during dialysis or more than one visit as markers of service levels for hemodialysis. The rates for the new codes were derived from prior dialysis procedure rates. All other visits to the dialysis patient on nondialysis days were handled as standard inpatient visits. These charges vary among localities and are updated similar to other physician procedures, based on more recent fee screens. According to HCFA, the new codes reduce or have no effect on the level of payment.

NOTES

1. Independent OPOs establish a standard rate annually with Aetna, the single intermediary for IOPOs. They bill the RTC at this rate. The IOPO is then paid by the RTC out of its Medicare acquisition payment. Hospital OPOs are generally associated with a single hospital RTC and submit claims to the intermediary serving the parent hospital.

2. Under the customary-, prevailing-, reasonable-charge system, the prevailing charge is adjusted by the Medicare Economic Index (MEI) when the MEI is less than the increase in the prevailing charge for that procedure for a carrier. In the case of kidney transplants, the prevailing charge is updated by the lesser of the MEI or the percentage change from one year to the succeeding year in the weighted average of the carrier's prevailing charge for a unilateral nephrectomy.this exception to Medicare policy for setting charges was established in 1973 because no historical charge data on kidney transplantation were available. This policy could be reviewed since such data now exist. It is unclear, however, whether current policy restrains the increase in the prevailing charge more than if the increase were based on the carrier's prevailing-charge data for kidney transplants. Furthermore, since policy is the lesser of the MEI or the percentage change in carrier's prevailing charges, the MEI may be the increase factor regardless of which prevailing-charge data are used (either unilateral nephrectomy or kidney transplant).

3. Medicare reimbursed 80 percent of the $138; the beneficiary's share was 20 percent of the $138, or approximately $28.

4. The HCFA justification for the different rates was that services were essentially the same, but that hospital units had higher overhead costs. HCFA found no basis for accepting the arguments that patient complexity or case mix differed in a discernible way, and chose instead to rely on exceptions requests to deal with such alleged differences. Different percentages were recognized in the composite rates for home dialysis patients: 23.5 percent for hospital-based facilities and 10.5 percent for independent units.

5. Effective October 1, 1986, the wage index consisted of a blend of 80 percent of the Bureau of Labor Statistics (BLS) wage index and 20 percent of the HCFA gross hospital wage index for the Metropolitan Statistical Areas (as designated by the Office of Management and Budget). The wage index revised for October 1, 1987, reflects a 60/40 BLS/HCFA split. The index has not been revised since 1987.

6. The exceptions review process generally coincides with payment policy changes and is typically open for a 180-day period. The last open period began December 1, 1989, and closed May 29, 1990.

7. Education costs were once used as an exceptions process criterion but no longer apply.

8. *National Kidney Patients Ass'n* v. *Otis R. Bowen*, Civil Action No. 88-3251 (D.D.C. December 22, 1988).

9. Under Method II, the cap for CCPD is 130 percent of the Method I rate. Therefore, some incentive for a facility to establish a supply company in order to bill under Method II continues to exist.

10. According to Joseph Eschbach, M.D. (University of Washington), early data from studies in progress in Europe show that daily subcutaneous self-administration of EPO corrects anemia in the majority of hemodialysis and CAPD patients at approximately one-third of

the dose administered intravenously three times a week during dialysis (personal communication, July 16, 1990).

11. For all other nonrenal-related services provided by a nephrologist, in either the home, the outpatient unit (hospital-based or independent facility), or an inpatient setting, the payment is determined on the reasonable-charge basis. In fact, most bills for outpatient services are denied, since such services are typically included within the MCP.

12. Reimbursement of the MCP is described in Section 1881.b.3.B of the Social Security Act; a description of reasonable charges is in Section 1842.b.

13. One manual listed these basic coding principles for admitting ESRD patients under the DRG system: (1) The principal diagnosis is the condition established after study to be chiefly responsible for admission of the patient to the hospital. (2) The underlying cause should be designated as the principal diagnosis when disease manifestations were a direct result of that condition. (3) Complications of treatment should be coded according to the nature of the complication whenever a specific code exists for the condition. (4) The principal procedure is the one most related to the principal diagnosis or the procedure performed for definitive treatment rather than for diagnostic purposes or for handling a complication. (5) Coding should be as complete as possible—i.e., code all diagnoses and procedures performed. (6) V-codes should be used only when a patient is admitted for purposes other than acute illness or for suspected conditions ruled out (Cobe Laboratories, Inc., n.d.).

14. Technically, since October 1, 1984, current policy provides additional payments to hospitals whose total discharges of Medicare ESRD beneficiaries having non-ESRD-related DRGs (excluding transplant patients) account for 10 percent or more of all their Medicare discharges. According to HCFA, however, no more than 12 hospitals per year qualify for this extra payment.

15. The physician payment for inpatient dialysis services may be updated and increased each year, whereas the outpatient MCP has remained constant since 1986. Over time, then, the one-thirtieth reduction corresponds to a small percentage of total Medicare payments for outpatient dialysis services.

REFERENCES

Cobe Laboratories, Inc. n.d. Hospital Reimbursement for ESRD Admissions Under the DRG System. Lakewood, Colo.

Community Psychiatric Centers. 1989. Proxy Statement, July 12, Laguna Hills, Calif.

FDA (Food and Drug Administration). 1989. Summary Basis of Approval for Epoetin Alfa. ELA #87-0535, PLA #87-0536. Washington, D.C., June.

GAO (General Accounting Office). 1985. Changes needed in Medicare payments to physicians under the Medicare End Stage Renal Disease program. Washington, D.C., February.

GAO. 1989. Payments for home dialysis much higher under reasonable charge method. GAO/HRD-90-37. Washington, D.C., October.

GAO. 1990. Medicare: Options to provide home dialysis aides. GAO/HRD-90-153. Washington, D.C., August.

Guterman S. 1986. A descriptive analysis of PPS outlier payment policy. Unpublished study.

HCFA (Health Care Financing Administration). 1989. Part 1 — Chapter 27: Reimbursement for ESRD Services and Transplant Services. Medicare Provider Reimbursement Manual: Transmittal No. 11. Baltimore, Md., July.

Jencks SF, Kay T. 1987. Do frail, disabled, poor, and very old Medicare beneficiaries have higher hospital charges? JAMA 257:198-202.

OIG (Office of Inspector General, U.S. Department of Health and Human Services). 1987. Organ acquisition costs: An overview. Washington, D.C., September.

OIG. 1988. Kidney acquisition costs: A management advisory report. Washington, D.C., November.

OIG. 1990. The effect of the interim payment rate for the drug Epogen on Medicare expenditures and dialysis facility operations. Draft report. Washington, D.C., May.

OTA (Office of Technology Assessment). 1990. Recombinant erythropoietin: Payment options for Medicare. OTA-H-451. Washington, D.C.: Government Printing Office.

REN Corporation-USA. 1989. Prospectus, November 28. Nashville, Tenn.

Rettig RA. 1980. The politics of health cost containment: End-stage renal disease. Bull NY Acad Med 56:115-138.

SSA (Social Security Administration, Bureau of Health Insurance). 1974. Alternative reimbursement method of monthly payments to physicians for services rendered to patients on maintenance dialysis. Intermediary Letter No. 74-29(A)(3). June.

Trude S, Carter GM. 1989. A description of expensive and long-staying patients. N-2998-HCFA. The RAND Corporation. Santa Monica, Calif.

10

Reimbursement Effects on Quality

OBRA 1987 asked this study to consider the effects of reimbursement on quality of treatment. This question arises from the need to understand the effects on patients of ESRD cost-containment efforts. Although there is substantial literature on reimbursement and growing literature on quality, the effects of the former on the latter have not been examined extensively in any area of medicine. An example of what is possible, however, is the recent set of reports from a group at Rand-UCLA-Value Health Sciences (Kahn et al., 1990a,b,c; Draper et al., 1990; Keeler et al., 1990; Rubenstein et al., 1990; Kosecoff et al., 1990; Rogers et al., 1990) examining the effects of the DRG-based Prospective Payment System on outcomes of care. No comparable assessment has been conducted for the ESRD program.

What can be said about the relationship of reimbursement to quality in the ESRD context? Studies in this areas are limited; neither the federal government nor providers have systematically monitored the effect of changes in Medicare reimbursement on indices of quality. However, useful albeit scattered studies of this relationship have been published. Moreover, the committee commissioned new studies in certain areas. This chapter reviews the available information on the effects of reimbursement on dialysis patient mortality, hospitalization, dialysis unit staffing, and innovation. The focus is entirely on dialysis; there are no studies of the effect of reimbursement on quality in transplantation.

EFFECTS OF REIMBURSEMENT ON MORTALITY

As noted in Chapter 4, gross (or unadjusted) ESRD patient mortality has been increasing over time. With adjustment for age and diagnosis, however, mortality rates have been stable. Although an upward shift in mortal-

ity is observed between 1982 and 1983, this is attributed to patient characteristics, data reporting, and unexplained factors.[1] In any case, these data
do not bear directly on whether changes in Medicare ESRD affect mortality.

The committee is aware of only two studies that attempt to assess this
question directly. Both focused on the effects of implementation of the
1983 ESRD composite rate, which significantly reduced reimbursement to
many facilities. The first, by Held and his colleagues at the Urban Institute
(1987),[2] noted a general increase in reported mortality, suggested that the
increasing age of the patient population might account for much of this
change, and observed that changing patient selection criteria might account
for some increase in the proportion of sicker patients. Specifically, with
respect to the effect of the composite rate on mortality, the study reported
that "evidence of a correlation between changes in mortality and the extent
of composite rate changes was not found, i.e., mortality did not rise more
where the composite rate changes were larger" (Held et al., 1987) The
authors noted, however, that further analysis was needed to draw firm conclusions.

This 1987 Urban Institute study was done under pressure of time. The
present IOM study subcontracted with the Urban Institute to perform further
analysis and to update its earlier study. More follow-up data were evaluated,
and an improved research design was used. This new report (Held et al.,
1990b) uses patient data from two nonconcurrent, prevalent cohorts of patients
who were in the system on January 1, 1982, and January 1, 1984. It uses
price data for the 1982 and the 1984-87 reimbursement rates adjusted for
area wage differences to capture the real resource costs across areas, an
adjustment not undertaken in the earlier study.

Two types of analyses ("models") are presented. The price-level model
analyzes whether mortality is associated with variations in price levels among
facilities at a given time. It analyzes whether mortality is higher at facilities
receiving lower standardized prices (payments) during a specific year. Data
from 1982 and from 1984 were analyzed in the new report. The first-difference
model uses each facility as its own control by comparing the mortality rates
in each facility at two different times. It examines whether the mortality at
a facility changed when the price it received changed.

Analyses from the price-level model suggest that there is an inverse
correlation between patient mortality and the standardized price that dialysis
facilities received. These data suggest that higher standardized prices tend
to be associated with lower mortality rates. Results from the first-difference
model, however, are less definitive. None of the correlation coefficients for
the five primary disease groups (diabetes, hypertension, glomerulonephritis,
other diseases, unknown) in the first-difference model is statistically significant. All five coefficients, however, consistently point in the same
direction, i.e., that a larger decrease in standardized payment to a given

facility between 1982 and 1984 correlates with a higher mortality rate in that facility. Since the level of statistical confidence in the results is low, evidence from this analysis must be regarded as inconclusive. Held and colleagues (1990b) caution in their report that the findings "do not definitively substantiate the conceptual model proposed," that is, that increased mortality was the result of reduced payments.

The committee regards the results of these two studies as suggestive but insufficient to establish firmly a direct effect of reimbursement on mortality. Since no other studies of this question are available, the committee concludes that the empirical evidence is not sufficient at present time definitively to support or to refute the hypothesis that past changes in reimbursement have adversely affected mortality directly.

There is some evidence supporting an indirect effect. Held and colleagues (1990a) examined the effect of the 1983 composite rate price change on treatment time and of treatment time on the mortality during a 2-year follow-up period of the 1982 and the 1984 incident patient cohorts. They found that average treatment time decreased by 6 percent (from 5.0 to 4.7 hours) in independent units and by 7.8 percent (from 5.12 to 4.72 hours) in hospital-based units between 1982 and 1987. The percentage of hospital units reporting less than 4.5 hours treatment time increased from 25 percent to 37 percent during this period. Analysis indicated that a decrease in treatment time from 4.5 hours to 4.0 hours resulted in an increase in the relative risk of death of 1.06 (6 percent higher per year) over the follow-up period (statistically significant, $P < .01$). Findings from the hospital-based units alone, however, were not statistically significant (beta = 0.99, $P = .48$).

Lowrie and Lew (1990) analyzed data on a sample of more than 12,000 patients treated in National Medical Care units who were alive at the end of 1988. Shorter treatment times were associated with higher mortality. After adjustment for differences in certain laboratory values, the relative risk of mortality was reduced but not eliminated.

The committee believes that these data suggest the possibility that decreases in reimbursement may have led to increases in mortality indirectly via an economic incentive to shorten treatment times, which in turn led to increased mortality. (Shortened treatment periods reduce costs by permitting nurses/technicians to treat more patients in a given shift.) The committee believes that no firm conclusion can be drawn, however, because factors other than changes in payments have probably influenced the trend to shorter treatment times.

Assessing the Effects of Reimbursement on Mortality

Although the use of mortality as an outcome measure represents an important step toward the objective quantification of outcomes, there are reasons to think that the emphasis in available studies on the effect of the 1983 composite rate change on mortality may be inappropriate. First, the interpretation of the indirect relationship mentioned above is complicated by the fact that clinical opinion, reinforced by patient preferences, may also have contributed to shorter treatment time.[3]

Second, as noted above, gross mortality has been increasing, but age-adjusted and diagnosis-adjusted mortality have been quite stable. This implies that the increasing age and complexity of the patient population may account for much of the observed increase in mortality. However, adjustment for ESRD patient complexity is somewhat crude at present, being limited to standardization for the effects of patient age, gender, race, and primary diagnoses. More refined means to adjust for patient complexity may be needed to detect significant mortality changes among subgroups of the patient population. (See Chapter 12.)

Third, the decrement in reimbursement due to the composite rate was small compared to the effects of inflation. Any mortality effects of the composite rate, therefore, might be expected to be small. From 1974 to 1982 the nominal payment rate of $138 per treatment remained unchanged; when adjusted for inflation using the gross national product (GNP) price deflator, it fell nearly 50 percent in constant dollars by 1982 to the equivalent of $74.50 in 1974 dollars. In addition, other changes in reimbursement occurred at about the same time as the composite rate for dialysis was implemented. Medicare-as-secondary-payer in the first year of an ESRD patients' eligibility was authorized in OBRA 1981 (see Chapter 7) and the Prospective Payment System was instituted in 1983. Moreover, providers had a long time to anticipate and prepare for the changes introduced by the 1983 composite rate.[4] The net economic effect of all these changes on hospitals and on independent facilities is difficult to assess and complicates attempts to determine the isolated effect of the composite rate on mortality.

Finally, there are reasons to think that providers have adapted to reimbursement reductions in ways that dampened the effects on patient mortality. Dialysis units can respond to economic constraints in many ways that protect their core activity of providing dialysis treatment to ESRD patients. For example, they can accept lower "profits" (the difference between revenues and expenses); they can replace equipment more slowly than previously; and they shop more actively for deals and discounts among suppliers. These types of responses presumably deliver dialysis of unchanged quality at lower costs.

On the other hand, they can replace higher-paid with lower-paid personnel, or they may cut services (presumably nonessential amenities first). These latter types of adaptations may be adequate to prevent or minimize increases in mortality but inadequate to avoid decreases in quality by other measures. For example, cutbacks in nutritionist and social worker staffing may increase morbidity and reduce patient quality of life, even though mortality does not increase.

In the mid-1980s, representatives of the provider community responded to the introduction of the 1983 composite rate and the observed increase in gross mortality by arguing that reductions in reimbursement were causing this increase. The committee's review of available studies of this issue, described in the preceding section, indicates that data in support of this contention are suggestive but by no means conclusive. On the other hand, when the Secretary of Health and Human Services, Dr. Otis Bowen, transmitted the 1987 Urban Institute report to Congress in December 1988, he interpreted the latter's cautious conclusions as showing no "negative effect on the quality of care provided to the Medicare beneficiaries receiving dialysis" (Bowen, 1988). The committee finds no basis for this definitive conclusion either.

EFFECTS OF REIMBURSEMENT ON HOSPITALIZATION

Another important outcome measure is ESRD patient morbidity. The only studies available have used hospitalization rates and lengths of stay as an index of morbidity. Data from Dialysis Clinic, Inc.-Cincinnati (DCI) on its entire historical patient population show that from 1976 to 1989 both the average and the median age of the patient population had increased, and patient severity, measured by the total number of ICD-9 diagnosis codes per patient at the time hemodialysis began, increased significantly (Pollack and Pesce, 1990). The number of hospital admissions for the prevalent 3-year patient cohorts increased substantially over the study years whereas the average duration of hospital stay declined more than 30 percent.

Held (Urban Institute, personal communication, 1990) analyzed data for ESRD admissions and length of stay for incident dialysis patient cohorts from 1979 through 1985. Using 1982 as a reference year, he found that when controlled for age, gender, race, diagnosis, and days at risk, relative hospital admissions fell steadily from 1.25 in 1979 (i.e., 1979 admissions/ 1982 admissions) to 0.86 for 1985. Relative days of hospitalization fell from 1.73 in 1979 to 0.70 in 1985. In general, more ESRD patients are hospitalized than ever, because of increased age and complexity, although the relative risk of hospitalization for all but the elderly ESRD patients may be declining.

What effect, if any, does reimbursement for outpatient dialysis have on the hospitalization of ESRD patients? The hypotheses to be considered are: First, the level of payment influences the level of resources available for dialysis (a lower price is hypothesized to reduce the quality of treatment, for example, by shortening treatment time or reducing well-trained person-nel); second, less adequate treatment will lead to increased morbidity, as evidenced by a higher rate of hospitalization and longer length of stay.

The 1987 Urban Institute report (Held et al., 1987) found that inpatient stays of a 1984 ESRD patient cohort were higher than those of a 1982 cohort. However, the study did not find an association between the reimbursement change introduced by the composite rate and greater patient morbidity as measured by in-hospital stays, at least in the first year after the rate was introduced.

The update of the Urban Institute study done for this committee (Held et al., 1990c) differs from the 1987 study in several respects. It includes patients in independent units only, in contrast to patients in all units in the earlier study. It is based on two nonconcurrent prevalent patient cohorts, as of January 1, for the years 1982 and 1984, whereas the 1987 study relied on incident cohorts for these years. Each cohort was followed for 2 years. It uses a first-difference model and a price-level model to measure how changes in price affect morbidity.

The study provides some evidence that the level of the dialysis price may affect hospital use by ESRD patients. The study design controlled for differences in the primary renal disease leading to ESRD, for known patient characteristics, and for the demographics of the region in which the dialysis unit is located. By the price-level model, the 1990 study found a significant inverse correlation between the dialysis price level and hospital admission rates as well as hospital length of stay (days). The analysis estimated that a decrease of $10 in the standardized dialysis price is associated with a 2 to 4 percent increase in hospitalization. These results were most conclusive for diabetic patients, an intuitively reasonable result, since these patients are clinically less stable and require extra care in management on dialysis. The persuasiveness of the conclusion is limited, however, because there was no correlation between price changes and hospital use when the data were analyzed by a different method in which each facility was used as its own control (first-difference model).

Evidence from Held and colleagues (1990c) suggests that average dialysis treatment time affects hospitalization rates and days. They estimate that an increase of treatment time by one hour is associated with a decrease of 4 to 11 percent in hospital days, with diabetic patients experiencing the largest effect.

Data on the effect of reimbursement on hospitalization of ESRD patients are limited. An earlier study by Held and colleagues (1987) showed no relationship between the introduction of the composite rate and hospitalization. The more recent study by the Held group (1990c) raises the possibility of an inverse relationship between the composite rate and hospitalization. One analytical method showed such an inverse association, but a second analytical method did not. Therefore, no firm conclusion can be drawn that there is a direct effect of reimbursement on morbidity (hospitalization).

As with mortality, there is the suggestion that there may be an indirect effect mediated via changes in length of dialysis treatments, i.e., that decreased reimbursement is associated with decreased length of treatment, which in turn is associated with increased hospitalization.

EFFECTS OF REIMBURSEMENT ON UNIT STAFFING

One important structural measure of quality is the level and compositi of dialysis unit staffing. In this section, the changes in staffing that ha occurred in the 1980s, and the causes and the consequences of these chang are discussed.[5]

Both qualitative and quantitative changes in dialysis unit staffing occurr during the 1980s. Evaluation of the effects of reimbursement on staffi and of staffing on patient outcomes has been hampered by the lack national statistics.

In 1989, however, Held and colleagues (1990a) compiled a data set th included national data on facility staffing as well as on dialysis time a reimbursement. Data were extracted from 1982 and 1987 statistical co forms for a sample of dialysis facilities. Using these data, they calculate medical staff hours per patient per week for independent as well as hospita based outpatient dialysis units, including total, registered nurse (RN), l censed practical nurse (LPN), technician, nursing assistant, social worke and dietitian hours. The results are shown in Table 10-1.

Between 1982 and 1987, hospital-based and independent units reduce total staff hours per patient-week. Hospital-based units changed more tha independent units: In 1982, they provided nearly 11 percent more tot staff hours per patient-week than independents, but by 1987 the differen was only 1 percent. A major difference between hospital and independe units is that the latter average 2 hours less RN time per patient-week tha hospital-based units, making greater use of LPNs, nursing assistants, an technicians. Hospital-based units, by contrast, report less social worker an dietitian time per patient-week.

Data submitted to the committee at its May 1989 public hearing in Chicag are consistent with these national data. Dr. Raymond Hakim (1989), representin DCI, the largest chain of not-for-profit dialysis providers, testified regardin staffing changes:

Even though patients are older and sicker, reductions in reimbursement and ir creases in labor costs have forced dialysis facilities to increase their patient to sta ratio. In 1981, the average patient-to-staff ratio at DCI was 3.9 to 1. However, i 1988, the average patient-to-staff ratio at DCI was 4.83 to 1.

Similar testimony was presented by Dr. Edmund Lowrie, President o National Medical Care (NMC). Lowrie (1989) testified that whereas NM(units once maintained patient/staff ratios of 3:1, "ratios greater than 4:1 ar now common." Furthermore, the ratio of licensed nursing staff to unli censed patient care staff has been reduced in many NMC facilities. Othe providers confirm this general trend.

Dr. Alan Kanter (1989), President of North Central Dialysis Centers (NCDC

TABLE 10-1 Outpatient Dialysis Units: Staff Hours per Patient-Week, 1982 and 1987

	Hospital-based Units			Independent Units		
	1982	1987	% Change	1982	1987	% Change
Total	9.88	8.22	-16.7	8.91	8.12	- 8.9
RN	5.76	4.94	-14.3	3.43	2.85	-17.0
LPN	1.25	1.12	-10.5	1.63	1.21	-19.4
NAS	0.41	0.22	-46.4	0.30	0.59	97.7
TECH	1.79	1.59	-11.4	2.76	2.69	- 2.6
SW	0.39	0.22	-43.7	0.48	0.44	- 8.6
DIET	0.28	0.14	-48.5	0.32	0.25	-22.0

NOTE: RN = registered nurse; LPN = licensed practical nurse; NAS = nursing assistant; TECH = technician; SW = social worker; DIET = dietitian.

SOURCE: Held et al., 1990a.

a four-unit proprietary organization in Chicago), presented the data on actual and projected staffing levels for 1986 through 1990 displayed in Table 10-2.

Several general trends in the staffing of outpatient dialysis units are evident from these sources. First, patient-to-staff ratios increased substantially during the 1980s. Second, units have shifted away from highly trained and well-paid registered nurses toward less well-trained, lower-paid staff, mainly technicians.

Third, patient hours with social workers and dietitians have also been reduced. Kanter (1989) described the NCDC experience:

In the first decade of operation, our social service personnel provided many hours of family counselling for our patients. More recently these sessions have been all but discontinued. Our social workers now spend much of their time in crisis management and in routine activities such as those involved in providing patient transportation. They are increasingly responsible for obtaining and maintaining insurance information. This latter activity, so necessary for NCDC's fiscal health, is a sad waste of their professional skills. We have not increased the number of these personnel. Each social worker and dietitian now has a patient load about 30 percent bigger than in 1986.

The use of LPNs and nursing assistants reveals no clear pattern or trend. It suggests, however, that facilities are searching for new staffing patterns. Kanter (1989) testified: "The increased number and percentage of licensed practical nurses in 1987 and 1988 produced inadequate economy of operation. We have started a new program to find and train experienced medical assistants and unlicensed immigrant nurses and physicians as dialysis technicians." Searching for an optimal mix that will deliver good care at the

TABLE 10-2   Staffing Changes, 1986-1990: North Central Dialysis
Centers, Chicago, Illinois

Category of Professional	Year				
	1986	1987	1988	1989	1990
RNs	30.5 (68.5)[a]	22 (48.9)	17.3 (38.2)	16 (36.4)	17 (37.0)
LPNs	12 (27.0)	22 (48.9)	27 (59.6)	19 (43.2)	11 (23.9)
Technicians	2 (4.5)	1 (2.2)	1 (2.2)	9 (20.5)	18 (39.1)
TOTAL FTEs	44.5	45	45.3	44	46

NOTE: RN = registered nurse; LPN = licensed practice nurse; FTE = full-time equivalent.

[a]Figures shown are numbers of full-time-equivalent employees. Figures in parentheses are the percentage with respect to each column.

SOURCE: Kanter, 1989.

lowest possible cost is desirable, and it can be quite constructive. Under the current resource constraints, however, the search is an empirical exploration not informed by analysis relating inputs to outcomes and running increasingly counter to professional judgment.

What Factors Are Causing These Changes?

Unit managers—medical directors, owners, hospital administrators—whose revenues are constrained must reduce costs if they are to continue to provide dialysis services. Since payroll costs constitute a large and growing portion of total unit costs, the level and mix of staffing is a logical, indeed a necessary target of managerial attention.

Held and colleagues (1990a), using a sample of dialysis units, analyzed the relation between the change in reimbursement introduced by the 1983 composite rate and unit staffing levels and composition. They found that independent units with higher standardized reimbursement rates in 1982 had higher levels of RNs and other medical staff (LPNs, nursing assistants, and technicians); social worker and dietitian hours per patient per week showed no clear pattern as a function of price differences. In 1987, there was a consistent relation between price and staff time per patient-week for other medical staff, including social workers and dietitians. The pattern for RNs was similar to that in 1982, although the inverse relationship between reimbursement and RN staffing was statistically less than that in 1982.

The data from hospital-based units revealed a different pattern. In 1987, hospital units with the highest standardized price did show the highest number of RN hours per patient-week. However, this relationship did not hold for other nursing personnel, social workers, or dietitians; their hours were stable regardless of standardized price. Moreover, 1982 data revealed no relationship between reimbursement and RN staffing.

The same research group (Garcia et al., 1990), in a related analysis of the effect of the reduction in reimbursement between 1982 and 1984, found that independent units with cuts of $15 to $30 per treatment reduced RN and social worker/dietitian time more than those with cuts of less than $15. The three units with price cuts of more than $30 showed the largest reductions of RN and other medical hours per patient-week. Hospital-based units showed no clear pattern of RN hours as a function of the size of price cuts; they did reveal a clear relationship between the size of price cuts and decreases in other nursing staff, social workers, and dietitians.

Held and co-workers (1990a) summarize the results of their analysis as follows:

The staffing of dialysis units is affected by the Medicare price of dialysis. Both hospital and freestanding [i.e., independent] units show impacts of the Medicare price level. The hospital units appear to respond to the lower prices by lowering the entire staff to patient ratio. Freestanding units, perhaps because their total staff to patient ratio was already substantially lower than the ratio for hospitals at the beginning of the period under study, respond to lower prices by reducing the RN hours per patient with less change in the total staff hours per patient.

What Are the Consequences of These Staffing Changes?

Does reimbursement affect staffing? Studies indicate with reasonable certainty that the answer is yes. Do the observed changes in the level and composition of staffing represent a deterioration in quality? The answer is more difficult to obtain. Changes in the number and composition of dialysis staffs do not by themselves indicate that patient outcomes, the key measure of quality, have deteriorated.

ESRD program data do not allow the relationship among structure, process, and outcomes to be analyzed definitively. The recent research by Held and colleagues (Garcia et al., 1990; Held et al., 1990b,c), however, does relate reimbursement (or price) to dialysis unit staffing (a structural measure), staffing to treatment time (a crude process measure), and treatment time to mortality (an outcome measure). On the relationship of reimbursement, staffing, and treatment time, they find that, for independent units, price affects RN hours per patient-week and dialysis treatment time. For hospital-based units, price affects total staffing hours but not RN hours or average dialysis treatment time. Although shorter treatment time has been correlated with patient mortality, staffing changes have not.

Again, the results are suggestive but not conclusive. Measures and data that permit the analysis of relationships among reimbursement, staffing, treatment, and patient outcomes are needed. In the absence of such data, it is useful to discuss the potential implications of staffing changes on the quality of care delivered to patients.

Nurses

The institutional base of dialysis nursing has shifted in the past decade from hospital-based to independent units, as the latter have grown in number and total capacity. In both settings, demands on nurses, especially RNs, reportedly have increased because of a reduction of their absolute numbers, higher patient/nurse ratios, greater patient complexity, increasingly sophisticated technology, and diminished scheduling flexibility. The involvement of more technicians and other non-RN staff in delivering dialysis treatments has increased the supervisory responsibilities of RNs. The decrease in social workers and dietitians has meant that some of their responsibilities have fallen on nurses.

Data on salaries of nephrology nurses are not available. There are suggestions that salary opportunities in other nursing fields make recruitment and retention in nephrology difficult. Reports from the American Nephrology Nurses Association (ANNA) indicate that support for educational programs, attendance at professional meetings, tuition reimbursement, and on-the-job orientation and training have declined. A 1984 survey reported low morale among dialysis unit head nurses (ANNA, 1985), but data on nursing satisfaction are not regularly collected by anyone.

What are the implications of changing patterns of nurse staffing and especially the substitution of technicians for nurses? It should be emphasized that nurses are broadly trained to care for patients and then obtain specialized training in dialysis delivery. Technicians, by contrast, are trained only to deliver dialysis treatments. Specific effects of the staffing changes, then, include the following: direct clinical supervision of patients is reduced; clinical information on specific patients is less readily available to physicians as they make rounds; crisis management capability is reduced; and the probability of errors in comprehensive patient management is increased.

The effect of substitution of technicians for nurses on patient management or patient outcomes has not been analyzed. At present the clinical judgment of unit medical directors and the policy of providers nevertheless indicate concerns about the effect of this substitution. NCDC, for example, recently adopted the policy that RNs shall constitute a minimum of 40 percent of all unit personnel.

Technicians

Dialysis technicians have increased substantially in numbers in recent years. However, they are responsible both for patient care and for purely technical procedures, such as equipment operation and maintenance, water treatment, dialysate preparation, and dialyzer reprocessing. As these technical demands have increased, technicians cannot be regarded as one-to-one substitutes for nurses in the direct delivery of treatment to patients. The total number of staff hours for direct patient care may actually be decreased.

Representatives of technicians identify the following problems that they and the provider community confront. First, no uniform, consistent definition of technician exists. Second, no standardized training and education is required of technicians.[6] Third, there is no official program to certify technicians.[7] Fourth, the implications of the increased use of technicians for the quality of patient care is a matter of growing concern. Finally, state laws and regulations vary widely in the extent to which they limit or allow direct patient care by technicians and to which they specify the relationship between nurses and technicians.[8]

Social Workers

Social worker time has declined and ratios of social workers to patients have increased in the past decade. Held and colleagues (1990a) found substantial reduction in social worker time from 1982 to 1987. In 1988, the Council of Nephrology Social Workers (CNSW) of the National Kidney Foundation (NKF) surveyed dialysis unit social workers.[9] They found that the average patient-to-social worker ratio was 102 to 1; the for-profit average was 111 to 1, the not-for-profit average, 95 to 1. The average patient case load included 20 diabetic patients, 3 nursing home residents, 3 patients who required ambulance transport, 10 with other transportation problems, 10 with inadequate social support, 17 who needed aid for medications, and 27 welfare/Medicaid recipients.

Ideally, social work services include patient education; supportive counseling for patients and their families about the effects of kidney failure and dialysis on marriage, family, work, and social life; crisis intervention; and the development of access to community resources. The effect of current social worker/patient ratios, however, has been to reduce social workers to arranging transportation and helping patients find coinsurance. They report that far less of their time is spent on counseling than they believe is appropriate.

Social workers are sometimes employees of, but often consultants to, dialysis units. Their status in dialysis units was set initially by 1976 Medicare regulations, which stated that social services were to be furnished by "a qualified social worker" (41 Fed. Reg. 22502, June 3, 1976). A qualified social worker was defined as one who is licensed, if applicable, in the relevant state and has a Master of Social Work (MSW) from an accredited graduate school.[10]

In recent years, some dialysis facilities have hired social workers without a master's degree, although there are no data on the extent of this practice. Facility managers, responding to continued economic pressures, have argued that such highly trained individuals are not needed for the routine functions now performed by many social workers. This practice has been questioned by the CNSW as contrary to the 1976 Medicare regulations. HCFA responded initially to the CNSW by suggesting that the "qualified" requirement could be met by a single MSW-trained social worker in a facility and as many non-MSW staff as needed as long as they were under the supervision of a qualified social worker (Smith, 1989). In 1989, the CNSW challenged HCFA's interpretation of the regulations (Klahr, 1989). HCFA has conceded that the NKF CNSW interpretation is correct but has announced its intention to issue new regulations on the subject.

The Director of the HCFA Health Standards and Quality Bureau, Thomas G. Morford, in a March 15, 1990, letter to Saulo Klahr, M.D., President of the NKF, stated the HCFA position clearly (Morford, 1990):

Our review of the social service requirements has led us to believe that they may now be overly restrictive to the ESRD facility. . . . We believe that to the maximum extent possible, Federal regulations should focus more on the adequacy of services provided (outcomes) and less on the structure and process of how the services should be provided.

Conceptually clear, the current HCFA position raises the question of how HCFA proposes to assess the outcome of social work without reference to process or structural aspects of care. Unless any new regulation includes a specific answer to this question, it will lead to the suspicion that the change in regulation is designed to reduce costs without addressing the implications of patient care.

In 1983, CNSW developed a formula for calculating the social worker resources needed for a given patient load, based on the percent age of patients who were socially disadvantaged, lacked family or community support, had diabetes mellitus, or were older than 60 years. This formula, although reasonable on its face, has never been formally evaluated for its implications for patient care. Pollack and Pesce (1990), at DCI-C, obtained data from 33 other units in the DCI chain, from 40 facilities in ESRD Network 9, and from DCI-C. Using the CNSW formula to define normatively the level of needed services, they calculated that during 1989 the number of social workers was 37 percent of need at DCI-C, 34 to 39 percent at DCI, and 40 to 46 percent at Network 9. Using a more conservative Medicare requirement, the available social workers were 67 percent of need at DCI-C, 62-72 percent in all DCI, and 72-84 percent in Network 9 units. Research is needed to definitively examine the relationship of social services to patient outcomes.

Dietitians

Data on patient/staff ratios for renal dietitians are scarce but ratios ranging from 140/1 to 200/1 are estimated by knowledgeable individuals. The importance of nutrition to patient outcomes in dialysis is increasingly recognized. The existing dietitian/patient ratios may limit implementation of suitable dietary programs. In a recent survey, members of the Council on Renal Nutrition of the NKF expressed great interest in quality assurance (CRN, 1989). The opportunity exists in nutrition to examine carefully the relationship of certain professional input to the treatment process to determine the effects on patient management and patient outcomes.

Implications of Changing Staff Patterns for Quality

The combined effect of declining real reimbursement rates and increasing salaries and wages provides strong incentives to dialysis units to alter staffing patterns. In the committee's judgment, current patterns have not been determined by professional judgment of requirements for adequate care but rather represent a response to increasing economic constraints. The practical effect has been that units that staff only for a routine treatment process may have inadequate staff for crisis management and may have reduced social worker and dietitian resources to a minimum.

If dialysis were simply an industrial production process, the search for appropriate staffing patterns would be determined largely by the homogeneity of inputs, opportunities for substituting capital for labor, and the balance between the routine and crisis demands of treatment. Dialysis units, however, confront a patient population ("input") that is growing more heterogeneous over time; treatment technology is unlikely to provide significant labor substitution opportunities in the near future (see below); and, as noted earlier, the limits of reductions in treatment time appear to have been reached.

Changing personnel patterns in dialysis units represent empirical adaptations to scarce resources that have been made without a clear understanding of their clinical implications. Moreover, these changes are occurring without any ongoing assessment of their implications for the quality of patient care. As discussed in Chapter 12, this situation should be changed.

EFFECTS OF REIMBURSEMENT ON INNOVATION

The committee also considered the effects of reimbursement on innovation. In general, economic discipline has encouraged cost-reducing, quality-enhancing technical change in the competitive dialysis equipment and supplies market. Such changes incorporate increased scientific and clinical knowledge about treatment as well as increased manufacturing knowledge. As a result, the equipment and supply (nonlabor) component of the total cost per dialysis treatment has fallen. Romeo (1984) estimated that the average price of all dialyzers purchased by hospitals from 11 manufacturers fell from an average of $20.10 in 1978 to $13.20 in 1983 when adjusted for inflation. Testimony before the February 1990 IOM public hearing indicated that the equipment and supply component fell from roughly one-third 15 years ago to one-fifth or less at present. Further cost-saving technical change, therefore, will afford smaller economic benefits to providers and payers.

Major clinical innovations, such as cyclosporine for preventing rejection of the transplanted kidney and erythropoietin for treating anemia in dialysis patients, have resulted from progress in basic scientific research. Such developments are not likely to be influenced by ESRD reimbursement policy. Major innovations with unequivocal clinical benefits, such as the two cited, will diffuse into practice; when necessary, HCFA has modified its reimbursement policy to encourage such major developments. On the other hand, targeted research and development efforts to improve the technical aspects of dialysis may be discouraged by the knowledge that they are unlikely to be used if they increase costs. In the past, reimbursement has not been increased to pay for small technical improvements.

The effect of Medicare reimbursement on innovation in the treatment of ESRD patients has not been examined systematically. It requires that distinctions be made between dialysis and transplantation, hemodialysis and peritoneal dialysis, incremental and major innovations, and periods of reimbursement policy. The IOM commissioned a paper (Levin et al., 1990) to assist it in this task, which, augmented by other sources, leads to the following appraisal.

Hemodialysis

Hemodialysis treatment systems have three major components: vascular access, surgically created, which allows the patient's blood to circulate repeatedly through the system; a semipermeable membrane blood path (known as the dialyzer) and connecting tubing; and a system that produces and monitors a dialyzing fluid (dialysate) to carry off toxins that diffuse from the blood through the membrane, that pumps blood through the dialyzer and monitors its pressure, and that operates alarms to protect against hazards in the operation of the dialysis system. Innovations have occurred in each of these elements over time.

Dialyzers have progressed from assembled structures of large volume and mediocre efficiency, to presterilized compact devices with much greater effectiveness. Geometries have included the coil, the flat plate, and hollow-fiber dialyzers, the last of which has dominated the market for more than a decade.

The development of high-efficiency polymer membranes, now termed "high flux" because of their rapid passage of water at low pressures, had to await the development of equipment capable of continuous monitoring and control of fluid removal since staff monitoring was unable to provide safe control. In addition, high rates of water and solute removal required a shift from acetate- to bicarbonate-based dialysate because the former, when used with high-flux membranes, caused discomfort or injury to the patient. In turn, systems were required to proportion the bicarbonate separately from other dialysate components since bicarbonate dialysate could not be stored for long periods. Dialysis machines are now usually computerized to control and monitor fluid removal and dialysate proportioning.

Initially, blood flow through the dialyzer was driven by the patient's own heart, but all current means of repeated dialysis use external blood pumps to drive blood through the system. The higher efficiency of water and solute transfer in the dialyzer has resulted in blood flow rates of 300 to 500 milliliters per minute (ml/min), up from the initial rate of 200 ml/min, with generally acceptable safety to and comfort for the patient.

Rapid dialysis treatments offer shorter time on dialysis, and thus more patient shifts per day. They also require staff that is able to respond to problems that develop quickly and demand immediate attention.

The prescription of dialysis therapy for each patient now spans a wider range of options than existed previously. Each prescription includes dietary instruction and monitoring, medications, and regular observation. Assessment of the actual and optimal amount of dialysis treatment administered in a session, a week, or a month is a source of controversy. The most accepted measure, based on urea removal by Kt/V calculation,[3] was developed through a clinical trial sponsored by the Artificial Kidney/Chronic Uremia program of NIH. This program was terminated before the study was completed and, consequently, further refinement of the method and validation in controlled circumstances did not occur.

The Interim Regulations of 1973 (38 Fed. Reg. 17210, June 29, 1973), which remained in effect for 10 years, appear to have affected innovation in several different ways. First, they imposed economic limits on all dialysis units and gave providers strong incentives to search for operational efficiencies. Provider incentives, in turn, encouraged manufacturers and suppliers to engage in substantial price competition in the competitive product market. In the main, the net effect appears to have been a period of useful cost-reducing, quality-enhancing technical change.

The Interim Regulations paid hospital-based outpatient units on a reasonable-cost basis not to exceed $138 per treatment unless an exception was granted. In fact, most hospital-based units received such exceptions and were being paid, on average, $159 per treatment by the early 1980s. This rate differential provided financial support for a limited amount of ESRD research in some academic institutions.

By the end of this period, the economic discipline imposed by a fixed payment rate stimulated many dialysis units to begin to reuse dialyzers. Dialyzer reuse reported to the Centers for Disease Control increased between 1983 and 1987 from less than 20 percent of facilities to more than 60 percent. Advances in the technology of dialyzer reprocessing allowed multiple uses of one dialyzer on a single patient to divide the dialyzer cost per treatment. Without reuse, the cost of the new polymer membranes would have precluded their widespread use. The hollow-fiber dialyzer configuration, which is compact and rigid, permits monitoring of reuse by uniform techniques.

Reuse was seen by some patients, however, as providers using second-hand goods to enhance profit, not patient care, and by others as potentially harmful. In most instances, open discussion between physicians and patients was effective in restoring confidence. Guidelines for the practice of reuse were developed by national consensus through the auspices of the Association for the Advancement of Medical Instrumentation (AAMI) and were a stimulus to ensuring quality control over reuse through standardized practices. AAMI guidelines were incorporated into regulations in 1988, and the reuse controversy receded.

The introduction of the composite rate in 1983 had several general effects on providers and, derivatively, on innovation. It increased the severity of the economic discipline on all providers, further encouraging the search for efficiency. It also reduced the differential between hospital-based and independent dialysis units substantially, thus eliminating any research support from this source.

Peritoneal Dialysis

The composite rate affected peritoneal dialysis differently than it did hemodialysis. Peritoneal dialysis had been used as therapy for acute renal failure since the 1960s, but despite its definition as a treatment for chronic renal failure by Tenckhoff and Schecter (1968), it was little used in the 1970s. Oreopolis and colleagues (1978) and Popovich and co-workers (1978) conceived of CAPD, which, despite its low efficiency, would be effective because of its continuous process and would require no hardware. The

FDA approved the use of CAPD in 1978. Baxter Laboratories introduced the first CAPD kit in 1979, the year following legislation that sought to encourage home dialysis.

CAPD appealed to HCFA as conceptually simple, possibly less costly than hemodialysis, and a way to encourage patients to dialyze at home. From 1979 until 1983, peritoneal dialysis was reimbursed on a cost basis. The composite rate, however, paid providers the same for an in-center and a home treatment, for both hemodialysis and peritoneal dialysis. The margins on CAPD fluids thus provided an economic incentive for its use, and as its clinical effectiveness improved, peritoneal dialysis became the treatment modality for more than 15 percent of patients.

Dialysis Research Support

The dialysis supply industry in the 1980s experienced substantial consolidation, consistent with the pattern that Romeo (1984) had anticipated earlier in the decade. The reduced sales volume resulting from reuse and the sustained pressure on prices left few resources for U.S. firms to pursue development of existing products or the discovery of new ones. In 1990, there were fewer firms worldwide than in 1980, and only a small number of these were American. Several U.S. firms have been acquired by European companies. Industrial investment in dialysis-related research and development has largely left the United States for Europe and Japan, where research costs are lower and where the industry has larger earnings.

Numerous innovations in membranes, dialysate, materials, and applications were supported from the mid-1960s to the early 1980s by the NIH Artificial Kidney/Chronic Uremia program mentioned above. That program was phased out in the 1980s, in part because NIH concluded that industrial research was supporting the development needs of clinical dialysis. From 1984 through 1989, the National Institute of Diabetes and Digestive and Kidney Diseases supported no clinical research in dialysis treatment. This has had several effects. First, the flow of research results and ideas into the dialysis clinical community effectively ceased. The quality control of medical practice that is exercised by clinical research and the example it sets were lost from that arena. For instance, just as the NCDS provided a rationale and method for prescription dialysis monitoring, the source of research support to test and validate the study's results dried up.

Second, the flow of research results to replenish the stock of ideas from which private firms draw inspiration for commercial products also ceased. The flow of results from publicly funded research results to private R&D and commercialization is complex, and the appropriate boundaries between the two sectors are never entirely clear. Yet the social rate of return on basic and applied research is estimated to exceed the return that private firms receive (Mansfield et al., 1977). This argues for public support of research. If no public research investment is forthcoming, industry is unlikely to make up the difference.

SUMMARY

1. Some data suggest that decreased reimbursement may increase mortality. This effect may be direct or indirect (decreased reimbursement led to shorter dialysis time, which in turn led to increased mortality). However, available studies are insufficient to conclusively establish either a direct or an indirect effect of reimbursement on mortality.

2. As with mortality, some studies suggest but do not prove a direct or indirect effect of decreased reimbursement to increase morbidity, assessed from hospitalization data.

3. Data strongly suggest that decreased reimbursement has led to decreased staffing in dialysis units, to shifts from nurses to technicians, and to important reductions in social worker and dietitian staffing. There is no evidence that these changes in staffing patterns have affected quality. However, professional opinion favors this contention.

4. Dialysis treatment time has decreased in the past decade. Studies indicate that decreased time may have adversely affected mortality and morbidity. The shorter times are attributable in part to economic pressure from decreased reimbursement. However, a clear relationship between quality and reimbursement cannot be established because clinical judgment and patient preference also have influenced shortening of dialysis times.

5. Reimbursement policy appears to have had mixed effects on innovation. Initially, payment policy encouraged cost-reducing technical change in equipment and supplies. More recently, reductions in reimbursement and elimination of support for dialysis research appear to be restricting further technical improvements. Reimbursement policy does not appear to have restricted the development of major new clinical innovations such as cyclosporine and erythropoietin. In these instances, policy has been modified to permit their use.

CONCLUSIONS

Taken together, available data suggest but do not prove conclusively that previous decreases in reimbursement may have adversely affected quality. Conclusive evidence is unlikely a priori. The question of reimbursement effects on quality has received little careful study. Existing data systems were not designed to measure reimbursement effects on quality. Moreover, because many other changes were occurring concurrently with changes in reimbursement (e.g., in the ESRD patient population and in professional opinion), only large effects of reimbursement would be detectable.

The lack of progressive improvement in age- and diagnosis-adjusted dialysis patient mortality over the past decade suggests the possibility that providers may have reached the limits of increasing efficacy in the application of current technology. It is possible that age- and diagnosis-adjusted mortality would have improved over the past decade, as has happened with other medical conditions, had reimbursement not been eroded by reductions and by inflation. Cuts in reimbursement may have limited the development and introduction of new techniques that require increased physician and staff time or capital investment.

Moreover, even if prior reductions in reimbursement had *no* effect, it does not follow logically that further decreases will not increase mortality. We may be at the edge of a "slippery slope," beyond which further cuts will have large effects because the ability of providers to absorb the effects of decreased resources without dangerously eroding quality have been reached. Because dialysis is a life-sustaining treatment, the committee concluded that it must give some weight even to imperfect data that point in the direction of adverse effects.

Taken together, the suggestive evidence deserves attention because all results point in the same direction (decreased reimbursement may have eroded quality). Changes in quality are related temporally to changes in reimbursement, and the underlying behavioral and physiological hypotheses are plausible. Although none of these studies constitute conclusive proof of the adverse effects of prior reductions in reimbursement on patient outcomes, none rule out such an effect and none suggest that reimbursement reductions are contributing to improved quality of care.

These data have important implications for reimbursement policy. Reimbursement issues are discussed and recommendations offered in Chapter 11.

NOTES

1. Inconsistencies in the reporting of HCFA data occurred simultaneously with this mortality shift and, consequently, the change is believed to be, in part, an artifact of the data system. The data in question involve mainly elderly patients and those for whom the primary diagnosis was missing. Although some of these problems can be controlled by statistical techniques, a residual difficulty remains in comparing patients' mortality risk in the years before and after this shift.

2. OBRA 1986, enacted in October of that year, in addition to limiting the HCFA-proposed $6 reduction in the composite rate to $2, also directed the Secretary of DHHS to request the National Academy of Sciences to propose a study "to evaluate the effects of reductions in the rates of payment for facility and physicians' services under the Medicare program for patients with end stage renal disease on their access to care or on the quality of care." This study was to be submitted to Congress by January 1, 1988. The combination of the time limits imposed by the statutory deadline and HCFA submission requirements (September 30, 1987) and the complexity of the subject led the Institute of Medicine to decline to do this study. HCFA then asked the Urban Institute to conduct the study. They did so

and submitted a final report to HCFA in December 1987. The Department of Health and Human Services publicly transmitted the report to Congress one year later on December 30, 1988.

3. A vigorous discussion about the adequacy (or the appropriate "dose") of dialysis treatment is occurring at present (Hull and Parker, 1990). This topic is not new, having been the subject a cooperative clinical trial conducted in the late 1970s, known as the National Cooperative Dialysis Study (NCDS). The NCDS reflected the desire of many clinicians to develop a quantitative approach to the prescription of an individualized dialysis "dose" and to develop clinical predictors of successful treatment. The NCDS published preliminary results in 1981 (Lowrie et al., 1981) and its major findings in 1983 (Lowrie and Laird, 1983).

The NCDS presented a complicated rationale and procedure for prescription dialysis that involved calculating and monitoring patients' nutritional status, the time-averaged concentration of urea (TAC_{urea}), and treatment time. The trial gave strong support to prescription dialysis and to a corollary message that sanctioned shorter treatment time. On the latter, the trial concluded that an adequate "dose" of dialysis could be achieved by calculating a patient-specific prescription and that the modeling required for such a prescription would "result in a smaller dose of therapy for a particular patient" than if it had not been done (Lowrie and Teehan, 1983). Although the other variables (nutrition, TAC_{urea}) were important, treatment time was the most easily controlled by clinicians.

Gotch and Sargent (1985) reanalyzed the NCDS data and developed their formulation for calculating adequate dialysis treatment: Kt/V, where K = dialyzer clearance, t = total treatment time at the prescribed blood and dialysate flow rates, and V = the estimated volume of urea as a function of patient muscle mass and body weight. They showed that the dialysis procedure could be performed more precisely and more efficiently to fit the needs of the individual patient and that shorter treatment time was adequate for some patients.

The findings of the NCDS and Gotch and Sargent coincided with the introduction of the composite rate in 1983 and the proposed reduction of 1986. Actual and proposed reimbursement policy encouraged the search for treatment efficiency and also intersected with the development of clinical opinion that, in effect, sanctioned shorter treatment time. Moreover, patient preferences, once shorter treatment became a clinical option, reinforced this development.

Entering the 1990s, prevailing clinical opinion about prescription dialysis, adequacy, and treatment time has been challenged. The papers by Held and colleagues (1990a) and Lowrie and Lew (1990) were cited in the text. The latter found that low serum albumin was associated most strongly with probability of death, suggesting that malnutrition, especially among older patients, may contribute to mortality. Lowrie and Lew conclude, among other things, that "short dialysis time should be prescribed with caution, and, if used with individual patients, the treatment should be carefully monitored and controlled" (Lowrie and Lew, 1990, p. 480).

In addition, Gotch and colleagues (1990) analyzed 101 transient patients treated by him in San Francisco and concluded that most prescription dialysis was empirical (i.e., did not use kinetic modeling), that half the prescriptions from these patients' home facilities were inadequate by NCDS criteria, and that length of dialysis was prescribed mainly as a function of BUN (with low BUN resulting in shorter treatment time). He described the relationship between the depressed appetite of dialysis patients, the poor nutrition of some patients, low BUN (which may follow from poor nutrition), and the consequent tendency to prescribe shorter treatment on the basis of BUN as a marker of adequacy as a "dangerous downward spiral."

Sargent (1990) examined the delivery of prescription dialysis for 297 patients in 48 treatment units and found that many dialyses "deviate significantly from the intended prescription," many falling outside NCDS guidelines because of poor treatment delivery. Two strategies for improving mortality, he concludes, are "(1) to aggressively monitor the delivery of treatment to assure that the intended dialysis is performed; and (2) to over-prescribe treatment to assure that even compromised dialyses still result in adequate therapy" (p. 509). Both strategies, it should be noted, have economic dimensions. The first requires greater clinical supervision; the second longer treatment times.

These developments make it imperative that the relationships among reimbursement, dialysis prescription (including treatment time), patients' nutritional status and preferences, and patient mortality be clarified in the 1990s.

4. The legislation of June 1978 called for a prospective reimbursement rate for outpatient dialysis. Although implementing regulations, proposed in 1980, were shelved by the new Reagan administration in 1981, OBRA 1981 restated the congressional requirement that HCFA establish a prospective rate. In February 1982, HCFA published a Notice of Proposed Rulemaking regarding the proposed reimbursement policy (47 Fed. Reg. 6556, February 12, 1982) and promulgated a final rule in May 1983 (48 Fed. Reg. 21255, May 11, 1983).

5. The committee hosted a workshop of nurses, social workers, and dietitians in November 1989 to discuss the implications of staffing changes. The participants in that workshop are listed in Appendix G. A draft paper was prepared and circulated for comment. Representatives of technicians also reviewed the document and provided useful information.

6. The State of California is an exception. Since 1982, it has required that dialysis units have a training and examination program, certified by the state, that includes fluids and electrolytes, kidney disease and treatment, dietary management, principles of dialysis, dialysis technology, and dialysis patient care.

7. The Board of Nephrology Nurses and Technicians offers a test to technicians who voluntarily choose to be examined. These test results, however, have no official status with any state regulatory body.

8. State health codes in Connecticut, New York, Texas, and elsewhere provide a focus for conflicts between nurses and technicians.

9. The survey was mailed to 1,576 facilities; responses were received from 345 social workers. Respondents' facilities included 6 for-profit hospital-based units, 113 not-for-profit hospital units, 163 independent for-profit units, and 41 independent not-for-profit units.

10. Individuals with experience in ESRD-related social work before 1976 but without MSW degrees were "grandfathered" into eligibility.

REFERENCES

ANNA (American Nephrology Nurses Association). 1985. 1985 head nurse survey results. ANNA Update. May-June.

Bowen OR. 1988. Report to Congress: Impact of the Changes in the ESRD Composite Rate. Washington, D.C.: Department of Health and Human Services. December.

CRN (Council on Renal Nutrition). 1990. CRN Membership Survey Results. New York: National Kidney Foundation.

Draper D, Kahn KL, Reinisch EJ, et al. 1990. Studying the effects of the DRG-based Prospective Payment System on quality of care. JAMA 264:1956-1961.

Garcia J, Held PJ, Cahn MA, Pauly MV. 1990. Staffing of dialysis units and the price of dialysis. Paper prepared for the Institute of Medicine ESRD Study Committee. Washington, D.C.: Urban Institute. January 18.

Gotch FA, Sargent JA. 1985. A mechanistic analysis of the National Cooperative Dialysis Study (NCDS). Kidney Int 28:526-534.

Gotch FA, Yarian S, Keen M. 1990. A kinetic survey of US hemodialysis prescriptions. Am J Kidney Dis 15:511-515.

Hakim R. 1989. Testimony presented to a public hearing of the IOM ESRD Study Committee. Chicago. May 5.

Held PJ, Bovbjerg RR, Pauly MV, Garcia JR, Newmann JM. 1987. Effects of the 1983 "Composite Rate" Changes on ESRD Patients, Providers, and Spending. Washington, D.C.: Urban Institute, December 21.

Held PJ, Garcia JR, Pauly MV, Cahn MA. 1990a. Price of dialysis, unit staffing, and length of dialysis treatments. Am J Kidney Dis 15:441-450.

Held PJ, Garcia JR, Pauly MV, Wolfe RA, Gaylin DS, Cahn MA. 1990b. Mortality and the price of dialysis. Paper prepared for the Institute of Medicine ESRD Study Committee. Washington, D.C.: Urban Institute. June 19.

Held PJ, Garcia JR, Wolfe RA, Gaylin DS, Pauly MV, Cahn MA. 1990c. Price of dialysis and hospitalization. Paper prepared for the Institute of Medicine ESRD Study Committee. Washington, D.C.: Urban Institute. June 19.

Hull AR, Parker TF. 1990. Introduction and Summary: Proceedings from the Morbidity, Mortality, and Prescription of Dialysis Symposium (Dallas, Tex., Sept. 15-17, 1989). Am J Kidney Dis 15:375-383.

Kahn KL, Rubenstein LV, Draper D. 1990a. The effects of the DRG-based Prospective Payment System on quality of care for hospitalized Medicare patients: An introduction to the series. JAMA 264:1953-1955.

Kahn KL, Rogers WH, Rubenstein LV, et al. 1990b. Measuring quality of care with explicit process criteria before and after implementation of the DRG-based Prospective Payment System. JAMA 264:1969-1973.

Kahn KL, Keeler EB, Sherwood MJ, et al. 1990c. Comparing outcomes of care before and after implementation of the DRG-based Prospective Payment System. JAMA 264:1984-1988.

Kanter A. 1989. Testimony presented to a public hearing of the IOM ESRD Study Committee. Chicago. May 5.

Keeler EB, Kahn KL, Draper D, et al. 1990. Changes in sickness at admission following the introduction of the Prospective Payment System. JAMA 264:1962-1968.

Klahr, Saulo, M.D., President, National Kidney Foundation. Letter of November 29, 1989, to Louis B. Hayes, Acting Administrator, Health Care Financing Administration.

Kosecoff J, Kahn KL, Rogers WH, Reinisch EJ, Sherwood MJ, Rubenstein LV, Draper D, Roth CP, Chew C, Brook RH. 1990. Prospective Payment System and impairment at discharge. JAMA 264:1980-1983.

Levin NW, Keshaviah P, Gotch FA. 1990. Effect of reimbursement on innovation in the ESRD program. Paper prepared for the Institute of Medicine ESRD Study Committee. New York: Beth Israel Medical Center.

Lowrie EG. 1989. Testimony presented to the IOM ESRD Study Committee. Chicago. May 5.

Lowrie EG, Laird NM, Parker TF, Sargent JA. 1981. Effect of the hemodialysis prescription on patient morbidity. N Engl J Med 305:1176-1181.

Lowrie EG, Laird NM (eds.). 1983. Cooperative Dialysis Study. Kidney Int 23(Suppl 13).

Lowrie EG, Lew NL. 1990. Death risk in hemodialysis patients: The predictive value of commonly measured variables and an evaluation of death rate differences between facilities. Am J Kidney Dis 15:458-482.

Lowrie EG, Teehan BP. 1983. Principles of prescribing dialysis therapy: Implementing recommendations from the National Cooperative Dialysis Study. Kidney Int 23(Suppl 13): S113-S122.

Mansfield E, Rapoport J, Romeo A, Wagner S, Beardsley G. 1977. Social and private rate of return from industrial innovations. Quarteerly J Econ 91(May):221-240.

Morford TG, Director, Health Standards and Quality Bureau, Health Care Financing Administration. Letter of March 15, 1990, to Saulo Klahr, M.D., President, National Kidney Foundation.

Oreopolis DG, Robson M, Isatt S, Clayton S, DeVeber GA. 1978. A simple and safe technique for continuous ambulatory peritoneal dialysis (CAPD). Trans Am Soc Artif Intern Organs 24:478.

Pollack VE, Pesce A. 1990. Analysis of data related to the 1976-1989 patient population: Treatment characteristics and patient outcomes. Report to the Institute of Medicine. Cincinnati: Dialysis Clinic, Inc.-Cincinnati.

Popovich RP, Moncrief JW, Nolph KD, et al. 1978. Continuous ambulatory peritoneal dialysis. Ann Intern Med 88:449.

Rogers WH, Draper D, Kahn KL, et al. 1990. Quality of care before and after implementation of the DRG-based Prospective Payment System. JAMA 264:1989-1994.

Romeo AA. 1984. The Hemodialysis Equipment and Disposables Industry. OTA-HCS-32. Washington, D.C.: Office of Technology Assessment.

Rubenstein LV, Kahn KL, Reinisch EJ, et al. 1990. Changes in quality of care for five disease measured by implicit review, 1981 to 1986. JAMA 264:1974-1979.

Sargent JA. 1990. Shortfalls in the delivery of dialysis. Am J Kidney Dis 15:500-510.

Smith, Wayne, Director, Office of Survey and Certification, Health Standards and Quality Bureau, Health Care Financing Administration. Letter of August 3, 1989, to Dolph R. Chianchiano, Associate Director, National Kidney Foundation.

Tenckhoff H, Schecter H. 1968. A bacteriologically safe peritoneal access device. Trans Am Soc Artif Intern Organs 14:181-183.

11

Outpatient Dialysis
Reimbursement Issues

This chapter deals with several of the controversial issues of outpatient dialysis facility reimbursement—the services covered in the composite rate, the rate-setting process, and payment policies. Issues of physician reimbursement for outpatient dialysis treatment are also briefly discussed.

The committee was guided in its deliberations by the criteria that ESRD payment policies and the rate-setting process should

- promote the appropriate level of care;
- ensure access to good quality care;
- encourage cost-effective delivery of care;
- recognize justifiable differences in costs among facilities, types of patients, and treatment modalities in the provision of ESRD services;
- facilitate the adoption of cost-effective new treatment technologies and procedures; and
- promote administrative simplicity.

COVERED SERVICES IN THE COMPOSITE RATE

The IOM committee considered two basic approaches to defining the services that should be included under the composite rate for outpatient dialysis:

- continued reliance on the current HCFA method of definition, which is basically empirical and implicit; and
- a more explicit, regular redefinition using a normative method and the services of a technical advisory committee.[1]

In general, under a prospective payment system, covered services must be defined before a rate can be established. From the outset of the ESRD program, the outpatient dialysis facility reimbursement rate has been an all-inclusive payment for a comprehensive "bundle" of institutional and home dialysis services, including nursing services, supplies, equipment, drugs, and administration associated with a dialysis treatment episode. Dialysis and kidney transplantation services covered by Medicare are currently specified in Chapter 27 of the *Medicare Provider Reimbursement Manual*, as "Reimbursement for ESRD and Transplant Services."[2] Chapter 27 includes instructions and procedures regarding payment for home and in-center dialysis treatment; the ESRD items and services included under the composite rate; other ESRD items and services that are separately billable, such as laboratory tests, injectable drugs, and blood furnished to dialysis patients; the calculation and payment of bad debt; recordkeeping and submission of cost reports; the exceptions process; and the appeals process.

An item or service included under the composite rate is paid for through the composite rate payment to the facility, unless specifically excluded. Inclusion of an item or service under the composite rate does not depend on how frequently it is needed or the number of dialysis patients who require it. Items or services not included under the composite rate are covered only if they are *not* part of a routine dialysis service and have been listed as billable.

The current HCFA approach to stipulating the services to be included within the composite rate is largely empirical and involves several steps. First, the *Medicare Provider Reimbursement Manual* (HCFA, 1989) lists the general services that are to be included in the composite rate in terms of those historically determined by providers as necessary; HCFA modifies the list over time as clinical knowledge and practice change. This list does not specify a quality standard regarding services to be delivered, but relies on providers to set an implicit standard, with the specific mix of services to be determined by each provider. Although Medicare regulations establish some structural standards for care, and state health code requirements set additional standards (mostly structural), none of these efforts attempts to describe what an adequate set of dialysis services includes.

Second, HCFA establishes the reimbursement rate on the basis of audited facility costs and proposes revisions on the basis of subsequent cost reports. Although the processes for revising the composite rate are controversial, as discussed below, they are relatively well understood. No formal processes exist for periodically relating changes in the services included under the composite rate to the reimbursement rate itself. Under such an arrangement, providers cannot be certain that reimbursement rates will be set at a level that is sufficient to meet the costs of a continually changing high-quality "bundle of services" that they consider necessary. On the other hand, there is currently no guarantee against some providers sacrificing the quality of services for economic reasons.

A normative approach, by contrast, would specify a detailed bundle of services to be included within the composite rate, with reference to an explicit quality standard. A payment rate would then be determined by pricing the services required for that bundle. The bundle of services would be revised periodically in response to clinical and technological changes, with the composite rate changed as appropriate. Under this approach, individual providers would have less freedom to allocate resources in accordance with their own judgments about what services were needed. The system also would be very complex, administered centrally, and would probably require a continuing expert advisory panel.

The concern of providers with how the services currently included in the composite rate are determined centers on the fact that these have changed over time as clinical practice and technology have changed. Although these changes are reflected to some extent by HCFA modifications to Chapter 27 of the *Provider Reimbursement Manual*, providers identify several objections with the process by which HCFA makes such changes.

First, since the introduction of the composite rate, some services previously billable by providers have been incorporated into the composite rate base. For example, intermediaries have disallowed separate reimbursement for mileage to transport blood for transfusions, drugs and blood products such as Benadryl and albumin, antibiotics for home patients, and a separate handling charge for drawing or collecting laboratory specimens at ESRD facilities.

Second, some services that have been introduced into the routine clinical treatment of dialysis patients since 1983 are not included in the composite rate. Examples are the use of urokinase to declot vascular access catheters and the administration of parenteral nutrition during dialysis. The supplies for these services are separately billable, but staff time to administer them is compensated under the composite rate. If a patient needs a subclavian catheter declotted, that service must be provided; if intradialytic parenteral nutrition is required, it must be provided. But the distribution of these demands on facilities varies as a function of patient complexity, and facilities are paid the same whether or not they are required to provide these services. In this way, necessary clinical decisions may impose an uncompensated cost on a facility. Data on the financial impact of such services on dialysis facilities, however, have not been collected.

Some providers believe that a serious problem has arisen because the type and amount of services required by dialysis patients have changed over time, but that HCFA's failure to modify the composite rate to reflect such changes constitutes an implicit rate reduction. However, other providers contend that the complaints are about items or services required by only a few patients, and that HCFA is justified in leaving the payment rate unchanged.

The current system creates an incentive for providers to unbundle the dialysis service package to the extent possible. For example, some services previously provided by an outpatient dialysis unit, such as physical therapy or counseling, are now provided to patients via non-ESRD-related outpatient services. Therefore, they can be billed separately from the composite rate. However, this may mean that ESRD patients will find it necessary to make multiple visits to various providers in order to obtain the full range of services that they need and to which they are entitled. If so, this may not be cost-effective and may be clinically deleterious. National data on such behavior do not exist.

It is difficult to evaluate these provider concerns, since data are not readily available to substantiate their views. However, DCI-Cincinnati (DCI-C) provided data on injections of medications administered to all the hemodialysis patients treated in its freestanding and hospital facilities over four consecutive 3-year periods: 1978-80, 1981-83, 1984-86, and 1987-89 (Pollack and Pesce, 1990). From 1978 to 1989, the average number of medications administered per patient increased dramatically by nearly ninefold, excluding erythropoietin (EPO), and over 17-fold including EPO (Table 11-1). Although the committee heard testimony that supports the data presented by DCI-C, aggregate data on medications do not exist.

Such increases in the number of injections, particularly of complex medications, result in part from the availability of new drugs developed in recent years. The use of these medications also reflects the increasingly complex needs of patients, both at the time they begin treatment and as they grow older on maintenance dialysis. The increase in injections places a growing demand on the time of unit personnel that significantly affects their work load.

The total bundle of services currently provided to dialysis patients has been determined in important ways by the expectation of providers that Medicare reimbursement in real dollars will be decreased each year. Thus, to survive economically, providers must provide care within diminishing real levels of Medicare reimbursement. They have done so partly by increasing efficiency and by innovations. However, these processes may not have adequately compensated for decreasing real resources. Core medical services needed to maintain life have been provided but some important support services such as nutrition education, physical therapy, and counseling have been reduced. (See Chapter 10.)

The committee is concerned that medical services may continue to decrease if the rate remains constant over time. Efficiency gains and service reductions lead to decreased costs reported to HCFA. Lower reported costs are then used to calculate a new, reduced base composite rate without reference to any quality standard.

TABLE 11-1 Injections for Per Year Complex Medications, Hemodialysis Outpatients, University of Cincinnati Medical Center and Dialysis Clinic, Inc.-Cincinnati, 1978-1989

	1978-80	1981-83	1984-86	1987-89
Patients treated	213	232 (8.9)[a]	258 (11.2)	299 (15.9)
Injections (total)				
Without EPO[b]	155	342 (120.6)	1,432 (318.7)	2,038 (42.3)
With EPO	155	342 (120.6)	1,432 (318.7)	3,879 (170.9)
Injections (average) per patient				
Without EPO	0.7	1.5 (102.6)	5.6 (276.5)	6.8 (22.8)
With EPO	0.7			13.0 (133.7)

[a]Figures in parentheses are percentage increase over the prior period.
[b]EPO = erythropoietin. EPO became available in the last half of 1989.

SOURCE: Pollack and Pesce, 1990.

THE RATE-SETTING PROCESS

The HCFA rate-setting process has been criticized on several grounds, including the timeliness of the cost data, the representativeness of the sample of facilities used to determine costs, the adequacy of Medicare cost accounting principles, the basis for calculating the facilities' average costs per dialysis treatment on which the rate is based, and the oversight of the process.

Timeliness of Cost Data

This issue involves technical as well as policy considerations. The lack of timely Medicare cost report data is due to the lag of 3 to 4 years between the audit year and the effective date of a new payment rate. The cost reports used to set the rate in 1983, for example, reflect resources consumed in 1977, 1978, and 1979.[3]

Technically, there are inherent limits on acquiring timely cost data. Cost reports are submitted by facilities to their fiscal intermediary each year within 90 days of the end of their accounting year. Facilities have accounting years, however, that do not necessarily coincide with the federal fiscal year. Even though submitted (reported) cost data can be available for audit analysis by HCFA within 6 months after the end of a facility's accounting period, assembling a representative sample of facilities will require more time.

The Prospective Payment Assessment Commission (ProPAC), dealing with a similar issue for the entire hospital sector, has suggested several ways to shorten the time required to generate Medicare audited cost report data. These methods may apply to dialysis facilities as well: shorten the 90-day intermediary processing period, reduce the time dialysis facilities are allowed for the preparation of cost reports, require facilities to submit cost reports in machine-readable form, collect cost report data from an "early returns" sample of facilities (those with accounting years closer to the federal fiscal year), or use the unaudited costs submitted by facilities.

In fact, the technical aspects are secondary. Electronic data submission, for example, does not increase the amount of data available for analysis or overcome the primary cause of delay in making data available. The basic policy problem that underlies provider criticism of HCFA is that *the current rate-setting process for dialysis facilities, unlike that for the hospital sector, makes no provision for adjusting the cost data between the audit period and the date that a new payment rate is adopted.* Unless this policy issue is addressed, the criticism will persist.

Sampling Versus the Universe

Another rate-setting issue involves sampling. HCFA audits a sample of approximately 120 dialysis outpatient units; as of April 1990, it had performed four separate national audits on these facilities. A letter from Bernadette S. Schumaker, HCFA Bureau of Policy Development, describing these four ESRD audits appears as Appendix 1 to this chapter. Technically, it is feasible to audit the cost reports of all 1,900 renal dialysis facilities. The PPS experience with the hospital sector is illustrative since the original PPS standardized amounts were computed using cost report information for all hospitals in 1981.

Using the cost reports of all dialysis facilities to determine the rate would eliminate questions about the representativeness of the sample and increase provider trust. Auditing all dialysis units would probably require facilities to submit their cost report information electronically, something that began to occur in 1987. At the very least, the sampling process should be explicitly described in proposed rules, with opportunity for providers to comment.

Medicare Part A Cost Principles

These cost principles govern the reporting of costs by facilities and the auditing of costs by fiscal intermediaries and by HCFA. Audited cost data are then used in rate setting. Controversy over the application of the Medicare Part A Cost Principles to ESRD providers focuses on which costs are allowable and which are not.

Medicare cost principles involve determination about which costs are necessary and proper and related to the care of beneficiaries. Medicare defines the allowable costs of dialysis services to include those that are directly attributable to the provision of dialysis services and the proportionate share of indirect costs, such as administration and occupancy (space, equipment, depreciation, and utilities) that are appropriately covered by its payments. These principles were developed in 1965 at the inception of Medicare to determine the reasonable costs of hospital medical services. From 1965 to 1983, when all hospitals operated under retrospective, cost-based reimbursement, it was necessary for Medicare to define carefully both what was meant by "reasonable costs" and how these were to be allocated to Medicare. With the advent of PPS in 1983, however, and reliance on DRGs as the basis for payment, these cost principles have become less important to hospitals, especially since the initial PPS cost base of 1981 has never been rebased, only updated. More frequent rebasing, of course, would increase the importance of the cost reports.

Renal providers argue that accounting rules designed for hospitals in 1965 are inappropriate for dialysis facilities in 1990. In general, dialysis providers believe that the Medicare definitions of allowable costs are too restrictive, unreasonable, or inconsistent with other federal government requirements. As indicated in Chapter 6, the dialysis provider community consists increasingly of independent rather than hospital-based units. In financial management terms, these facilities operate much like businesses.

A number of renal providers who testified at the committee's February 1990 rate-setting public hearing argued that generally accepted accounting principles (GAAP) should be used rather than Medicare Part A Cost Principles. GAAP rules and procedures are widely used by most private businesses for preparing and reporting financial information to management, owners, the Internal Revenue Service, the Securities and Exchange Commission, and other regulatory agencies. The use of GAAP, proponents argue, would result in a more comprehensive presentation of independent dialysis unit operations than does reliance on the Medicare Part A Cost Principles.[4]

HCFA responds that requiring all dialysis facilities to report costs according to Medicare cost principles allows it to compare costs across independent and hospital-based units in a standard way. The use of GAAP, however, would make it impossible to compare the costs of independent and hospital-based facilities, since the hospitals' statements report total operations and not individual departments.

Any accounting system, in fact, is a set of conventions for reporting financial transactions to multiple users—managers, directors, shareholders, or public officials. Such systems provide consistency on certain matters, flexibility on others; all have their arbitrary features. Some accounting practices are very technical; many involve policy considerations.[5]

Clearly, Medicare must apply the same accounting principles to all health care providers with which it deals—hospitals, skilled nursing facilities, and independent renal treatment units. Moreover, any accounting system requires that prior policy decisions be made about allowable and nonallowable costs. Finally, conflict is inherent in the relationships of payers and claimants in any accounting system.

Notwithstanding these general comments about accounting systems, several examples of substantive conflict between HCFA and ESRD providers have been identified. These include the allocation of utility costs on the basis of the square feet occupied rather than on actual use; the depreciation of capital assets over an 8-year period, whereas the Internal Revenue Service permits varying depreciation rates depending on the nature and effective life of the asset; and the reporting of pension costs, where ERISA requires that employers escrow funds for future employee pension benefits on an accrual basis, but Medicare recognizes such costs only when they are actually spent.

Procedural issues include variation in the application of Medicare rules across fiscal intermediaries; the limited recourse that providers have to correct errors in reported costs or to challenge the results of audited costs;[6] and the limited incentives of ESRD providers, save the large chains, to report costs accurately since payment is not contingent on such data and the likelihood of being included in an audit sample is low.

The Calculation of Cost per Treatment

The 1983 composite rate was based on the per-treatment cost of the median dialysis facility in the HCFA audit sample. This did not account for differences among facilities in number of patients or treatments. In 1986, therefore, HCFA proposed to calculate the rate on the basis of the median cost per treatment for all facilities, thus across the entire sampled patient population. HCFA's rationale was that costs per treatment were more accurately reflected by the median costs of all treatments rather than by those of the median facility.

This proposed change, however, became enmeshed in the controversy surrounding the 1986 proposal to reduce the base composite rate on average by $6. Providers argued that the underlying motivation for the HCFA proposal was an effort to reduce the program expenditures by $100 million in response to the Office of Management and Budget. The strong negative reaction led Congress to limit the reduction to $2 and leave unchanged the methodology of the 1983 composite rate as the basis for calculating the cost per treatment.

Regarding the proposed 1986 methodology, a composite rate calculated on the basis of the median costs of all treatments encourages facilities to search for economies of scale. Although this would adversely affect smaller facilities, no major policy issue is raised by this proposed methodology save for rural units whose size is limited by low population density.

Oversight of the Rate-Setting Process

The committee believes that the process by which HCFA revises ESRD reimbursement rates needs to be open and reviewable. HCFA had previously taken the position that methodology changes required notice and comment, but rate changes per se required only formal notice. The law now requires HCFA to use full notice-and-comment rulemaking procedures when modifying rates, a requirement that the committee endorses.

During the course of this study, especially at the February 1990 public hearing, various proposals for oversight of the Medicare ESRD rate-setting process were suggested. Most of these recommended the involvement of an objective, competent third party, such as an independent body consisting of major accounting firms, an "ESRD ProPAC," or ProPAC itself assuming periodic, but not necessarily annual, advisory responsibility for ESRD rate-setting similar to its hospital-sector responsibilities.

The committee, deliberating in 1989 and 1990, regarded the ProPAC option as the most attractive alternative, especially since its mission was being expanded to include the reimbursement of hospital ambulatory care as well as inpatient care. In fact, after the committee's final meeting in October 1990, Congress, in OBRA 1990, directed ProPAC to study the cost, services, and profit associated with dialysis treatment modalities. The statute directed ProPAC to consider the conclusions and recommendations of this study. ProPAC was also to recommend the method of payment for the facility component of outpatient dialysis services for fiscal 1993 and the methodology for updating payments in subsequent years.

FACILITY PAYMENT POLICY ISSUES

This section examines the following issues of outpatient dialysis payment policy: the level of payment, the dual rate for hospital-based and independent facilities, rebasing and updating the rate, and the labor portion of the rate.

Level of Payment

Although the outpatient dialysis reimbursement rate has fallen steadily over time (in real dollars), treatment units have remained financially solvent by obtaining lower equipment and supply costs from competition in the product market and by dialyzer reuse; achieving unit operational efficiencies including reduction in the duration of dialysis treatment; changing staff size and mix; reducing noncritical services such as nutrition and counseling; and realizing economies of scale in treatment units, chains of units, and vertically integrated firms.

In February 1990, at the IOM public hearing on rate setting, many providers indicated that they are at the point where the quality even of core medical services is threatened because further economies and efficiencies are limited or impossible. For example, Community Dialysis Center (CDC), of Cleveland, Ohio, a not-for-profit independent facility then operating 41 stations, 4 patient shifts per day, with a census of 335 patients, testified to this effect (DeOreo, 1990):

As long as continued productivity increases are feasible, it is reasonable to have a relatively fixed rate. In recent years, however, it is clear that the potential for productivity increases has been restricted substantially by (1) our past success in obtaining efficiencies, (2) the increasingly more difficult mix of patients, (3) restrictions on primary care access outside the dialysis system, (4) the slowing of the evolution of technology, (5) limits to the physical process of dialysis. Declining payment coupled with additional cost increases from waste disposal, regulatory procedures and requirements with regard to normal activities, plus the introduction of erythropoietin, EPO, have put our future financial stability in some question.

HCFA, however, has consistently maintained that the costs of dialysis treatment units fall below their payments. HCFA provided the IOM with 1985 reported (unaudited) and audited cost data and 1987 reported cost data for the sample of treatment facilities on which the composite rate is based. An analysis of these data for 1985 goes far to explain the HCFA point of view.

The HCFA data for 1985 audited costs, reported costs, and facility-specific composite rates for the 124 treatment units in the audit sample (62 hospital-based and 62 independent facilities) show the following: dialysis facilities provided treatment at an audited cost, on average, that is lower than their facility-specific composite rate, the mean difference exceeding $8 (Table 11-2).

The differences between audited costs and facility-specific composite rates, however, vary greatly among the sampled facilities. Twenty-five percent of the facilities had rates that were $30 above their audited costs, and 10 percent had rates nearly $50 greater than costs. At the other end of the distribution, however, 10 percent had rates that were almost $30 below their costs.

Independent and hospital-based outpatient units also differ substantially. Rates exceeded audited costs for nearly all independent units, on average, by $29 per treatment (Table 11-2). For hospital-based units, however, on average, the cost per treatment was $12 greater than their Medicare rate (Table 11-2). For only about 40 percent of these units did rates exceed audited costs.

TABLE 11-2 Outpatient Dialysis Facilities, 1985: Distribution of Differences (in dollars) Between Facility-Specific Composite Rates and Audited Costs

Facility Group	Number in Sample	Mean Difference	Percentile 10th	25th	50th	75th	90th
All facilities	124	8.38	-28.97	-7.67	14.09	30.10	47.64
Hospital units	62						
Center + home	62	-12.46	-49.11	-23.92	-5.04	10.76	21.12
Center only	62	-16.83	-62.18	-28.98	-8.99	7.33	19.22
Home only	37	5.23	-62.42	-3.10	18.26	26.98	38.18
Independent units	62						
Center + home	62	29.21	6.88	17.32	28.50	44.66	53.39
Center only	62	28.69	5.08	14.18	28.65	46.34	55.76
Home only	35	25.84	-9.69	10.24	33.07	44.53	50.86

SOURCE: Health Care Financing Administration, Bureau of Policy Development. HCFA cost report data from 124 audit sample facilities.

If reported (unaudited) costs of the sampled facilities are compared to facility-specific composite rates, the 1985 data show that the average facility lost about $2 per treatment (Table 11-3). However, the distribution by independent and hospital-based units is again substantial: payments exceed reported costs in over 50 percent of independent units, but in less than 40 percent of hospital-based units.

The differences between reported and audited costs are also substantial, especially between independent and hospital-based units. On average, Medicare disallowed more than 15 percent of the reported costs of independent facilities. By contrast, on average, the reported costs of hospital-based units were adjusted *upward* by more than 2 percent.

On the basis that audited costs reflect true costs, HCFA claims that the majority of outpatient dialysis treatment units are doing well financially, i.e., their facility-specific composite rates exceed their audited costs. HCFA argues that independent units are doing quite well and that hospital-based units reflect inefficiencies.

Providers respond with several arguments. First, on the cost side, they contend that audited (or allowable) costs, defined by HCFA in accordance with Medicare Part A Cost Principles, significantly and deliberately understate their true costs. Second, on the revenue side, they argue that HCFA, which pays 80 percent of the composite rate, assumes that facilities receive 100 percent payment while making it very difficult to collect bad debt under the Part A Cost Principles.[7]

Finally, and more fundamentally, providers argue that the imperatives of economic survival as business enterprises force them to maintain costs that are equal to or lower than their revenues or face bankruptcy. To the extent that the Medicare payment rate determines their revenues,[8] which it does in large measure, their reported costs will always fall below the composite rate. Many providers also contend that reimbursement rate reductions have forced compromises over time in treatment methods and staffing in order to maintain costs at or below revenues. They are victims, they argue, of a vicious cycle that cannot be interrupted: Declining real reimbursement rates force providers to reduce their expenditures (costs); these translate into lower reported and, ultimately, audited costs; lower audited costs, in turn, are used as the basis for proposed rate reductions.

The differences between HCFA and the providers cannot be resolved, then, simply by the examination of cost report data done by the committee. If audited costs do not reflect true costs, then careful attention to the accounting issues is necessary. If audited costs do reflect true costs, it is still necessary to relate payments and costs to patient outcomes. Such efforts will require adequate measures of quality, which are unavailable at present.

The limited data currently available suggest that prior reductions in reimbursement may already have affected patient outcomes adversely. (See

TABLE 11-3 Outpatient Dialysis Facilities, 1985: Distribution of Differences (in dollars) Between Facility-Specific Composite Rates and Reported (unaudited) Costs

Facility Group	Number in Sample	Mean Difference	Percentile					
			10th	25th	50th	75th	90th
All facilities[a]	124	-1.79	-37.10	-20.11	5.71	21.04	35.62
Hospital units	62	-14.28	-44.26	-29.72	-7.05	12.44	34.06
Independent units	62	10.71	-14.43	-5.1	12.43	25.86	35.89

[a]Data include in-center dialysis costs only; home dialysis cost data were not available.

SOURCE: Health Care Financing Administration, Bureau of Policy Development, 1985, cost report data for 124 sample facilities.

Chapter 10.) If data are acquired that systematically relate costs to outcomes, then two possibilities must be considered. First, if the data show that providers can deliver high-quality care at low cost, there is every reason for public policy to reflect this in lower reimbursement rates. On the other hand, if providers reporting low costs are delivering poor quality of care, there is no reason to permit that to continue. The committee (Chapter 12) recommends that HCFA examine high- and low-cost units in relation to the quality of care they are providing.

Dual Composite Rate

OBRA 1981 required that separate composite rates be established for hospital-based and independent outpatient dialysis units. Currently, the average base rates are $125 and $121, respectively. HCFA determines the rate differential for hospital-based units by adjusting the median cost per treatment for all units for two factors: an overhead cost differential of $2.10 for hospitals above that for all facilities; and a 5 percent add-on to adjust for possible deficiencies in the data and to mitigate the effects of the composite rate on hospitals. These adjustments are not based on an assessment of the cost data for each type of facility and were probably derived after the $4 differential was determined.

The HCFA 1985 data indicate that the reported (unaudited) and audited costs per treatment for hospital-based units were significantly higher than for independent facilities. Mean audited costs were $144 and $99 for hospital-based and independent units, respectively (Table 11-4). Reported costs for hospital facilities were adjusted upward 2 percent in the audit, whereas they were adjusted downward 15 percent for independent units. Audited costs were $112 at the 10th percentile and $185 at the 90th percentile for hospital-based facilities, compared to $71 and $124 for the same percentiles for independent units.

On average, hospital-based facilities provided dialysis at an audited cost $17 above the Medicare payment (composite rate) per treatment; independent units, by comparison, provided dialysis at an audited cost of $29 below the Medicare rate. Obviously, based on this audited cost information, very different rates would result if the rates for hospital-based and independent facilities were calculated separately rather than on the basis of pooled data.

The differences between the costs of outpatient dialysis treatment in independent and hospital-based units are not fully understood. However, not all hospital-based units are the same. Some provide backup services that are essential to the safe and effective performance of independent units, which are not equipped to care for very unstable or acutely ill patients. Others are simply hospital-owned outpatient facilities, often physically separate from the parent hospital, that provide the same services as independent units.

TABLE 11-4 Outpatient Dialysis Facilities, 1985: Comparison of Differences Between Reported (unaudited) and Audited Costs (in dollars)

Facility Group	Number in Sample	Average Costs per Treatment		Differences Between Reported and Audited Costs		Average Composite Rate
		Reported	Audited	Dollars	Percentage	
All facilities	124	131.18	123.46	-7.72	-6	129.39
Hospital-based	62	145.61	148.16	2.55	2	131.33
Independent	62	116.75	98.77	-17.98	-15	127.46

NOTE: Data include in-center dialysis costs only; home dialysis cost data were not available.

SOURCE: Health Care Financing Administration, Bureau of Policy Development, 1985 cost report data for 124 audit sample facilities.

There is no apparent basis for different payment rates for the same service, such as chronic dialysis, based on ownership of the facility. Further study is needed to justify existing payment differences.

However, it is appropriate to pay a higher rate to hospital backup units, althought this is not currently done. Hospital backup units care for inpatients as well as outpatients. Most of their patients receive routine care in another outpatient facility and receive only transient care for special problems in the hospital unit. Caring for new ESRD patients, pediatric patients, and unstable or acutely ill patients is an essential service that permits the provision of safe and efficient outpatient service in independent units. Backup facilities must maintain the capacity to deal with such problems. Thus, they cannot sustain the efficient utilization of stations, and their costs per dialysis treatment are higher. The overhead costs associated with an acute-care hospital providing a wide range of services add to an increased cost per dialysis in this setting. If expenses are incurred for the training of physicians and other clinical personnel, these must be reimbursed if the service is to continue. Some definition of backup units providing these higher levels of care is necessary to fairly reimburse them for their treatment and to support independent units.

HCFA should provide separate rates for special services, however, or for patients who require additional services. In this category, *the IOM committee calls attention to the extra medical, nursing, nutrition, and counseling services required for adequate care of children and supports a rate differential for pediatric patients.*

Rebasing and Updating

The implications of rebasing or updating the composite rate need to be clarified. *Rebasing* means revising or recalculating the existing reimbursement rate using more recent cost data. The current base composite dialysis rates, established in 1983 and later modified by OBRA 1986, OBRA 1989, and OBRA 1990, are derived from 1977, 1978, and 1979 cost data. They have never been rebased, although adoption of the 1986 HCFA proposal would have done so. *Updating* refers to adjusting the base rate annually by some factor to account for changes in input prices, patient complexity (case mix), or scientific and technological advances that occur in the years in which the rate is not rebased. Neither the composite rate nor its predecessor has ever been updated.

By comparison, although the Medicare prospective payment rates have also never been rebased from their original 1981 cost data, they are updated annually to adjust for inflation, patient case mix, and scientific advancement. Each of these factors is discussed below.

Inflation (or Market Basket)

Historically, HCFA has not adjusted the ESRD composite rate for inflation. The absence of such an adjustment may have had a larger economic effect over time than specific rate reductions in withdrawing real resource inputs from dialysis providers.

HCFA was criticized, for example, for failing to inflate the 1982 cost data in establishing its 1986 rate reduction proposal. It responded that no adjustment was made because no evidence existed that the overall cost of furnishing dialysis followed general price inflation. HCFA further stated that some inputs to the dialysis service appear to have increased in price (e.g., salaries), but other inputs have decreased (e.g., dialyzer prices have decreased by between 30 to 50 percent).

HCFA's response does not reflect an explicit analysis of input prices over time. The policy issue, therefore, is whether HCFA should develop a specific market-basket index for ESRD dialysis services that would take into account cost increases as well as decreases. If it chooses not to develop a dialysis index, it would seem logical to apply the same index as a basis for public policy. *Absent empirical data to support the view that the cost of an adequate "bundle of dialysis services" can be expected to decrease each year enough to compensate for annual, real-dollar decreases in payment rates, failure to update can only be regarded as arbitrary.*

Patient Complexity (Case Mix)

No adjustment is made in the dialysis payment rate for patient complexity. Respondents to the 1986 proposed rate reduction argued that the patient mix was then more expensive to treat than the 1982 patient population: For example, there were more aged patients, more diabetic patients, and increasing numbers with HIV infection and AIDS, requiring isolation.

Currently, there are no adequate means to adjust for patient complexity or severity. (See the discussion in Chapter 12 on a strategy to address this situation.) Although all signs point in the direction of increased patient complexity, the claims of providers to this effect cannot be strongly supported because adequate measures have not been developed, and supporting data have not been collected. HCFA, in 1986, rejected the argument of increasing severity as a consideration for rate revision.

The exceptions process, by which facilities seek adjustment to their composite rate, does acknowledge patient complexity in a minimal way. The exceptions criteria include atypical service intensity (patient mix), extraordinary circumstances, isolated essential facilities, self-dialysis training costs, frequency of dialysis, and education costs. To establish atypical service intensity, providers must show that they provide more intense services for patients referred from another facility for stabilization, pediatric patients who require more intensive staff services, or patients with medical conditions not commonly treated by ESRD facilities and which complicate dialysis treatment (48 Fed. Reg. 21279, May 11, 1983).

The burden of proof for demonstrating an atypical patient mix falls on the provider. No formal measures of patient severity or complexity exist. However, informal, unpublished criteria screens are used to determine whether an exceptions request should be reviewed. These screens, which are quite inadequate as adjusters for severity or complexity, include comparisons of a unit's patient population to the entire patient population in terms of age, percent diabetic, days of hospitalization, and mortality.

Technological Advances and Productivity

HCFA makes no adjustment to the composite rate for scientific and technological advances. For example, high-flux dialysis and prescription dialysis may improve quality but may also increase cost. Similarly, Gotch (Levin et al., 1990) has argued that the use of kinetic modeling as the basis for prescribing dialysis has been inhibited because its cost is not compensated in the composite rate.

HCFA selectively recognized technological change in its rationale for the 1983 composite rate. This decreased rate was justified, it stated, "because increased efficiencies in the technology and delivery of services have offset the cost increases of some components of the services" (48 Fed. Reg. 21259, May 11, 1989). A more systematic acknowledgment for such change, which may increase or decrease costs, is warranted.

Methods for Rebasing and Updating

Substantial differences in the composite rate will result depending on the approach used for rebasing and updating. The rate also will depend on the base year selected. For example, the IOM project staff used the 1985 cost data to develop a base rate for 1988, with varying assumptions about bases and updating factors (Table 11-5). The hypothetical 1988 average composite rate for all dialysis facilities varied from a low of $101.19 to a high of $148.06, a spread of $47—depending on the base rate and update factor used. The analysis in Table 11-5 does not calculate separate rates on the basis of different costs of hospital-based and independent facilities. Were calculations of separate rates made on the basis of the audited costs of these two groups of facilities, they would differ dramatically from the current dual rates, which permit only a fixed $4 differential.

TABLE 11-5   Results of Alternative Scenarios for Rebasing and Updating
the ESRD Composite Rate for All Dialysis Facilities

Scenarios	1985	1986	1987	1988	1989
Current rate	129.39	129.39	127.39	127.39	127.39
Base = Current rate Updated by:					
CPIU[a]	129.39	131.85	136.59	142.20	149.02
Hospital MB[b]	129.39	133.40	138.07	144.56	152.37
PPS update factor[c]	129.39	130.04	131.53	133.28	134.45
PPS payments/case[d]	129.39	133.79	139.94	148.06	NA
Base = Costs Updated by:					
CPIU	121.01	123.31	127.75	132.99	139.37
Hospital MB	121.01	124.76	129.13	135.20	142.50
PPS update factor	121.01	121.62	123.01	124.65	125.75
PPS payments/case	121.01	125.12	130.88	138.47	NA
Base = Independents' rate Updated by:					
CPIU	98.24	100.11	103.71	107.96	113.14
Hospital MB	98.24	101.29	104.83	109.76	115.68
PPS update factor	98.24	98.73	99.87	101.19	102.09
PPS payments/case	98.24	101.58	106.25	112.42	NA

[a]CPIU = Consumer Price Index, Urban - all areas.
[b]Hospital MB = hospital market basket.
[c]PPS update factor = Prospective Payment System update factor.
[d]PPS payment/case = Prospective Payment System payments/case.

SOURCE: Data on current rate are from Health Care Financing Administration, Bureau of
Policy Development.

Labor Portion of the Composite Rate

The labor portion of the base composite rate has remained unchanged
since the 1983 composite rate was introduced and is calculated as approximately 40 percent of the rate.[9] The labor share of treatment costs, however,
has been increasing relative to the costs of equipment and supplies. In a
recent study, for example, Held and colleagues (1990) estimated that the
labor portion of dialysis costs was 75 percent.

Providers often characterize the present situation as one in which reimbursement has not been adjusted upward to account for noncovered services.
However, the underlying reality appears to be that the number of labor-
intensive services has increased. The increased number of medications
administered to patients (Table 11-1) reflects this intensity. Even though
the wage index adjustment reflects wage increases across the various re-

gions, it does not necessarily account for changes in staff mix or increases in work intensity. In light of the growing intensity required in dialysis treatment, which in turn alters the labor and nonlabor shares of this treatment, the labor percentage of the rate to which the area wage index is applied should be reassessed.

PHYSICIAN PAYMENT POLICY ISSUES

A decade-long discussion of dialysis payment policy has defined facility reimbursement as the primary issue. Physician reimbursement policies generally have been overlooked, including the effect of such policies on the provision of treatment and the quality of care provided. Nor has this study addressed these issues at any length.

Many physician payment issues mirror those of outpatient dialysis units: the definition of the bundle of covered services included under the monthly capitation payment (MCP); the process for calculating the MCP; and the payment policies (level, differential rates). The discussion of these issues would be similar to those described above for facility providers.

Originally, the monthly capitation payment was a comprehensive fee for the primary care of patients on dialysis. Indeed, it has been suggested that the implied agreement between Medicare and the physician community was that nephrologists and dialysis units were to provide primary care to dialysis patients.

Changes in staffing patterns and the composition of the patient population have increased the range of services provided to ESRD patients by the renal community, and the primary-care role of the nephrologist has expanded over time. Ideally, nephrologists should coordinate the care of their dialysis patients, not only monitoring their outpatient care but also participating in the treatment of other serious health problems such as cardiovascular diseases, endocrine disorders, and infectious diseases.

Although dialysis patients increasingly require more primary care and additional specialized care, the MCP has not been adjusted to reflect any of these changes. It has not been changed since 1986, when it was reduced on average by nearly $12 from the 1983 payment rate. As a result, current physician reimbursement may adversely affect the actual scope and nature of physician services. Moreover, physicians may have an incentive under current payment policy to decrease contact with patients and diversify their practice away from dialysis treatment to include general nephrology, hypertension consultation, and general internal medicine.

The nephrology community anticipated some reprieve with the adoption of the Medicare Fee Schedule (MFS), scheduled to take effect on October 1, 1991. Nephrologists presumed that under MFS the MCP rate would increase, because the MFS will increase payments for cognitive services. However,

HCFA announced in 1990 that the MCP will not be included in the MFS. Consequently, it is unclear what payment policy changes, if any, can be expected to apply to the MCP for physician outpatient dialysis services.

CONCLUSIONS AND RECOMMENDATIONS

The committee discussed at length the implications for dialysis reimbursement policy of the information it had reviewed regarding (1) the effect of reimbursement on quality of dialysis care and (2) future needs for dialysis in the light of projections of growth in the size and diversity of the dialysis patient population over the next decade (Chapter 4). Two approaches to reimbursement policy emerge in the discussion. Broadly framed, these may be termed the "implicit" and the "explicit" approaches.

Historical and current policy has taken the implicit approach. Rates are set by determining what providers actually spend to deliver dialysis to patients. These reported costs, adjusted in accordance with Medicare Part A Cost Principles as to what costs are allowable (audited costs), are the basis for periodic proposals to review the rates. This approach has a number of virtues, most important that it minimizes governmental involvement in clinical practice. Providers are free to use their judgment in deciding how to maximize quality within the limits of their income. In theory, if a broad consensus exists among providers that expenditures must be increased to provide adequate quality, they will increase incurred costs in the expectation that these increases will lead to increased reimbursement in subsequent rate adjustment cycles. Historically, this implicit rate-setting process succeeded for many years in financing adequate care for patients. It fostered progressive reduction in costs and promoted the development and use of technical innovations. It developed an economic and administrative climate in which dialysis capacity grew appropriately to meet increasing patient need. (The arguments in favor of a continuation of this policy are presented in detail in the dissent to this chapter by C.R. Neu [see Appendix 2].)

On the other hand, the committee came to believe, based on its review of the data assembled in this report, that the current reimbursement system needs modification if it is to serve dialysis patients and society well in the future. Concern about the implicit rate-setting method arose primarily because it makes no connection between reimbursement and quality. The focus of the committee's concern is that implicit rate-setting may have generated a "vicious cycle," in which rate reductions lead to unmonitored system-wide quality reductions; the lower cost of these inferior services then constitutes the basis in the rate-setting process for a cut in reimbursement.

The evidence, reviewed in Chapter 10, that quality has already deteriorated is suggestive rather than conclusive. Given the lack of a comprehensive ESRD program for quality assessment and assurance and the difficulty of isolating the effect of any limited change in rate from ongoing changes in patient demographics and provider clinical opinion, the absence of conclusive evidence on this key point was to be anticipated. For a life-sustaining treatment, however, the committee feels it must give weight even to suggestive evidence that quality has deteriorated. Moreover, these previous effects, arguable in themselves, may signal the potential for a "slippery slope" on which further cuts may lead to larger decreases in quality. *Therefore, the committee recommends against any cuts in dialysis reimbursement at this time.*

Two arguments against the thesis that rates have been reduced excessively were discussed at length. The first is that the continued growth in national dialysis capacity in proportion to need indicates that reimbursement has been adequate to attract and retain providers. In simple terms, this argument is that if providers were not making a profit (or at least breaking even), they would go out of business rather than expanding capacity. The committee concluded that at least three explanations may account for the discrepancy between provider complaints that reimbursement is inadequate and the maintenance and, indeed, the growth of dialysis capacity.

First is the vertical integration of large chains, which can operate dialysis units at break-even or even at a small loss because they can generate profits from other related activities such as manufacture of dialysis equipment or supplies or performance of laboratory tests needed for the care of dialysis patients. The committee found no evidence that quality of care in large chains is inferior to that in smaller units but has reservations about any reimbursement policy that permits only large chains ultimately to survive.

The second explanation is that physician-owned units may be able to operate at break-even or less because physicians earn offsetting income from professional fees for care of patients treated in the unit. Hospitals may operate dialysis units even at a loss because it is part of a full-service program or because they can subsidize losses from other income, including income from admissions of dialysis patients. Obviously, these mechanisms for survival despite financial loss, perhaps adequate for some units in the past, cannot be expected to suffice if real rates are reduced progressively.

Finally, the most troublesome explanation of *survival and growth* of dialysis units is that they have been achieved to an important degree by progressive reduction in quality. This explanation finds at least some support from the data in Chapter 10. It cannot be ruled out since quality has not been monitored systematically.

The other important argument against the thesis that rates have been reduced excessively derives from the HFCA data reviewed in this chapter (Tables 11-2 and 11-3). These data indicate that, in most independent dialysis units and many hospital units, payment rates exceed even reported (unaudited) costs. Again, the committee is concerned that, absent quality assessment, these data may indicate merely that faced with progressive decreases in real payment rates, units survive by reducing overall services to patients, possibly to the point of erosion of adequate standards.

The committee recommends two stages for reimbursement policy. For the immediate future, as noted earlier, rates should not be decreased. Moreover, until a quality assessment program is in place, annual rates should be adjusted for inflation by some appropriate factor. Although earlier in its evolution, dialysis treatment benefited from the cost reductions typical of new technology, this pattern cannot be expected to continue indefinitely. During nearly 20 years of increasing technical efficiency, the proportion of dialysis costs attributable to supplies and equipment has fallen drastically. There is little reason to assume that future gains in this area will offset inflationary increases in personnel and other costs, especially in view of the increasing age and comorbidity of the dialysis patient population.

During the initial phase of the proposed rate-setting policy, the committee recommends that a quality assessment and assurance program be implemented, guided by the principles and examples discussed in Chapter 12. The committee noted the research opportunity inherent in the data showing wide variations in costs among dialysis units. Analysis of the relationship between cost and quality may reveal techniques by which the least costly units have maintained quality or, on the contrary, that low costs have been achieved only at the price of unacceptable decreases in quality.

Once a quality assessment program is in place, HCFA may wish to revert to an "implicit" rate-setting process. Should that process lead to rate reductions, HCFA will be in a position to monitor its effects in patients. The committee discussed at some length the alternative of recommending an "explicit" rate-setting process. In essence, this calls for the development of a detailed "bundle of services" needed for the adequate care of dialysis patients. The sum of the prices of these individual components would constitute the basis for rate setting. However, the committee decided against this alternative because it would unduly involve government agencies in setting detailed and potentially rigid standards of clinical practice. On the other hand, the committee felt strongly that some mechanism for continuing review of rate setting was appropriate. It recommends, therefore, that ProPAC, which has been mandated to review ambulatory care, also review rate setting in the ESRD program.[10] In addition, the committee recommends that HCFA establish an expert committee to advise it on potential additions to the "bundle of services" needed for dialysis patients as innovations arise and clinical practice changes.

The committee recommends that Congress and HCFA adopt the following payment policies for dialysis facilities:

Do not reduce the composite rate at this time.

Do not, at present, rebase (recalculate) the rate using recent cost report data because there is reason to believe that current costs reflect prior payment reductions rather than provider decisions about the services needed for appropriate medical care.

Follow general Medicare payment policies in setting dialysis payment policies:

1. Update the rate yearly, as is the practice for the rest of Medicare.

2. Rebase the rate only when an ESRD quality assessment program is in place and HCFA rebases the other parts of Medicare governed by the Prospective Payment System. Ultimately, predicate rebasing of outpatient dialysis reimbursement on efficacy and quality studies that determine the components needed for appropriate dialysis care. Because these components will change as clinical and technical knowledge advance, HCFA should establish an expert advisory body to review periodically the services that Medicare should reimburse.

3. The Prospective Payment Assessment Commission, consistent with its recently expanded charge to examine Medicare outpatient as well as inpatient reimbursement, should periodically review ESRD payment policy.

Adopt the following specific ESRD reimbursement policies:

1. Evaluate the justification for the rate differential between hospital-based and independent facilities, especially in terms of patient complexity (see Chapter 12), and retain or eliminate the differential on the basis of that analysis.

2. Establish a separate rate for hospital backup units that treat inpatients as well as outpatients and that provide support to independent units in the care of complex outpatient cases.

3. Establish a separate rate for ESRD pediatric patients.

4. Evaluate the need for a separate rate for rural facilities.

The committee also recommends that HCFA review the MCP physician payment policy in light of its exclusion from the Medicare Fee Schedule, regarding the effects of this policy on the quality of care provided.

NOTES

1. Discussion of this approach was stimulated by the controversy that followed the introduction of the 1983 composite rate and the proposed, but limited, 1986 rate reduction.
2. In addition to Chapter 27 of the *Medicare Provider Reimbursement Manual*, covered services are currently specified in 42 CFR §§ 410.50 and 410.52 [which recodify 42 CFR §§ 405.231(o) and (p), and 405.2163]; and in HCFA Publication 13-3, Section 3165.
3. The acquisition of cost data from dialysis providers was hindered in the 1970s by the refusal of proprietary facilities to submit cost data to the Bureau of Health Insurance of the Social Security Administration and, from 1977 onward, to HCFA. They agreed to do so only after a federal district court upheld the authority of HCFA to obtain such data (Rettig, 1980).
4. Subsequent to the IOM ESRD study committee's February 15, 1990 hearing on rate-setting, Dialysis Clinic, Inc., Nashville, Tennessee, compared the average cost per dialysis treatment calculated according to GAAP and Medicare cost reporting principles for the year ending September 30, 1989. For 51 facilities, urban and rural, the GAAP costs were $141.44 compared to Medicare costs of $119.53 (personal communication from Ed Attrill, February 16, 1990). North Central Dialysis Centers, Chicago, Illinois, provided similar data. Their GAAP costs for 1987 were $121.32 compared to Medicare costs of $107.42; for 1988, the figures were $127.96 and $113.04, respectively (personal communication from Myron P. Nidetz, February 20, 1990).
5. For example, the decision by the Financial Accounting Standards Board, which establishes GAAP procedures, to require that private corporations account for the pension liabilities of their retirees reflects both the technical and the policy aspects of accounting (FASB, 1985). The lengthy phase-in of this rule, as well as the postponement of certain aspects of it, reflects corporate resistance.
6. Providers can seek review of HCFA's decisions on allowed costs through the Provider Reimbursement Review Board or the federal courts only when an exception is not granted.
7. Bad debts are defined by HCFA as "the deductible and coinsurance amounts for which beneficiaries are liable and which, when uncollectible, result in providers being reimbursed less than costs" (48 Fed. Reg. 21273, May 11, 1983). HCFA allows the recovery of bad debt by a facility only when its revenues from the Medicare portion (80 percent) of the composite rate *plus* the other deductible and copayment collectibles are less than its audited costs. The allowable bad debt is then limited to the lesser of the unrecovered Medicare cost (up to the amount of the audited costs) or the uncollectible deductible and coinsurance amounts.
8. The revenue picture is clouded, however, by several factors. The precise effects of the Medicare-as-secondary-payer provision are not known, nor is the income derived from auxiliary sources, such as management by independent units of hospital inpatient dialysis units on a contract basis. Finally, there is no information about whether physician-owners are willing to accept losses on facility revenues in order to maximize income from physician reimbursement. See discussion p. 257.
9. This compares to the labor portion of the standardized amount under PPS, which is 74 percent.
10. The committee discussed this recommendation during 1989 and 1990. In the Omnibus Budget Reconciliation Act of 1990 [Public Law 101-508, Section 4201(b)], Congress directed ProPAC to "conduct a study to determine the costs and services and profits associated with various modalities of dialysis services provided to end stage renal disease patients" under Medicare. ProPAC was also directed to consider the conclusions and recommendations of this study.

REFERENCES

DeOreo PB. 1990. Testimony before the IOM ESRD Study Committee public hearing on dialysis reimbursement rate setting. Washington, D.C. February.

FASB (Financial Accounting Standards Board). 1985. Statement of Financial Accounting Standards No. 87: Employers' Accounting for Pensions. Norwalk, Conn.

HCFA (Health Care Financing Administration). 1989. Medicare Provider Reimbursement Manual, Part 1-Chapter 27: Reimbursement for ESRD and transplant services. Baltimore, Md.

Held PJ, Dor A, Pauly MV. 1990. The Medicare cost of training for self-care dialysis: An estimation by statistical cost function. Washington, D.C.: The Urban Institute, April.

Levin N, Keshaviah P, Gotch FA. 1990. Effect of reimbursement on innovation in the ESRD program. Paper prepared for the Institute of Medicine ESRD Study Committee. New York: Beth Israel Medical Center.

Pollack VE, Pesce A. 1990. Analysis of data related to the 1976-1989 patient population: Treatment characteristics and patient outcomes. Report to the Institute of Medicine ESRD Study Committee. Cincinnati: Dialysis Clinic, Inc.-Cincinnati.

Rettig RA. 1980. The politics of health cost containment: End-stage renal disease. Bull NY Acad Med 56:115-138.

APPENDIX 1

DEPARTMENT OF HEALTH & HUMAN SERVICES	Health Care Financing Administration
	6325 Security Boulevard
APR 1 9 1990	Baltimore, MD 21207

Richard A. Rettig, Ph.D.
ESRD Study Director
Institute of Medicine
National Academy of Sciences
2101 Constitution Avenue
Washington, D.C. 20418

Dear Richard:

This is in response to your letter concerning the procedures the Health Care
Financing Administration (HCFA) used and is currently using to compute base
composite rates for dialysis treatments under the End Stage Renal Disease (ESRD)
Program. We are enclosing copies of the 5 Federal Registers (Enclosure 1) that were
published concerning the composite payment rate system. For the most part, these
notices should answer your questions or provide you with our rationale for policy
decisions. The first 3 notices developed the payment methodology and the base
rates currently in effect. Effective October 1, 1986, these base rates were reduced
by $2.00 as mandated by the Omnibus Budget Reconciliation Act of 1986 and
superseded the rates published in the 1986 notice. Summarized below are the
sampling procedures used to select facilities for the 4 national ESRD audits.

FIRST AUDITS--1978 & 1979 COST DATA

The Office of Research and Demonstration (ORD) has designed all of the audit
samples. The original audit sample was developed in February of 1980. The
universe included all renal facilities that had submitted a Renal Disease Facility Cost
and Statistical Questionnaire, Form HCFA-9734. All certified renal facilities were
required to submit a copy of this form at the end of their fiscal year to report their
costs. At that time the Office of Special Program maintained a computer file that
contained this information. As of January 1980, there were 825 of these forms on
file. These facilities were divided into 4 frames: 1) rural independent, 2)rural hospital,
3) urban independent and 4) urban hospital. The purpose of this strategy was to
calculate 4 payment rates based on facility type and location. This is explained on
page 64009 of the September 26, 1980 notice.

Each frame was stratified by the amount of reported costs. Facilities with no
reported costs were placed in separate strata. Enclosure 2 summaries this process.
The overall sample sizes within the four major groups were assigned to the strata
using optimum allocation techniques. Sample facilities were identified using
systematic selection with fractional sampling intervals and random starts within each

2

stratum. The sample design required a sample size of 110 facilities to produce a relative precision of about 7 percent. There were 70 hospital facilities and 40 independent facilities selected. On page 6562 of the February 12, 1982 proposed notice, we explained why only 67 hospital and 38 independent renal facilities were used in calculating base rates. The chart summarizes the cost questionnaires that were audited by their fiscal year end.

FISCAL YEAR END	HOSPITAL	INDEPENDENT
1976	1	0
1977	6	0
1978	51	13
1979	9	23
1980	0	2
TOTAL	67	38

On August 13, 1981 Congress enacted section 2145 of Pub.L. 97-35 requiring us to develop a prospective reimbursement system for outpatient dialysis that promotes home dialysis. The original audits only verified outpatient costs; they did not attempt to verify home cost data. On page 6563 of the proposed notice, we described the 25 entities selected to compute home dialysis costs. The cost data included 19 facilities with fiscal years ending in 1980 and 6 with fiscal years ending in 1981. These facilities were not audited. Instead the Office of Inspector General auditors prepared home cost data from these facilities' books and records.

The sampling strategy ignored training costs and medical educations costs. However, facilities selected for audit included ones that had incurred these costs. Training costs were never exacted from any set of audits, since these costs are disregarded in computing base rates. In establishing base composite rates, we did not eliminate medical educational costs. These costs were included in the May 11, 1983 and August 15, 1986 Federal Register notices.

In calculating base composite rates, we added routine laboratory costs to a facility's audited costs when it was not reported. In addition, if a facility did not report equipment costs for home hemodialysis treatments, we added $12.00 per treatment to its audited costs. This was particularly true where a facility had purchased equipment under the 100% agreement and no equipment costs were reported. These adjustments are explained in both final notices.

SECOND AUDITS--1982 & 1983 COST DATA

The second round of audits were conducted in 1983 and the results were used in the 1986 Federal Register notices. Cost reports with fiscal years ending between July 31, 1982 and June 30, 1983 were audited. These reporting periods were prior to the effective data of the composite payment rate system; and therefore, did not include composite payment rate data.

This sample was also designed by the ORD. The universe consisted of all certified renal facilities providing outpatient dialysis treatments. The frame contained 1147 facilities. Of this total 7 were deleted, since they had no outpatient stations. The universe was first separated by type of facility either hospital or independent. This list was arrayed based on the number of certified outpatient dialysis stations from low to high. Within each frame, three strata were formed on the basis of the number of dialysis stations and the method described by William Cochran on page 129 of Sample Techniques. Enclosure 3 summarize the results of this process. Sample facilities were systematically selected with independent random starts in each stratum and fractional skip interval were used. In addition, we selected 17 target rate facilities that were audited to compute home dialysis costs. Prior to the composite payment rate system, there was no requirement that facilities furnish all services needed to perform home dialysis. Under the target rate agreement, facilities agreed to furnish all services, equipment and supplies required to perform home dialysis for a set fee. These facilities were selected for audit to ensure, that we had captured all costs needed to furnish home dialysis. In addition, since these facilities were furnishing all components of home dialysis for a fixed fee they were functioning in a manner similar to the composite rate system.

Starting in 1981, renal facilities were required to submit newly issued cost report forms as opposed to the cost questionnaires previously submitted. Independent renal facilities were required to submit Form HCFA-265, while hospitals were required to submit Supplement Worksheet I as part of their HCFA-2552 to report their outpatient dialysis costs.

On page 17539 of the May 13, 1986 proposed notice, we explained the sample design and the reason we did not use all 143 (126 + 17 target rate facilities) facilities in computing new base rates. In the final notice on page 29411, we decided to use the audit results of 4 facilities that were previously excluded in the proposed notice. We originally excluded these facilities because of their low treatment count. It was felt that these 4 facilities were outliers and not representative of renal facilities in furnishing maintenance dialysis treatments.

4

To compute new base composite rates in the 1986 notices, we calculated the median costs of a dialysis treatment as opposed to the median costs of a dialysis facility. This was accomplished by weighing the median audited labor and non labor cost per treatment (CPT) by the number of treatments in each frame. Using treatments as opposed to facilities recognize costs of the larger more efficient facilities, in particular independent facilities.

Outpatient treatments in each frame were calculated from the 1984 ESRD Facility Survey, form HCFA-2744. This is an annual survey form which every certified renal facilities files with the Bureau of Data Management. Each calendar year, facilities are required to report treatments and patient information on this form. For the prior 4 years, this form has shown that 50 percent of certified renal facilities have accounted for 82% of all dialysis treatments.

THIRD AUDITS--1984 & 1985 COST DATA

In 1986 we audited 63 hospital cost reports with fiscal years ending in 1984 and 1985 and 63 independent cost reports with fiscal years ending in 1985. As in previous years, the ORD designed the sample.

The universe consisted of renal facilities that had filed form HCFA-2744 in 1984. This definition include all certified renal dialysis facilities. From this list, we excluded VA hospitals, children hospitals, facilities in Guam, the Virgin Islands, American Samoa and Saipan and facilities providing fewer than 600 treatments. VA hospitals were deleted since these facilities do not file a Medicare cost report. Children hospitals were deleted since these facilities have exceptions to their payment rate and they usually report a low volume of treatments. The renal facilities located outside the U.S. did not have a wage index to adjust their audited labor costs. Facilities furnishing fewer than 600 treatments are not representative of a renal facility operating in an efficient manner. The resulting universe contained 1,174 facilities.

The frame was separated into hospital and independent renal facilities. Within each type, facilities were stratified on number of outpatient maintenance dialysis treatments performed in 1984. Facilities were, first, arrayed by number of treatments from low to high. Secondly, facilities were divided into 3 groups such that the cumulative number of treatments in each group was nearly equal. (See enclosure 4). Equal sample sizes of 21 facilities were allocated to each of the resulting 6 strata. Random numbers were take from A Million Random Digits with 100,000 Normal Deviates by the Rand Corporation. Facilities were assigned sequential number from

1 to N within each stratum, where N is the number of facilities in each stratum. Facilities chosen were those whose sequential number corresponded to the 21 unique random numbers.

Although 126 facilities were selected for audit, we received only 124 audit reports. A hospital facility in stratum 1 was not audited because its intermediary was terminated. An independent facility in stratum 1 was not audited because its books and records were incomplete.

A separate sample was not used to compute home dialysis costs. From this audit sample, 37 hospital facilities and 34 independent renal facilities reported home dialysis costs. As with previous audits, we added routine laboratory costs and equipment costs where a facility failed to report these costs. In addition, we adjusted CAPD home supply costs for 6 independent facilities.

FOURTH AUDITS--1988 & 1989 COST DATA

For the most part, this sample design was the same as the third set of audits. The universe was defined as all facilities that had filed an ESRD survey form, HCFA-2744, for 1988. This definition included all certified renal facilities. From this list, we excluded the same facilities as in the third round of audits. Facilities in the universe were separated into two categories hospital or independent. Outpatient treatments were arrayed from low to high. Facilities were then divided into three groups such that the cumulative number of treatments in each group was nearly equal. Equal sample sizes of 21 facilities were allocated to each of the resulting six strata. The facilities were selected systematically using fractional intervals with random start in each stratum. A separate sample was not designed for home costs. Of the 126 facilities selected for audit, 48 hospital and 38 independent renal facilities report that they were providing dialysis services to home patients.

ADDITIONAL CONCERNS

There was no plan to audit the same facilities each year. However, since the sample design selects a high proportion of facilities in the third strata, there is a high degree of probability that some of these same facilities would be selected during the fourth round of audits.

Regarding the composite rate table in your letter, there are some minor changes. In setting the initial base rates, our chart shows that mostly 1978 and 1979 cost data were used. Although payment rates were published in the 1986 Federal Register, they were superseded and no claims were paid using these rates. The $2.00

reduction mandated by OBRA of 1986 became effective for service on or after October 1, 1986 and not November 1, 1986. In addition, these payment rates were computed using 80% of the BLS wage index and 20% of the HCFA wage index. The payment rates effective October 1, 1987 were computed using 60% of the BLS wage index and 40% of the HCFA wage index. This was the last time revised composite payment rates were published.

The payment rates currently in effect were based on the original audited data and have never been rebased. A facility receives its composite payment rate for each completed dialysis treatment furnished to a Medicare beneficiary. The rate is a per treatment rate as opposed to a facility rate or a discharge rate.

If you have any questions concerning our response, please call Dan Driscoll at (301) 966-4555.

Sincerely yours,

Bernadette S. Schumaker
Director
Division of Dialysis and
 Transplant Payment Policy
Bureau of Policy Development

Enclosures

APPENDIX 2

Dissenting View of C.R. Neu[*]

I dissent from the committee's suggestions regarding how reimbursement rates for dialysis services should be set. The committee recommends the establishment of a "technically qualified advisory panel" to "advise the Health Care Financing Administration (HCFA) about the elements needed for appropriate [dialysis] care" and to "review periodically the 'bundle of services' that Medicare should reimburse." The majority further recommends that HCFA base its rate-setting methods "on efficacy and quality studies that determine the components needed for appropriate dialysis care." In my view, these recommendations come close to constituting a call for a detailed, official description of "appropriate" dialysis care and for setting Medicare reimbursement rates by "pricing out" this officially sanctioned "bundle of services."

I believe that this approach to dialysis rate setting would be unwise for four reasons:

First, it would be contrary to the long-established policies of the Medicare program that reject the idea that the government should tell health care providers how to provide care. I recognize that Medicare is slowly being dragged away from absolute adherence to this principle, but I do not believe that it is in the interests of patients, the provider community, or society at large to hasten this process.

Although Medicare does require that certain minimum, general standards be met by Medicare-certified providers, neither detailed standards for care nor a specifically defined "bundle of services" are found anywhere in the Medicare program. In setting rates for other Medicare-covered services, HCFA relies on an implicit definition of what constitutes adequate care. No attempt is made, for example, to develop or to enforce a definition of adequate care for coronary artery bypass patients. Instead, HCFA continually monitors the costs that hospitals incur in performing bypass operations and adjusts DRG payments accordingly. To argue that a different approach should be adopted for outpatient dialysis requires that one also argue that dialysis is fundamentally different from other clinical services. I have yet to hear a convincing argument on this point.

Second, explicit, officially promulgated standards for care are likely to stifle desirable innovation. Any definition of adequate care adopted for federal reimbursement rate-setting purposes would, I believe, become a "gold standard" from which individual dialysis providers could deviate only at great peril to themselves. In these litigious times, any adverse outcome

---

[*]The views expressed here are those of the author only. They do not necessarily reflect the views of the RAND Corporation or of the sponsors of any of its research.

resulting from nonstandard patterns of care could prove financially disastrous for a provider or its insurer.

Advances in the quality of care available to dialysis patients, though, will be achieved only by changing the way that care is delivered. Similarly, any hopes of cost containment in the ESRD program must be based on finding new, less costly ways of delivering services. To further rigidify the system by introducing a new set of official standards—even standards intended only for rate-setting purposes—seems to me unwise. Those who argue that officially sanctioned standards could be made sufficiently flexible or adjusted frequently enough to allow the development of better and less costly alternatives have, I believe, misunderstood the lessons of the past 40 years of U.S. regulatory history.

My third reason for opposing the establishment of detailed standards for care is that I believe that any expert panel charged with recommending such standards will be put in an impossible position. Any proposed advisory panel will necessarily be made up of experts in renal medicine who, as competent and dedicated professionals, will and should seek to set a very high standard for care. But the Medicare program is not intended to reimburse the very highest standard of care. Rather, Medicare policy makers face the almost impossible task of ensuring that Medicare beneficiaries receive adequate care at a reasonable cost—to themselves and to the taxpayers. The desire for higher standards of care, therefore, may sometimes conflict with an obligation to control costs.

An expert advisory panel charged with defining adequate dialysis care in the Medicare context will have to confront this dilemma head on. It is essential that we have proponents of ever higher standards of care, and any advisory panel on appropriate renal care should be composed of such proponents whose primary concern is patient welfare. But is it reasonable to ask members of this panel to serve not only as scientists and advocates of better care (difficult enough tasks) but also as guardians of the public purse? The kind of experts we would want on such a panel will have no expertise in this last task. How then could such a panel balance between standards and costs?

Finally, I argue that the best mechanism for determining the costs of adequate dialysis care will be to observe the care that is actually being provided by the dialysis provider community at large and what this care is costing. These providers, by definition, deal with the full range of dialysis patients and work every day to balance the conflicting demands of quality of care and cost containment. Who better to define adequate care? What better method of defining it than by their actions? We can and should always aspire to higher standards of care, but the kind of care that is being provided in real-life situations is in fact the commonly prevailing standard of care and should constitute the basis for Medicare rate-setting. In the absence of any clear indication that a large fraction of dialysis patients are receiving care that is in some meaningful sense worse than that being provided to other Medicare patients or that they are receiving care that produces outcomes widely viewed as unacceptable, I see no reason to adopt anything other than an implicit approach to defining the "bundle of services" to be covered by Medicare reimbursement.

This approach to defining adequate care leads to a relatively straightforward method for setting rates for prospective reimbursement of dialysis care. On a regular basis, HCFA should survey dialysis providers to determine the per-treatment cost of dialysis care as it is actually being provided. The basic national reimbursement rate would be calculated by averaging (or calculating the median of) these costs, after adjustment is made for differences in local labor costs and other factors. As patterns of care change (in ways that may either increase or decrease costs), reimbursement would be adjusted—with some delay, to reflect these changed costs. Separate calculations might be done for hospital-based and freestanding units, urban and rural units, and so on as recommended by the committee.

To minimize the delay in adjusting reimbursement rates for changes in patterns of care, I recommend that reimbursement rates be recalculated (the majority report calls this "rebasing" reimbursement rates) annually. The DRG weights for Medicare-covered hospital services are "recalibrated" every year on the basis of the most recent cost data available. Dialysis providers are already required to file annual cost reports with HCFA,[1] and I see no reason that an annual recalculation of costs for a much smaller number of ESRD cases would not be feasible. When practice patterns or costs change dramatically, it would be appropriate to calculate an immediate rough adjustment to reimbursement rates. A rough adjustment is probably all that is needed. In 2 or 3 years, data will show how costs have actually changed, and any mistake in our rough calculation will be corrected.

The delay inherent in this approach to adjusting reimbursement for changing practice patterns, changing standards of care, or new technologies is not necessarily bad. Few changes in medical practice are obviously good ideas at the moment that they are introduced. Some time is typically required before the consequences of new techniques, equipment, and so on are fully understood. Immediate adjustment of dialysis rates to reflect all proposed changes in patterns of care would risk ratifying by bureaucratic means some changes that will ultimately prove undesirable. If numerous providers are willing to adopt changes in their styles or standards of care at some initial cost to themselves, then the case for adjusting payments to reflect these changes is presumably strong. Similarly, the fact that providers may make money on cost-saving innovations, at least until most other providers adopt similar practices and HCFA gets around to reducing rates accordingly, will provide a modest incentive for providers to find lower-cost ways to provide care.

Inevitably, cost data used to calculate reimbursement rates would be somewhat out of date. Next year's reimbursement rate would have to be calculated on the basis of costs incurred last year or the year before. In calculating reimbursement rates, we would recognize and attempt to correct for the fact that the general price level may have risen since the most recent cost data were gathered. This adjustment too needs to be only approximate. Any over- or underadjustments for past inflation in calculating next year's reimbursement rate will become apparent in a year or two when the actual costs are determined, and suitable corrections can be made. Errors will not be self-propagating.

I am suggesting only that inevitably out-of-date data be adjusted to account for inflation. I am distinctly not recommending an annual inflation adjustment for dialysis reimbursement rates. Dialysis costs may or may not rise at the same rate as general prices. I am also suggesting that we do the best we can on a regular basis at estimating the actual costs of dialysis care and that we set reimbursement rates to cover costs.

In the scheme that I am proposing for updating payment rates, worthwhile but cost-increasing changes in practice patterns will come about only if most dialysis providers are people of good will with the interests of their patients at heart and have the financial means to incur some extra costs for a couple of years until reimbursement rates are adjusted. Based on my discussions with other committee members and the testimony presented in public hearings, I believe that we need not worry too much about the motivations of the provider community. The same testimony also suggests to me that many (perhaps most) dialysis providers have the financial strength to absorb modest costs for improving care for short periods. If we want to make certain that this is the case, it might be wise to increase reimbursement rates by a couple of percent above the rates calculated by the method described above to allow some margin for providers to work with. I would not embrace this policy without further evidence that dialysis providers are hurting financially, but such a margin could be built into the payment scheme without changing the basic structure.

The committee argues that existing patterns of dialysis care should not form the basis for rate setting. They argue that years of declining real (or price-adjusted) reimbursement for dialysis care have forced dialysis providers to reduce the quality of care that is offered. To base rates on the costs of prevailing care patterns, they conclude, would be to lock dialysis care into patterns that some believe to be inadequate.

I find these arguments unpersuasive. The fact that reimbursement levels for dialysis care have been declining in real terms does not in itself constitute evidence that current reimbursement levels are too low to cover the costs of adequate care. The history of almost every technological process is that real costs decline over time, as experience is gained and better and more efficient ways are found to achieve the desired end. We should expect that the real cost of dialysis care has fallen since the beginning of the Medicare ESRD program. Similarly, the fact that dialysis unit staffing levels and patterns have changed over the years is not necessarily a sign that care quality is declining. The number and skill levels of the staff required to carry out most complex processes decline over time. It would be surprising if the same were not true of dialysis.

In 2 years of diligent searching, neither the Institute of Medicine ESRD Study Committee nor its highly capable staff were able to discover any convincing evidence that the quality of care provided to Medicare ESRD patients has declined. To a large extent, this lack of evidence may be explained by the simple fact that no one has been looking. I readily admit that there may in fact have been a major deterioration in the quality of care for ESRD patients, and we simply do not know it. I agree fully with the majority view that a concerted effort to assess the quality of dialysis care is necessary. But it is equally true that the quality of care for ESRD patients may have been improving over the years, and we do not know this. Where my view seems to differ from that of the majority is about how to set reimbursement rates today, in the absence of clear measures of changes in the quality of care.

Because they fear that the quality of care may have suffered in the past or may be about to suffer, the committee recommends against a recalculation of ESRD payment rates on the basis of costs of current practice. They suggest that future recalculations should reflect the costs of some officially specified "bundle of services" that may be rather different from current care patterns. Because I see dangers in this approach and because I see no evidence that current care patterns are inadequate, I argue that the correct course is to recalculate the true costs of providing dialysis care today and to set reimbursement rates to cover these costs. Some rough estimates by committee staff suggest that such a recalculation would lead to a reimbursement rate not much different from what Medicare is currently paying.

None of my views should be interpreted as supporting a complacent view about the quality of care for ESRD patients. ESRD patients, like all patients, deserve the benefit of strenuous programs of research aimed at devising new and better methods of care and assessing the effectiveness of current treatment practice. The results of this research should be widely disseminated to the renal community, and leaders in the renal community should work aggressively to encourage their colleagues to adopt the treatment practices that are understood at any particular time to result in the best patient outcomes. When and if the dialysis community at large changes its patterns of care in response to new research findings, then Medicare reimbursement should be adjusted (up or down, as the case may be) to reflect the costs of the newly prevailing patterns of care. In my view, no useful purpose is served, and some significant risks are assumed, by trying to short-circuit this process—by having some panel of experts define appropriate care, having some team of accountants price out the components of this care, and making that the Medicare reimbursement rate.

Finally, I recognize that some of the interest within the dialysis community for the establishment of an expert panel to play a key role in setting dialysis reimbursement rates stems from a long-standing distrust of HCFA. In my view, though, it is naive and possibly disingenuous to suggest that whatever problems currently exist within HCFA can be remedied by the creation of yet another official body, whether it is advisory or executive. Neither will problems be solved by passing responsibility to some already existing advisory body such as the Prospective Payment Assessment Commission. Some group of policy makers will always be needed to weigh the renal community's admirable desire to provide more and better care against the benefits that might result from using public funds for other purposes. These policy makers will never and should never provide the renal community with everything it wants. Today, the policy makers responsible for making these judgments are found mostly at HCFA. If there is dissatisfaction with how well they are doing their jobs, the right course would seem to be to work to make HCFA more effective, not to call for yet another group of policy makers who, facing the same agonizing choices, may perform no better.

Note

1. There is considerable controversy over whether HFCA's current concepts of allowable costs are realistic. Certainly this issue should be reexamined, but it is naive, I believe, to think that different standards for allowable costs could be applied to dialysis providers than are applied to other Medicare providers.

12

Quality Assessment and Assurance

The OBRA 1987 legislation asked the IOM to address "the quality of care provided to end-stage renal disease beneficiaries, as measured by clinical indicators, functional status of patients, and patient satisfaction." This charge cannot be fully addressed using existing data.

However, quality assessment and assurance are very important in the ESRD program, and this chapter responds to Congress in the following way: First, the principles of quality assessment and quality assurance are briefly discussed. Second, the management of ESRD quality assurance by the federal government is described. Finally, a strategy for quality in the ESRD program is suggested that is oriented to the treatment-unit level and to improving patient management.

This report refers to both quality *assessment* and quality *assurance*. Quality assessment deals with the measurement of quality and with the development of instruments and measures; it implies a need for research to develop, validate, and interpret these measures. Quality assurance (QA) typically involves the monitoring of care (usually through discharge abstracts, chart reviews, or patient reports) to identify instances of poor-quality care by physicians and institutions; providing feedback of information to the appropriate physicians and health care institutions; devising remedies for identified problems, including the education of providers or the application of sanctions; and reviewing issues to see if they have been solved or that no new ones have been created.

All of medicine is being asked for evidence that patients are receiving medical care of good quality. Nephrology confronts this same demand, but formidable obstacles exist to the use of QA in the ESRD setting. First, like many physicians, nephrologists resent the loss of public trust in their ability and willingness to deliver good-quality care (Starr, 1982). Second, neither the tradition nor the formal systems of QA are well developed in nephrology: Many nephrologists are skeptical that quality can be measured, the design and development of ESRD-specific QA measures and instruments has been minimal, and few good examples of ESRD QA exist. Third, many nephrologists see QA as a requirement imposed on treatment units by the federal government, which is to be delegated to a QA coordinator for paper compliance and shielding the unit from adverse effects. Fourth, the conceptual expertise regarding quality assessment generally resides in the health services research community, not in medical specialties. If effective ESRD QA systems are to be developed, the nephrology community will need to avail itself of this expertise.

Notwithstanding these obstacles, the committee is persuaded that more systematic approaches to QA are needed and possible in the ESRD arena. To be successful, however, QA systems will have to be seen by physicians, patients, and other ESRD clinicians as a way to improve routine, everyday patient management and patient outcomes at the treatment-unit level.

PRINCIPLES OF QA

A recent IOM report, *Medicare: A Strategy for Quality Assurance*, requested by Congress in OBRA 1986, presents a comprehensive picture of quality assessment and assurance in health care, especially for the Medicare program (Lohr, 1990). It deserves careful review by all.

The IOM Quality committee defined quality of care as *"the degree to which health services for individuals and populations increase the likelihood of desired health outcomes and are consistent with current professional knowledge"* (Lohr, 1990, p. 4). Building on that definition, "health services" in the ESRD context includes the full spectrum of medical, social, and rehabilitative services used in the care of the ESRD patient; "desired health outcomes" include reducing mortality and morbidity and maintaining and improving the health status and well-being of ESRD patients; and "consistent with current professional knowledge" implies that physicians remain abreast of changing clinical knowledge, that they not be expected to exceed that knowledge in their practice, that they be judged only on the basis of what is known and can be done, and that medical research contribute strongly to the clinical knowledge base.

The purposes of QA programs, as they have evolved over time, have been (1) to identify providers whose care is so substandard that immediate sanctions are needed to remove them from practice or to ensure that third-party payers no longer reimburse them; (2) to identify providers whose practices are unacceptable, but who may respond to information and education to correct their problems; (3) to improve the average level of quality of care provided by a community of providers; and (4) to motivate and assist providers to achieve high levels of quality. In recent years, the emphasis has shifted to the latter two objectives.

For the Medicare program, Congress has authorized the creation of external review bodies—first, the Professional Standards Review Organizations (PSROs) in 1972 and later the Utilization and Quality Control Peer Review Organizations (PROs). These efforts have been intended, in part, to guarantee that Medicare beneficiaries receive care of acceptable quality and, in part, to control costs. However, the QA orientation of the PSRO and PRO programs has been primarily to policing poor-quality care. The Joint Commission on Accreditation of Healthcare Organizations, formerly the Joint Commission on Accreditation of Hospitals, fulfills a QA role that is broader in scope than that of Medicare-certified facilities, but its activities intersect strongly with Medicare. It has moved beyond its survey-based accrediting function within the past 5 years, mainly through its "Agenda for Change," which embraces the improvement of care, the motivation of physicians, and an emphasis on clinical indicators (JCAHO, 1987, 1988).

In response to these external efforts, many providers have created internal QA systems for monitoring their own performance. As these systems have developed, a tension has emerged between meeting regulatory requirements and improving patient-care management at the treatment-unit level. Not surprising, these tensions also exist in the ESRD setting.

The purposes of ESRD QA systems vary considerably across four levels of potential users. First, the federal government agencies of the Public Health Service (PHS), Centers for Disease Control (CDC), Food and Drug Administration (FDA), National Institutes of Health (NIH), and the Agency for Health Care Policy Research (AHCPR) are engaged in public health and safety, education, and research; the Health Care Financing Administration (HCFA) is involved in provider oversight. Second, at the regional level, state survey agencies perform regulatory oversight of providers. ESRD networks, on the other hand, support medical care review and collect data from providers in order to establish regional and national norms for providers. At the third level of users, nephrologists and other ESRD clinicians comply with federal ESRD regulatory requirements, provide data through ESRD networks at HCFA, and independently deal with quality in their treatment facilities. The need for compliance with HCFA requirements shapes the view that many ESRD clinicians have of QA. However, partly in response to the IOM quality study, ESRD providers have begun recently to recognize the significance of continuous quality improvement oriented to systematically raising the average quality of care on a continuing basis at the treatment-unit level (RPA, 1990).

Fourth, ESRD patients are also potential users of QA information. Such information can indicate how their care compares to regional and national norms and can help them participate in decision making about their own care. This participation can provide valuable expression of patient preferences and important guidance for physicians and other clinicians. In addition, some evidence exists that patient involvement in clinical decision making actually results in better health outcomes (Kaplan and Ware, 1989; Kaplan et al., 1989).

In any event, the ultimate "guarantors" of quality care are the members of the clinical team. It is they who can make QA systems serve patient management and who implement practices to improve patient outcomes. Physicians must exercise QA leadership consistent with their professional duties to patients. Nurses, technicians, social workers, and dietitians must join them as members of a clinical team and reflect a corresponding commitment to patient well-being.

THINKING ABOUT QUALITY

Many years ago, Donabedian (1966) articulated the basic framework for assessing the quality of medical care in terms of structure (or resource inputs), processes, and patient outcomes. The Medical Outcomes Study offers a graphic interpretation of this framework as shown in Figure 12-1 (Tarlov et al., 1989).

Structure

Structure, or the basic inputs to care, consists of system, provider, and patient characteristics. *System characteristics* include the organization of the provider community (as described in Chapter 6). *Provider characteristics* are those of physicians and facilities. Physician characteristics include education, experience, and credentials, including board certification. Treatment-unit characteristics include the numbers, training, experience, and roles of nurses, technicians, social workers, and nutritionists; physical equipment and treatment technology (machines, dialysate, membranes, and software); and amenities.

Patient characteristics include demographic, clinical, and functional status. Baseline measures, against which processes and outcomes are later judged, should include primary diagnosis (and its severity), comorbid conditions (and their severity), functional status (physical, social, and mental functioning) patient perceptions of their own health, and patient preferences.

Process

The processes of care include both the technical and the interpersonal aspects of care. In dialysis, these involve

(1) the diagnosis, prescription, and delivery of treatment to the patient by physicians and other clinicians;

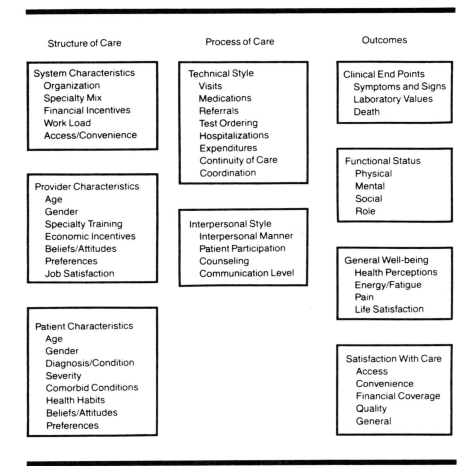

FIGURE 12-1   Conceptual Framework of the Medical Outcomes Study
SOURCE: Tarlov et al. (1989). Copyright, 1989, American Medical Association.
Used with permission.

(2) the biological interactions of the patient with the technology of vascular access, membrane, dialysate, machine, and prescription;

(3) the technical support of water purification and monitoring, dialysate concentrate handling, reprocessing of dialyzers and blood tubing, infection control, and equipment maintenance; and

(4) the vital personal interactions between patients and clinicians.

The actual use of the dialysis system for purifying the blood, usually three treatments per week, involves the following: pretreatment patient assessment; initiation of needle placement or other vascular connection; monitoring during dialysis; review of the dialysis prescription to confirm or alter it; termination of the dialysis session; and end-of-treatment assessment. Patient care also involves periodic chemistry and hematology monitoring, patient instruction, correction of identified problems, and periodic complete evaluations (physical examination, x rays, electrocardiogram, echocardiogram, and other tests).

This complex array of processes requires, at minimum, the treatment of complications and related conditions such as hypertension, anemia, infection, and bone disease. For patients treated by continuous ambulatory peritoneal dialysis (CAPD), special infection-control procedures associated with fluid exchange are required.

The validity of process measures, however, is often unsupported in the literature (Audet et al., 1990); they bear a presumed but seldom documented relationship to outcomes. The effectiveness of many tests, procedures, medications, and even counseling has not been critically demonstrated in medicine. For chronically ill patients with complex medical and social conditions, the relationships between process and outcome measures are even less well understood than for acute-care patients. Dialysis is no exception, despite the limited scope and recurring nature of most processes. Even the optimal prescription of dialysis treatment, for example, is far from agreed upon in the renal community.

Outcomes

The IOM quality study emphasizes patient-care outcomes (Lohr, 1990), as does this study. Outcomes of care may be categorized in terms of

(1) mortality;

(2) proximate or intermediate clinical outcomes (e.g.,infection rates, hematocrit levels, clinical and laboratory values, results of hypertension control, and results of prescription dialysis);

(3) morbidities (e.g., abnormal observed clinical signs, physiological laboratory measurements, and patient-reported symptoms, such as complications or adverse treatment effects);

(4) disease-specific and general functional-status effects; and

(5) patient well-being, satisfaction, and quality of life.

Several comments about these outcome measures are warranted. First, although ESRD patient mortality is essential (and has received much attention in recent years), other outcome measures are needed to assess patients with a complex clinical conditions (such as ESRD) who undergo treatment that extends over long periods of time and involves numerous prolonged contacts with many medical care providers.

Second, proximate clinical outcome measures guide patient management decisions as much as any other outcomes and are easily linked as endpoints to the relevant process measures. They include such measures as blood chemistries, hematocrit, and blood urea nitrogen.

Third, validated measures of functional status (physical, mental, and social functioning, including rehabilitation, general well-being, and patient satisfaction) have been developed at a brisk pace in the past decade, largely within the health services research community (Lohr, 1989). These measures have been used mainly for research purposes but are now being adapted for use in clinical practice (Patrick and Bergner, 1990). Unfortunately, this literature is not widely known to practicing physicians.

Outcomes *and* Process *and* Structure

In recent years, quality assessment and assurance have shifted from an emphasis on structure and process to widespread agreement that such measures are important only as they are related to outcomes (Lohr et al., 1988; Lohr, 1988). Although this increased emphasis on outcomes has led some to reject process and structural measures of quality as unimportant, it is important to underscore at both the conceptual and the practical levels the need to link outcome measures to process measures (Lohr, 1990). Nor should structural measures of quality be ignored, especially if no other measures exist, as the discussion of personnel in the previous chapter suggests. Structure provides the institutional, physical, and human framework that influences the range of possible outcomes and the nature and scope of the processes of care.

Proximate Clinical Indicators

Proximate clinical indicators include both process and outcomes. Outcomes, resulting from the patient-provider encounters, include, for example, infection rates, hematocrit levels, and the outcomes of prescription dialysis. Many factors affect such outcomes, including the initial functional and health status of the patient. The task of QA, and the supporting assessment function, is to identify those aspects of medical care that are under the control of providers, as distinct from other factors that affect outcomes, such as patient characteristics.

The criteria for selecting a proximate outcome measure include the following: the *time interval* between the receipt of care and the measurement of outcome must be chosen carefully to measure a cause-effect relationship; *comorbidities* must be acknowledged in the indicator or measure, minimally by their presence and preferably by their severity; the indicator or measure must be related to *standards* or norms of care, based on the literature, data aggregation, direct observation, or other means of ascertaining expert opinion; and the indicator must pertain to treatable medical factors.

Process statements, or instructions about diagnostic and treatment intervention, codify knowledge from the medical literature, expert judgment, and direct observation of patients into norms of practice, guidelines, indications for appropriate use, or algorithms (Audet et al., 1990). These statements guide physician and nurse behavior in the appropriate management of individual patients. Although these process measures must be validated, they provide a reasonable way to critically assess patient conditions and to improve the quality of practice.

There are at least three criteria for selecting a process measure. First, the measure must bear a putative relationship to outcomes that is supported by clinical studies of efficacy or, at least, by expert opinion. Second, its use must be feasible, that is, data about it can be found in the medical chart. Third, the measure must have a high degree of specificity regarding application; for example, it specifies that a patient with a temperature of 102 degrees F, due to an identified infection, should be treated in a particular way.

Proximate clinical indicators combine outcome and process measures. Typically, a discussion of one leads to a discussion of the other, since the two interact continuously in the clinical setting. For example, a low hematocrit, say, less than 20 percent, is an outcome (or perhaps an initial baseline measure); the administration of EPO under various protocols is a process; and a high hematocrit following treatment is a resulting outcome. The treatment of anemia, as an example of a proximate clinical indicator, is presented in Appendix 1 of this chapter for consideration by renal providers. This candidate indicator has been developed from the literature and from informally solicited expert opinion. Although empirical research is needed to validate it so that it can be used to distinguish between good and bad care, it illustrates the meaning of this section.

Functional- and Health-Status Assessments

Proximate clinical indicators are necessary but not sufficient for assessing quality of care. More important than the presence or absence of signs, symptoms, or laboratory test values is the patient's response to how treatment affects his or her life. Thus, functional- and health-status assessments are also necessary. *Functional status* refers to how well patients function. *Health status*, sometimes referred to as health-related quality of life, concerns itself not only with the health-related physical, social, and psychological functioning of patients but also with how patients perceive their well-being. It focuses attention on what the patient brings to the treatment situation, including his or her financial, social, family, and emotional resources-factors that powerfully affect the outcome of care of chronic-disease patients. That baseline status influences all subsequent internal and external assessments.

Health status assessment has developed strongly within the past decade. Several important summaries of the field have been published recently (Katz, 1987; Lohr, 1989; Lohr and Ware, 1987). The major conclusions emerging from that literature are the following: First, substantial progress in measurement has occurred in the past decade. Second, measures of the health status of pediatric patients need to be developed (Lewis et al., 1989), a need of ESRD pediatric patients also (Evans et al., 1990a).

Third, generic health status measures,[1] when supplemented by disease-specific measures, permit comparisons across groups and sites of care and are sensitive to the changes in the clinical status of patients that are of interest to physicians (Patrick and Deyo, 1989; Temkin et al., 1989). Generic measures have been used in research on ESRD patients (Hart and Evans, 1987; Julius et al., 1989). ESRD-specific measures have yet to be developed. Thus, a direct comparison of generic and ESRD-specific measures has not been made.

Fourth, health status assessment has begun to be used in clinical research, most extensively by pharmaceutical firms for clinical trials of new drugs and biologicals (Kazis et al., 1989; Luce et al., 1989). Both U.S. and Canadian clinical trials of erythropoietin (EPO) used such measures (Canada Erythropoietin Study Group, 1990; Evans et al., 1990b).

Fifth, health status research has shown that the physician-patient interaction affects the health status of patients. Ascertaining patient preferences has become a central concern, especially where the choice between two treatments does not turn clearly on scientific knowledge or the clinical skill of the physician but on how patients assess the different probable outcomes (Kaplan, et al., 1989; Kaplan and Ware, 1989).

Finally, health status assessment has only begun to be used in clinical practice. For such use to proceed further, the clinical utility of health status information must be demonstrated and then shown to have an effect on patient outcomes (Nelson and Berwick, 1989). Patrick and Bergner (1990) argue that two major challenges of clinical application must be confronted in the next decade. First, short, reliable, self-administered comprehensive measures that are sensitive to variations in health care organization and medical practice must be developed. Second, disease-specific health status measures must be developed to supplement generic ones.

The development of short patient survey instruments is necessary to adapt research instruments to patient management use by clinicians. The Medical Outcomes Study 36-item short-form Health Survey, for example, has been validated, takes 6 minutes to complete, can be self-administered by a patient or easily administered by a nurse (Tarlov et al., 1989). These short forms will need to be validated for use on special populations. Anecdotal reports suggest that, for the most part, patients are pleased at the attention implied by a survey. As short instruments are developed, their high information content and usefulness to clinicians for patient management and improving patient outcomes can become clear.

Patient Satisfaction

Mention of "patient satisfaction" in the OBRA 1987 ESRD legislation reflects recognition by Congress that a critical test of quality is how patients assess the care they receive. Patient satisfaction constitutes an important way to assess the amenities and interpersonal aspects of care and whether patients believe that they are treated with dignity and respect (Davies and Ware, 1988). It can be validly and reliably measured.

Quality of Life

The literature regarding the quality of life of ESRD patients intersects strongly with health status assessment (Evans et al., 1990a; Quevedo, 1991). Evans and his colleagues (1985, 1987, 1989, 1990b) have conducted three major quality-of-life studies in dialysis and kidney transplantation from 1981 to the present; other studies are in progress. These studies have focused on modality-specific quality of life and on longitudinal studies of the same patient group. All the studies have involved objective[2] (functional ability, employment, and health status) as well as subjective[3] (well-being, life satisfaction, psychological affect, and happiness) measures of quality of life. Case-mix adjustment was based on sociodemographic characteristics of patients and medical characteristics (primary diagnosis, the presence and number of comorbid conditions, duration of current treatment modality, and percentage with failed transplant).

The major findings are these: Transplant patients generally have greater functional ability, are in better health, are more likely to return to work, and have higher levels on all scales than patients on any form of dialysis. A failed transplant may adversely affect the quality of life of an ESRD patient, but most such patients continue to prefer transplantation to dialysis. Diabetes adversely affects the quality of life of transplant recipients. Longitudinal studies show that the quality of life of transplant recipients, diabetic or not, improves over time.

Among dialysis patients, home hemodialysis patients generally enjoy a higher quality of life than in-center hemodialysis or CAPD patients. External observers, using "objective" measures, tend to rate the quality of life of dialysis patients relatively low. Dialysis patients themselves, however, report satisfaction with their lives.

Studies of EPO have shown that it enhances the quality of life of dialysis patients (Evans et al., 1990b). Although, in the 10 months they were studied, these patients were no more likely to return to work than other dialysis patients, it would be premature to weigh these findings too heavily, since other factors affect employment.

Bremer and colleagues (1989) basically confirm the findings of Evans and colleagues in rank-ordering successful transplantation, home hemodialysis, CAPD, and in-center hemodialysis relating to quality of life, but found that a failed transplant reduces quality of life in objective as well as subjective terms. Julius and colleagues (1989) found that transplant patients fared better than dialysis patients on activities of daily living (ADL) Sickness Impact Profile when scores were adjusted by analysis of covariance for all factors in the analyses. Similarly, in-center hemodialysis patients did better than CAPD patients. The only statistically significant differences were between living-donor-transplant recipients and CAPD patients. The strongest explanatory factors for both high dependency in ADL and high physical dysfunction were older age, diabetes as primary cause of ESRD, and a greater number of comorbid conditions.

Finally, the objective-subjective distinction in these ESRD quality-of-life studies raises the question of what clinicians are to do when patients evaluate their own quality of life more highly than do "objective" observers. This is basically the same issue as that discussed in Chapter 3 regarding the initiation or termination of treatment. The appropriate response is that health-status and quality-of-life measures can provide useful information to clinicians for assessing individual patients. Such information may predict treatment outcomes, but it should be discussed with the patient and his or her family when major treatment decisions are being made.

ESRD quality-of-life studies have been used for *research* about the effectiveness of different treatment modalities. They have not been used for improving patient management. However, they have laid an important foundation for the future use of functional- and health-status measures in nephrology.

Adjustment for Patient Complexity

Adjustment for patient differences serves several purposes. For reimbursement issues, case-mix control or severity adjustment is done to predict resource use (Cretin and Worthman, 1986; Jencks and Dobbins, 1987). In quality assessment, it is used to compare treatment outcomes across institutions, as in the HCFA use of hospital mortality data (Green et al., 1990). For patient management purposes, adjustment for patient complexity is required to evaluate variation in outcomes by modality of treatment, site of care, length of treatment in years, and other factors, as well as to predict resource needs.

This report uses *patient complexity*, a comprehensive term, to encompasses both case mix and severity. *Case-mix control*, as used in the ESRD program, is limited to age, gender, race, and reported primary diagnosis leading to ESRD. *Severity-of-illness* measures specific to ESRD have yet to be developed, but severity is often used synonymously with case mix. Patient complexity refers to the following patient characteristics: demographic status, primary diagnosis, clinical severity of illness, as well as socioeconomic, social support, and functional and health status. Validated measures may exist for some variables and may need to be developed for others in the ESRD setting; similarly, data may be available for some measures and need to be collected for others. However, if outcome data are to be interpreted in a way that avoids the inappropriate attribution of causality, then the more comprehensive the basis for adjusting for differences among patients, the better. The measurement of patient complexity, then, represents a hoped-for future state, not a present reality.

In the development of measures of patient complexity, the most immediate practical need of clinicians is to develop adjusters for the *clinical severity* of ESRD patients. The simplest approach to this task uses patient-specific case-mix data found in Medicare data bases. A second approach builds on this data base with additional data about the accuracy of the primary diagnosis and the frequency of comorbid conditions. To this end, the USRDS is analyzing a retrospective sample of 2,500 patient abstracts (USRDS, 1990). The USRDS Scientific Advisory Committee has recommended to the National Institute of Diabetes and Digestive and Kidney Diseases (NIDDK) that a prospective study be done.

A third approach, not yet attempted in the ESRD patient population, reflects that used by the Medical Outcomes Study (Kravitz et al., 1991). A scaling and scoring approach was developed to assess the severity of the primary diagnosis in clinical- as well as functional- status terms for office-practice patients. This approach was extended to assess the severity of comorbid conditions in the same way. Severity scores for primary diagnosis as well as for comorbid conditions were then combined into a scale that has been shown to differentiate among patients and can be used to adjust for outcomes in terms of the baseline clinical severity of patients. This allows patients to be compared within units, across units, and across modalities. This group provides an example of this approach applied to diabetes mellitus (Kravitz, 1991).

In the ESRD population, disease severity and comorbidities affect health status so strongly that they must be assessed at the baseline in a systematic way. Only then can they be used for predicting outcomes of care. Developing means to adjust for clinical severity is a necessary first step toward creating a full set of measures of patient complexity.

RESPONSIBILITIES OF FEDERAL AGENCIES

The U.S. Department of Health and Human Services (DHHS) exercises responsibility for quality assessment and assurance in the ESRD program through both the PHS and HCFA.

Public Health Service

Within the PHS, CDC, FDA, NIH, and AHCPR, respectively, exercise broad authorities related to infection control, equipment and device safety, basic and applied medical research, health services research, technology assessment, and practice guidelines. Relative to ensuring the quality of care delivered to ESRD patients, their contributions are indicated below.

Centers for Disease Control

The CDC surveys dialysis facilities for dialysis-related problems, including hepatitis infection (Alter et al., 1983a,b; 1986), hepatitis vaccination, AIDS infection, extent of dialyzer reuse (Alter et al., 1988), and prevalence of pyrogenic reactions (Gordon et al., 1988). The survey, first conducted in 1976, has been done annually since 1982, being included with the annual HCFA facility survey since 1981. Although compliance with this survey is voluntary, CDC achieves a very high response rate. Results are reported annually within the DHHS (Alter and Favero, 1988) and in the clinical literature.

CDC, through its infection control program, investigates problems of water treatment and contamination as well as dialyzer reuse. These detailed, professional inquiries, often in cooperation with HCFA and FDA, permit rapid analysis of poorly understood but dangerous problems and allow appropriate remediable action by providers. However, their scope is limited. The multiagency efforts sometimes become disconnected, and the reports to the provider community are not systematically or widely distributed. Nonetheless, the agency has a well-earned reputation for scientific integrity, and most providers acknowledge the utility of the information that CDC collects.

Food and Drug Administration

The FDA responsibilities related to ESRD include ensuring the safety and efficacy of drugs and biologicals, medical devices, food additives, and manufacturing process standards. Basically, all currently used dialysis equipment resembles devices that existed before enactment of the 1976 Medical Device Amendments. Consequently, recent innovations in dialysis-related medical devices have been granted FDA approval under the "grandfather" clause of the 1976 amendments, and manufacturers have not been required to generate clinical trial evidence of efficacy.

FDA authority for the safety and efficacy of dialysis equipment and supplies includes devices such as the dialyzer membrane; proportioning and monitoring machines; subsystems for water purification and dialysate concentrate labeling and handling; and dialyzers and blood tubing.

However, FDA has gone beyond these regulatory limits to develop, with the renal provider community, educational materials—videotapes on human factors in dialysis treatment, infection control, water processing, and dialyzer reuse. It has also prepared a water treatment manual. These materials have been uniformly well received.

In addition, FDA contracted in 1990 with Dialysis Management, Inc., to produce a report, "A Quality Assurance Program for Hemodialysis Facilities." That report, expected in early 1991, will deal with water treatment, delivery systems (e.g., dialysate proportioning, temperature control, conductivity control, and monitoring), dialysate, dialyzers, other supplies and equipment, anticoagulation in dialysis, vascular access devices, hemodialyzer reuse, infection control, and toxic chemicals handling. It is expected to review the pertinent literature regarding risks and hazards, existing standards, routine and long-term monitoring, preventive maintenance, staff training, and patient education.

Hemodialysis equipment and systems are becoming more sophisticated and require more monitoring and maintenance. ESRD patients are also presenting with greater disease severity. Therefore, it may become appropriate in the future for FDA, or another agency, to assess the implications for safety and efficacy of the education and skill levels of technicians.

National Institutes of Health

NIH is seldom seen as a quality assessment or assurance agency. This view overlooks the critical role of clinical research and clinical trials in providing the scientific underpinnings of clinical practice. It also ignores the standard-setting role that academic investigators often exercise for a much larger group of practitioners.

NIH, through the National Institute of Allergy and Infectious Diseases (NIAID) and the NIDDK, supports transplant immunology and kidney disease research. Early in the 1980s, as indicated in Chapter 10, NIDDK terminated the Artificial Kidney Chronic Uremia contract research program in clinical dialysis and transplantation, which had existed since 1965. Since then, the agency has not supported the clinical study of dialysis to any appreciable extent (Levin et al., 1990). Thus, little was done in the 1980s, for example, to deepen scientific knowledge about the adequacy of dialysis, a critical treatment issue during a time when facilities were under increasing reimbursement-related pressures. The committee believes that the resumption of active support of clinical dialysis research by NIDDK would contribute greatly to the quality of clinical practice.

Agency for Health Care Policy and Research

OBRA 1989 created a new PHS organization, AHCPR. The new agency subsumes the health services research and technology assessment functions of the National Center for Health Services Research and adds new functions related to the dissemination of research results, the development of practice guidelines, and data base development. AHCPR administers the DHHS Medical Treatment Effectiveness Program (MEDTEP), which consolidates outcomes and effectiveness research. If adequately funded over the long term, AHCPR will provide an important focus of research addressed to what works in clinical practice.

Health Care Financing Administration

HCFA is responsible to the public for prudently managing the resources it administers, including ensuring that acceptable quality of care is delivered to Medicare beneficiaries. The HCFA responsibility for QA has been addressed historically through the PSROs and, more recently, the PROs. Since 1987, it has issued periodic hospital mortality reports, attempted to make Medicare data more accessible to researchers and practitioners, and advocated during 1987-89 an Effectiveness Initiative (Roper et al., 1988). This latter effort provided one major impetus for the creation of AHCPR and its MEDTEP program.

These general QA efforts provide the context for this committee's recommendations regarding the responsibility of HCFA for quality assessment and assurance of the ESRD program. The ESRD QA function has been exercised by the Health Standards and Quality Bureau (HSQB), primarily through the conditions of coverage, state survey agencies, and the ESRD networks.[4]

Conditions of Coverage

The 1976 regulations set forth conditions of coverage for renal transplantation centers and renal dialysis facilities and centers as requirements for participation in Medicare (41 Fed. Reg. 22502-22522, June 3, 1976). These are listed in Table 12-1. Several of these conditions may be considered indicators of quality because they stipulate standards that represent structural measures and some process measures of quality.

The most important conditions for QA purposes in dialysis facilities are 405.2137, 405.2138, 405.2161, 405.2162, and 405.2163. Condition 405.2137 requires that each treatment facility maintain a written long-term program and long-term patient care plan "to ensure that each patient receives the appropriate modality of care and the appropriate care within than modality." The patient, or his or her parent or guardian, is to be involved in planning that care. Condition 405.2138 requires that each facility establish a written statement of patients' rights and responsibilities and inform patients of this statement.

Condition 405.2161 specifies the responsibilities of a medical director, who must be a qualified physician. The most important are:

TABLE 12-1 Conditions of Coverage for ESRD Providers

405.2131	provider status: renal transplantation center or renal dialysis center
405.2132	fulfillment of service needs in network
405.2133	furnishing data and information for ESRD program administration
405.2134	membership in a network
405.2135	compliance with federal, state, and local laws and regulations
405.2136	governing body and management
405.2137	patient long-term program and patient-care plan
405.2138	patients' rights and responsibilities
405.2139	medical records
405.2140	physical environment
405.2160	affiliation agreement or arrangement
405.2161	director of a renal dialysis facility or renal dialysis center
405.2162	staff of a renal dialysis facility or renal dialysis center
405.2163	minimal service requirements for a renal dialysis facility or renal dialysis center
405.2170	director of a renal transplantation center
405.2171	minimal service requirements for a renal transplantation center

NOTE: Encoded at Title 42, Part 405 of the *Code of Federal Regulations.*

- participating in the selection of a suitable treatment modality for all patients;
- ensuring adequate training of nurses and technicians in dialysis techniques;
- ensuring adequate monitoring of the patient and the dialysis process;
- ensuring the development and availability of a patient-care policy and procedures manual and its implementation; and
- when self-dialysis training is offered, ensuring that patient teaching materials are available for patient use during training and at times other than during the dialysis procedure.

This statement is the most extensive ESRD QA requirement set forth in federal regulations.

Condition 405.2162 deals with standards for registered nurses, on-duty personnel, and self-care dialysis training personnel. Condition 405.2163 stipulates standards for laboratory services, social services, dietetic services, self-care dialysis support services, and participation in a recipient registry. The most important of these standards are:

- *Registered nurse.* At least one full-time qualified nurse must be responsible for nursing services.
- *On-duty personnel.* Whenever patients are undergoing dialysis, other than self-care dialysis, one currently licensed health professional (e.g., physician, registered nurse, or licensed practical nurse) experienced in ESRD care is to be on duty to oversee ESRD patient care. An adequate number of personnel

must be present to meet patient needs and medical and nonmedical emergencies.

• *Social services.* To support the patient's social functioning and adjustment, social services are to be provided to patients and their families. These services are to be furnished by a qualified social worker responsible for psychosocial evaluations, team review of patient progress, and recommendation of treatment changes based on the patient's current psychosocial needs. In addition, the social worker is to identify community social agencies and assist patients and families in using them.

• *Dietetic services.* Patients are to be evaluated for nutrition needs by the attending physician and by a qualified dietitian. The dietitian, in consultation with the attending physician, is responsible for assessing the nutrition and dietetic needs of each patient, recommending therapeutic diets, counseling patients and their families on prescribed diets, and monitoring adherence and response to diets.

These conditions do not establish staffing requirements; instead they specify the types of personnel with given training who are to provide treatment. Some state health codes prescribe staffing patterns in much greater detail. These federal standards represent structural measures of quality and have never been related to either process or outcome measures. They are based on the judgments of health professionals about necessary services, not on a demonstrated relationship to outcomes.

HCFA reimbursement policies reinforce staffing patterns that have the lowest economic cost (e.g., one licensed practical nurse and the rest technicians, with special training for each shift) without regard for patient complexity. Pressures from Medicare ESRD reimbursement, as discussed in Chapter 10, have led treatment units to depart from these Medicare-specified staffing standards. With respect to social services, HCFA announced in 1990 its intention to issue a Notice of Proposed Rulemaking that would move away from input standards and focus on outcomes. This outcome orientation is commendable, and presumably it will be accompanied by proposed outcome measures. HCFA should also relate these outcomes to the structural and process requirements to achieve them.

State Survey Process

HCFA contracts with state health departments to survey all Medicare-certified facilities, including ESRD treatment units. Although these state surveys have potential for measuring structural and some process measures of quality in dialysis units, providers frequently complain about the inconsistency of the surveys from state to state and the variability in the level of training of surveyors. The present system is characterized by poor support, inadequate training, and inconsistent oversight. It produces surveys that vary widely in approach, thoroughness, and perceived fairness. Consequently, they are seldom accepted as valid by clinicians.

Several simple steps can be taken to address these issues (personal communication, Douglas L. Vlchek, January 12, 1990). First, HCFA should rewrite the "Interpretive Guidelines" manual for surveyors to conform with the current conditions of coverage of End-Stage Renal Disease Services (42 CFR Part 405, Subpart U) and describe the context of its use. Second, all ESRD facility surveyors should be required to attend a training program that uses a standard curriculum. Third, all surveyors should be required to pass a certifying examination after completing the training program. Fourth, all surveyors should be required to attend a periodic refresher course, followed by an examination. Finally, HCFA should consider putting in place a broader, more effective quality control method than it currently uses.

The committee endorses efforts to strengthen the competence of state survey agencies to fulfill their responsibilities. The committee also believes that an effective ESRD QA program requires the integration of the state surveys with other QA activities. State surveys can make an important contribution to QA, but they cannot be the centerpiece of a QA system.

HSQB and the ESRD Networks

Quality assurance within the ESRD program derives from the 1972 statute that vested authority in the Secretary to regulate reimbursement and included the requirement of "a medical review board to screen the appropriateness of patients for the proposed treatment procedures." Regulations of 1976 (41 Fed. Reg. 22052, June 3, 1976) required that each ESRD network have a medical review board to monitor the effectiveness of the patient long-term program; oversee the evaluation of the performance of physicians, nonphysicians, and facilities; coordinate the medical care evaluation studies of network facilities (at minimum, one annually for each facility); and provide written recommendations to physicians and facilities about possible improvements in the care of patients.

The ESRD network medical care review function has been performed with varying degrees of effectiveness by different networks. As originally conceived, it was to depend on data from an ESRD medical information system that did not exist until several years after HCFA was created in 1977. Furthermore, networks struggled for survival during much of the 1980s, fending off repeated but unsuccessful attempts by HCFA to eliminate them. The circumstances were hardly suitable for putting together a sound QA system at the ESRD network level.

In OBRA 1985 and OBRA 1986, Congress directed the Secretary of DHHS to consolidate the 32 existing ESRD networks into 17 networks, later increased to 18. Under OBRA 1986, each network was to include a medical review board whose functions were to include "reporting on facilities and providers that are not providing appropriate care" and "conducting on-site reviews of facilities and providers . . . utilizing standards of care established by the network organization." Networks existed in administrative limbo until the issue of their liability for medical review was resolved in 1989. Since then, they have followed the lead of HSQB in QA efforts.

In March 1990, HSQB centralized the design of the medical review function. It distributed the "National Medical Review Criteria Screens" and "Medical Case Review Procedures" for public comment to implement Sections 9335(d)-(h) of OBRA 1986 regarding the establishment of criteria and standards related to the quality and appropriateness of patient care (HCFA, 1990a,b). The proposed review process requires ESRD networks to use screens[5] to review, through the Network Medical Review Boards, a random sample of medical records. Records that fail the screens are then reviewed by network personnel with the local facility personnel. Opportunities are provided to the facility for discussion, written comment, the development of a Corrective Action Plan, specific educational activities, or sanctions.

HSQB began pilot testing the review process during 1990-91, focusing on "validity and meaningfulness of screens, availability and ease of collection of data elements, sensitivity and specificity of data elements as flags, and controllability of underlying causes of variances from indicators." It plans to review the screens periodically and modify them to reflect evolving clinical knowledge.

The HSQB effort clearly represents one plausible approach to QA in the ESRD program. However, it reflects several problems. First, the objectives of the endeavor remain unclear. Although characterized as a pilot program designed to improve care, the plan also refers to sanctions, which are surely premature for a pilot effort. The approach further presumes that the provision of high-quality, comprehensive, and appropriate medical care to patients in ESRD facilities can best be ensured by a top-down monitoring system as opposed to QA activity rooted at the treatment-unit level.

Second, the HSQB proposal was designed rapidly by a small number of professionals drawn exclusively from the nephrology community without benefit of any expertise from the quality assessment community. A broader group, augmenting the expertise of the nephrology community with that of the quality assessment community appears warranted. The current initiative appears to underestimate the need for an investment in QA design. Third, allowing only one year for design and pilot testing may be too ambitious both technically and for the wide-scale learning that must accompany effective implementation. Adequate time is needed for system design, training and education of the provider community, and review and redesign. Although uniformity on a national scale for a common set of data elements is desirable, several competing approaches using these common elements might be considered in the pilot-test phase as a way to identify the appropriate elements of a national system.

Fourth, the effort imposes financial costs on providers and networks. The requirements of random chart review are labor intensive, expensive, and exceed the number of experienced ESRD reviewers.

Fifth, the random chart review methodology depends on criteria sets and exceptions that have yet to be validated. It represents a flagging system that is more likely to reveal the quality of documentation than the quality of care. Moreover, it overlooks more readily available flags such as mortality and hospitalization and appears to overlook the fact that existing data could guide focused case review.

The random chart review method also assumes that an individual patient record can be meaningfully evaluated against an untested universal clinical indicator of quality. Also important, this review strategy does not assess the quality of treatment units; facilities characterized by high mortality, low transplant referral, low home dialysis referral, and other measures of unit performance, for example, are completely overlooked. In this context, it does little to move outlier units toward the average level of quality and little to improve performance for those grouped around the mean.

Finally, the HSQB approach misses an important opportunity to QA oversight functions that it could exercise in concert with the Bureau of Policy Development (BPD) and the Office of Research and Demonstrations (ORD) using existing Medicare data bases. These opportunities are discussed below.

Opinion is divided in the renal community about the usefulness of ESRD networks. Defenders tout their potential; others tolerate their existence on the grounds that some institutional framework is better than none; still others argue that they should be eliminated. The utility of the networks can be realized if they implement a well-designed QA strategy and develop the supporting data systems. Responsibility for the articulation of such a strategy resides with HCFA.

Bureau of Policy Development

In Part IV, this report has examined ESRD reimbursement policies, the effects that such policies have had on quality, and several controversial reimbursement issues. Indirectly, all these chapters show that ESRD reimbursement policies have been developed without sufficient attention to their implications for quality. The atypical service intensity criterion for reimbursement rate exception requests, for example, is a category for classifying requests and not a decision rule (or criterion) in the technical sense of that term.

On the other hand, the HCFA coverage and reimbursement decisions regarding the use of EPO for the treatment of anemia in dialysis patients offer an interesting alternative perspective. The coverage decision was made promptly in 1989 within weeks of FDA approval of the compound. The reimbursement policy, although criticized by many providers, has clearly been transitional.

Congress, in OBRA 1990, modified Medicare policy on EPO to provide for self-administration of EPO by home dialysis patients and dose-related reimbursement for inpatients. HCFA, before this legislation, had initiated a review of EPO, the equivalent of a Phase IV trial protocol, that involved collecting data on EPO dosage and hematocrit response. It recently awarded a contract to evaluate these data to the Johns Hopkins University School of Public Health. The review may provide the basis for a dosage-related payment policy that is related, in turn, to proximate clinical outcome data—the effect of EPO on hematocrit levels. Outcome measures may perhaps be expanded to include measures of energy, employability, employment, functional and health status, and quality of life. The HCFA attempt to relate reimbursement to an observed proximate clinical outcome, then, suggests a QA approach for the entire ESRD program.

The committee believes that ESRD reimbursement policy has reached the point where it is essential that HCFA establish adequate measures, data, and systems to predict and monitor the consequences of all future reimbursement policy changes. The EPO experience may point in the appropriate direction.

Office of Research and Demonstrations

Within ORD, the Office of Research (OR) has established a basis for contributing to ESRD QA functions. It has been instrumental, with the Bureau of Data Management and Strategy (BDMS), in developing the ESRD data bases now widely used by the research community, including this committee. It has supported ESRD quality-of-life studies. Its staff have conducted many cost and epidemiologic analyses, prepared an annual ESRD Research Report since 1984, contributed to the literature, and conducted numerous internal analyses. Eggers (unpublished data, 1990), for example, analyzed ESRD ambulance use and showed that ESRD patients accounted for 8 percent of all Medicare ambulance expenditures, and that three-quarters of this 8 percent were generated by one percent of the ESRD patients. (Good functional status measures might predict such use.)

OR has an increasing capability to conduct analyses that link quality and cost data. It also has the technical capability to generate facility-specific ESRD mortality and other data on a time-series basis. Investigating the high-and low-mortality outliers among treatment units would be useful in its own right and might stimulate a demand by providers for development of validated measures, methods, and data in this area.

OR has not supported external research related to ESRD severity adjustment or health status assessment to any appreciable degree. Nor has it dealt with adapting generic functional- and health-status assessment instruments and measures for use in ESRD clinical practice. In short, OR has the data base and the analytical capability to enter more forcefully into the ESRD QA function, but it needs to do so with a coherent research agenda and in concert with other HCFA organizational units.

Coordination Within HCFA

Much greater coordination is needed within HCFA to develop a coherent agenda for QA in the ESRD program. Such an agenda would involve:

- relating major conditions of coverage to patient outcomes;
- developing measures of patient complexity to guide state surveys, assist network-based medical review, and help facilities with QA efforts;
- standardizing state surveys and integrating them within a broader QA strategy;
- distinguishing between oversight efforts to identify poor-quality providers and the aggregation of regional and national data to help develop norms of practice and improve the quality of care;
- assessing its QA efforts for their financial burden on facilities;
- analyzing reimbursement policy for its effects on quality; and
- supporting QA-related research.

Operationally, such coordination would require that the major bureaus within HCFA—BPD, HSQB, ORD, and BDMS—cooperate to develop such an agenda and pursue it in a systematic and credible way. In this context, the question asked by OBRA 1987 about the effects of reimbursement on quality is a very important question. How might it be answered? The EPO case suggests one way; that is, reimbursement policy could be analyzed in terms of patient outcomes. Not all aspects of dialysis or transplantation offer the opportunity to relate inputs and patient outcomes so directly. But the EPO case points in an appropriate direction.

HCFA might also consider the following issues, which join reimbursement and quality:

- The HCFA cost data analyzed in Chapter 11 indicate substantial variation among facilities on the basis of reported costs, audited costs, and "margins."[6] HCFA could easily identify the low- and high-cost outlier facilities (say, at the 10th and 90th percentiles of the audited-cost distribution), or those with high- and low-revenue margins, and devise a "quality audit" (that included mortality) to clarify the relationships between resources and quality.
- Available data permit HCFA to examine mortality on a facility-specific basis. It could identify low- and high-mortality treatment units and

conduct a "quality audit" that included payment and cost data to determine what factors might account for differences among units.

• If patient-complexity adjusters were developed, they could clarify the relationships among payment, treatment characteristics, and patient characteristics. Results could be analyzed for high- and low-cost units to clarify the utility of mortality as a quality measure.

• Hospital-based and independent outpatient dialysis units report quite different costs per treatment. Hospitals argue that these differences reflect greater patient severity. No compelling data have been presented, however, to support that claim. HCFA should design a pilot effort to examine prospectively the complexity differences between a random sample of patients drawn from hospital-based units and a random sample drawn from independent facilities as a way to resolve this decade-long issue.

Although none of the above proposals can be implemented immediately, all could be done soon if preceded by an appropriate investment in research design. Although existing data bases can provide substantial assistance in addressing these questions, some new data will be required. Most important, an agenda that includes the above issues would require a commitment from both HCFA and the provider community to engage these issues in a cooperative way. Absent such cooperation, the future is likely to be as fractious as the recent past.

Quality Assessment and Assurance Data Needs

The OBRA 1986 legislation authorized the creation of a National End-Stage Renal Disease Registry, discussed at length in Chapter 13. The registry has three identifiable functions: epidemiologic research, cost analyses linked to epidemiologic data, and data acquisition and analysis related to quality. Regarding the last function, the registry is "to assemble and analyze the data reported by network organizations, transplant centers, and other sources on all end stage renal disease patients" and determine "patient mortality and morbidity rates, and trends in such rates, and other indices of quality of care."

NIDDK established the USRDS on a contract basis in 1988, in a manner consistent with the OBRA 1986 legislation. USRDS receives the core of its data from HCFA; this includes all of the ESRD Program Management and Medical Information System (PMMIS) data and selected data on transplant follow-up and Medicare Parts A and B services. The ESRD networks are instrumental in collecting and processing PMMIS data and, through several consultative mechanisms, USRDS, HCFA, and the networks cooperate in data collection policies and procedures.

The committee attaches great importance to the establishment of an effective QA system for the ESRD program. What is needed is a system to collect data on selected measures of quality from treatment units. These data could then be aggregated to generate regional and national norms. National, regional, and facility-specific data should then be fed back promptly to individual treatment units by HCFA, on a nonpunitive basis, for unit review and evaluation. Where unit behavior deviates sharply from such empirically derived norms, HCFA mechanisms for investigating this variation can be established.

Given the establishment of the USRDS and its strong initial performance, it is essential that DHHS find a satisfactory way to facilitate the development of an effective QA data system implied by the OBRA 1986 legislation. This will undoubtedly require cooperative working relationships among NIDDK, HCFA, the ESRD networks, and the USRDS in the collection and analysis of quality-related data. Data support for ESRD QA is presently more of a hope than a reality. This situation should not be permitted to continue.

In addition to the data acquisition and analysis capability described above, a separate capability for the design of a QA system, including instruments, measures, and data elements, is needed. HCFA should be responsible for this capability, although it could be established either within the government or through a contractor. In any case, it requires an expert advisory group reflecting clinical, measurement, and quality assessment expertise and support for a staff that includes clinical and quality assessment professionals.

CONTINUOUS QUALITY IMPROVEMENT

Within the past 5 years, a literature has emerged dealing with the application of industrial quality control concepts to medicine and health. This nascent effort, known as the continuous quality improvement (or QI) model of quality assessment and assurance, has already gained many adherents. This section summarizes very briefly this literature. [A more extend summary can be found in Lohr (1990).]

The model originates with quality improvement in manufacturing and has been variously described as "total quality control," "total quality improvement," "quality improvement process," and "continuous improvement." In medicine, it is a facility-level approach to QA that represents an alternative to the top-down approach of HCFA. The best top-down system always risks becoming a paper compliance system and overloading treatment units with costly data requirements.

A facility-level approach is justified, however, as a way to incorporate the commitment to quality care into the unit philosophy and to focus on improving patient management and outcomes. Effective QA systems at the treatment-unit level can also help providers analyze the effects of reimbursement policies on patient management and outcomes. In fact, top-down and facility-unit-level QA approaches can be complementary, if HCFA and the provider community agree on the shared values and common purposes of QA.

The QI literature in health includes, first, by reference, the extensive literature on management and statistical quality control principles and applications, in which W. Edwards Deming and Joseph M. Juran are prominent (Garwin, 1986). Second, it includes the writings of a number of physicians regarding the attractiveness of the QI model for application in health (Berwick, 1988, 1989). Bataldan and Buchanan (1989), for example, provide an overview of the principles that have guided Hospital Corporation of America as it has pioneered in this area. Third, an applications literature has begun to emerge, much of which is still found in handbooks, conference notebooks, and applications manuals.

There are four core assumptions of continuous improvement. First, the individuals who deliver health care work mainly in organizations and QI, and therefore must use the energy and lines of accountability of these organizations to accomplish the purposes of QI. Second, health care workers—from physicians to technicians—wish to perform to the best of their ability, and QI challenges them to do so. It seeks to create a supporting environment and a progressively advancing set of quality benchmarks. Third, the failure of workers to perform at their best is usually a function of organizational systems, not of personal motivation. Fourth, the interactions among individuals, organizations, and systems of service delivery create situations that can always be improved.

The major principles that underlie the philosophy and rationale of the QI model are these. First, successful continuous improvement requires the commitment to quality of the highest leadership of a treatment unit or organization. This commitment must permeate the values and behavior of the entire organization. QI cannot be delegated to a peripheral "QA unit" or to a "QA professional," but must be primary to how the unit understands its clinical objectives and strategy.

Second, QI objectives are defined by an organization's orientation to its several "customers"—patients, employees, external payers, and policymakers. The patient is clearly the primary "customer" for health organizations, including ESRD treatment units, although not the only one.

Third, the commitment of a QI system is to *continuous* quality improvement, not to meeting *static* standards of care typical of traditional QA systems.

Fourth, QI emphasizes the systems or processes of care—how care gets delivered. All structures and processes of the organization that occur before the delivery of benefit to the patient must be engaged in a systematic, cooperative search to improve care. The QI activities of "planning, doing, checking, acting," therefore, are cyclic and iterative, and improvement occurs by integrating customers' views and the processes of care into the regular redesign of service and care.

Fifth, QI uses practical statistical techniques developed for industrial quality control to facilitate the search for improved quality. The instruments used for data collection and analysis follow from the organizational leadership's commitment to quality; they do not precede it. These include flow charts, fishbone diagrams, and run charts. Finally, the organizational commitment to continuous improvement is consistent with the professional values of physicians and the other clinicians who care for ESRD patients. It also provides the framework for integrating the clinical, technical support, administrative, and financial management aspects of a treatment unit.

The Dialysis Facility: Practical Considerations

Treatment units seeking to implement a QA system will have to address several practical problems. First, the unit philosophy of quality assessment and assurance must result from the careful deliberation and endorsement of the organization's board of directors, CEO or administrator, and medical director. These individuals must invest enough time to understand their QA strategy and adopt it in a deliberate, not superficial, way.

Second, relationships between medical directors and attending physicians should be clearly stated, preferably in writing, regarding adherence to unit or organization practices, including QA policies. Similarly, relationships between the medical director, the head nurse, and other professional members of the clinical team should be clearly articulated. These written statements should be the subject of training and education regarding both philosophy and implementation. They should state the organization's commitment to quality as a primary function, not as a delegated task of a QA professional.

Third, a commitment to QA underlines once again the importance of the careful monitoring of the dialysis prescription for the adequacy of treatment. The importance of monitoring water quality, dialysate concentrate, and dialyzer reprocessing is also emphasized by this orientation. Finally, a serious facility-level approach to QA must link process data to a critical review of patient outcome data, as discussed above.

Examples of ESRD Quality Assurance

In the ESRD context, the QI model has great potential applicability, both for clinical care and for the "industrial substrate" of dialysis. Although the committee is unaware of specific examples where individual ESRD providers have formally adopted the QI model, as defined by its foremost advocates, many providers have undoubtedly incorporated aspects of this model into their unit's routine practice and procedures. The principles of this model should be seriously considered by all ESRD providers.

Appendix 2 describes three ESRD provider organizations currently engaged in QA efforts that approximate some elements of the QI model, although none has explicitly characterized its efforts in this way. The examples are Dialysis Clinic, Inc., Cincinnati; Greenfield Health Systems, a division of Henry Ford Health System; and National Medical Care, Inc. They include not-for-profit and for-profit, independent and hospital-based organizations, ranging from a single unit to a large corporation.

What they have in common is a leadership commitment to quality and to using quality assessment and assurance for improved patient care and outcomes. They also rely extensively on strong data and measurement systems that are integral to the management of patient care and costs. The critical review of such data leads to process alterations and follow-up. These QA systems are not paper compliance efforts responding to the federal government. Presently, all focus on proximate clinical indicators, both process and outcome. None has yet to introduce measures of patient functional status and well-being to assess quality.

The committee has no systematic data about the extent of similar treatment-level QA systems within the ESRD provider community. These examples are hardly exhaustive and not necessarily representative. They do suggest the future direction of quality assessment and assurance for ESRD providers.

CONCLUSIONS AND RECOMMENDATIONS

Are quality assessment and assurance feasible and desirable within the ESRD program? The committee believes that they are. Substantial progress has been made on conceptual and measurement issues related to quality assessment, and the renal community should take advantage of that progress. The evolution of computer technology has made large-scale data collection, manipulation, and analysis feasible.

The challenge in the ESRD context is threefold. First, it is necessary to develop meaningful process and outcome indicators that are valid for ESRD patients in the ESRD treatment setting. Second, it is necessary to demonstrate to physicians that these measures have value for patient management and that they will benefit from incorporating them into their clinical practice. Third, it is essential that practicing clinicians adopt effective treatment-unit QA systems that reduce the QI philosophy to useful practice. The committee believes that the clinical community is prepared to engage in QA that permits them to do their jobs better and that genuinely helps patients.

Currently, a disjunction exists between federal QA systems, which are regulatory in character, and treatment-level systems that physicians and other clinicians use to improve patient care. This disjunction must be bridged in a mutually satisfactory manner if the maximum benefit of both approaches is to be realized.

As long as national and regional QA systems emphasize regulatory objectives, however, the medical community will respond with ambivalence. Providers generally accept the need to police those few among them who willfully trade quality for financial gain or simply disregard quality standards. They also value the opportunity to compare their own performance against national or regional norms. But they resent burdensome paperwork, are skeptical of the quality of QA programs, and remain suspicious of government motives.

The specific recommendations made by the committee are recapitulated here. They are that HCFA:

Improve the Medicare ESRD state survey system by developing uniform training and certification requirements for surveyors and by integrating the state system with other ESRD QA efforts.

Evaluate all policies, including reimbursement policies, for their quality effects on patients.

Provide adequate financial support to facilities for QA by incorporating facility QA costs in reimbursement for both dialysis and transplantation.

Coordinate the efforts of the Health Standards and Quality Bureau, the Bureau of Policy Development, and the Office of Research and Demonstrations; link existing data bases for the development and operation of ESRD QA oversight systems, and integrate the ESRD networks and state surveys into a coherent national QA strategy.

Establish an advisory group of nephrology professionals and experts in QA to design and develop ESRD-specific QA systems.

Support the regional and national data systems necessary for an effective QA system.

Modify the patient data intake to provide a basis for assessing patient complexity.

Support a continuing program of ESRD QA research.

NOTES

1. Generic instruments for assessing the functional and health status of individuals include the Sickness Impact Profile, the Quality of Well-Being Scale, Functional Limitations Index, the General Health Ratings Index, the Medical Outcome Study 36-item short form, the Health Utility Index, and the Patient Utility Measurement Set.
2. Objective refers to the assessment of patients by external observers.
3. Subjective refers to the patient's own assessment of his or her quality of life.
4. The ESRD networks were created in 1974, established by regulation in 1976, authorized by law in 1978, and consolidated by law in 1985 and 1986. Their development during the 1970s is described by Rettig and Marks (1980).
5. The screens, developed by a panel of nephrologists, are described as "clinical measures of quantifiable aspects of patient care to guide professionals in monitoring and evaluating patient care quality and appropriateness." Screens are not standards but, rather, triggers for identifying areas of patient care needing further evaluation.
6. It is uncertain whether this observed variation for one cross-sectional snapshot is volatile or stable over time. The factual situation should be easily determined by HCFA and analyses of quality adjusted accordingly by using multiyear data.

REFERENCES

Alter MJ, Ahtone J, Maynard JE. 1983a. Hepatitis B virus transmission associated with a multiple-dose vial in a hemodialysis unit. Ann Intern Med 99:330-333.

Alter MJ, Favero MS. 1988. National Surveillance of Dialysis-Associated Disease in the United States. Atlanta, Ga.: Centers for Disease Control.

Alter MJ, Favero MS, Petersen SM, Doto IL, Leger RT, Maynard JE. 1983b. National surveillance of dialysis-associated hepatitis and other diseases: 1976 and 1980. Dialysis Transplant 12:860-865.

Alter MJ, Favero MS, Maynard JE. 1986. Impact of infection control strategies on the incidence of dialysis-associated hepatitis in the United States. J Infect Dis 153:1149-1151.

Alter MJ, Favero MS, Miller JK, Coleman PJ, Bland LE. 1988. Reuse of hemodialyzers: Results of nationwide surveillance for adverse effects. JAMA 260:2073-2076.

Audet A-M, Greenfield S, Field M. 1990. Medical practice guidelines: Current activities and future directions. Ann Intern Med 113:709-714.

Bataldan PB, Buchanan ED. 1989. Industrial models of quality improvement. In: Goldfield N, Nash DB (eds.). Providing Quality Care: The Challenge to Physicians. Philadelphia, Pa.: American College of Physicians.

Berwick DM. 1988. Measuring health care quality. Pediatr Rev 10:11-16.

Berwick DM. 1989. Continuous improvement as an ideal in health care. N Engl J Med 320:53-56, 1424-1425.

Bremer BA, McCauley CR, Wrona RM, Johnson JP. 1989. Quality of life in end-stage renal disease: A reexamination. Am J Kidney Dis 13:200-209.

Canada Erythropoietin Study Group. 1990. Association between recombinant human erythropoietin and quality of life and exercise capacity of patients receiving haemodialysis. Br Med J 300:573-578.

Cretin S, Worthman L. 1986. Alternative Systems for Case Mix Classification in Health Care Financing. R-3457-HCFA. Santa Monica, Calif.: The RAND Corporation.

Davies AR, Ware JE Jr. 1988. Involving consumers in quality of care assessment. Health Affairs 7(1):33-48.

Donabedian A. 1966. Evaluating the quality of medical care. Milbank Memorial Fund 44(July, Pt 2):166-203.

Evans RW, Manninen DL, Garrison LP Jr, et al. 1985. The quality of life of patients with end-stage renal disease. N Engl J Med 312:553-559.

Evans RW, Garrison LP, Jr, Hart LG, Manninen DL. 1987. Health Care Financing Special Report: Findings from the National Kidney Dialysis and Kidney Transplantation Study. Baltimore, Md.: Health Care Financing Administration.

Evans RW, Manninen DL, Thompson C. 1989. A Cost and Outcome Analysis of Kidney Transplantation: The Implications of Initial Immunosuppressive Protocol and Diabetes. Seattle, Wash.: Battelle Human Affairs Research Centers.

Evans RW, Manninen DL, Dugan MK, et al. 1990a. The Kidney Transplant Health Insurance Study. Seattle, Wash.: Battelle Human Affairs Research Centers.

Evans RW, Rader B, Manninen DL, and the Cooperative Multicenter EPO Clinical Trial Group. 1990b. The quality of life of hemodialysis recipients treated with recombinant human erythropoietin. JAMA 263:825-830.

Garwin R. 1986. A Note on Quality: The Views of Deming, Juran, and Crosby. 9-687-001 (Rev. 6/87). Boston, Mass.: Harvard Business School.

Gordon SM, Tipple M, Bland LE, Harvis WR. 1988. Pyrogenic reactions associated with the reuse of disposable hollow-fiber hemodialyzers. JAMA 260:2077-2081.

Green J, Winfield N, Sharkey P, Passman LJ. 1990. The importance of severity of illness in assessing hospital mortality. JAMA 263:241-246.

Hart LG, Evans RW. 1987. The functional status of ESRD patients as measured by the Sickness Impact Profile. J Chronic Dis 40 (Suppl1):117S-130S.

HCFA (Health Care Financing Administration. 1990a. National Medical Review Criteria Screens. Health Standards and Quality Bureau. Baltimore, Md. March.

HCFA. 1990b. Medical Case Review Procedures. Health Standards and Quality Bureau. Baltimore, Md. March.

JCAHO (Joint Commission on the Accreditation of Healthcare Organizations). 1987. Agenda for Change. Update 1:1,6.

JCAHO. 1988. Agenda for Change. Update 2:1,5.

Jencks SF, Dobbins A. 1987. Refining case-mix adjustment: The research evidence. N Engl J Med 317:679-686.

Julius M, Hawthorne VM, Carpentier-Alting P, Kneisley J, Wolfe RA, Port FK. 1989. Independence in activities of daily living for end-stage renal disease patients: Biomedical and demographic correlates. Am J Kidney Dis 13:61-69.

Kaplan SH, Ware JE, Jr. 1989. The patient's role in health care and quality assessment. In: Goldfield N, Nash DB (eds.). Providing Quality Care: The Challenge to Clinicians. Philadelphia, Pa.: American College of Physicians.

Kaplan SH, Greenfield S, Ware JE, Jr. 1989. Assessing the effects of physician-patient interactions on the outcomes of chronic disease. Med Care 27(3, Suppl):S110-S127.

Katz S (ed.). 1987. The Portugal conference: Measuring quality of life and functional status in clinical and epidemiological research. J Chronic Dis 40:459.

Kazis LE, Anderson JJ, Meenan RF. 1989. Effect sizes for interpreting changes in health status. Med Care 27(3, Suppl):S178-S198.

Kravitz RL, Greenfield S, Rogers WH. 1991. Patient-mix in the practices of general internists, family physicians, cardiologists, and endocrinologists: results from the Medical Outcomes Study. In process.

Laffel G, Blumenthal D. 1989. The case for using industrial quality management science in health care organizations. JAMA 262:2869-2873.

Levin N, Keshaviah P, Gotch FA. 1990. Effect of reimbursement on innovation in the ESRD program. Paper prepared for the Institute of Medicine ESRD Study Committee. New York: Beth Israel Medical Center.

Lewis CC, Pantell RH, Kieckhefer GM. 1989. Assessment of children's health status: Field test of new approaches. Med Care 27(3, Suppl):S54-S65.

Lohr KN. 1988. Outcome measurement: concepts and questions. Inquiry 25(Spring):37-50.

Lohr KN (ed.). 1989. Advances in health status assessment: Conference proceedings. Med Care 27(3, Suppl).

Lohr KN (ed.). 1990. Medicare: A Strategy for Quality Assurance. Washington D.C.: National Academy Press.

Lohr KN, Ware JE, Jr (eds.). 1987. Proceedings of the advances in health assessment conference. J Chronic Dis 40(Suppl 1).

Lohr KN, Yordy KD, Thier SO. 1988. Current issues in quality of care. Health Affairs 7(1):5-18.

Luce BR, Weschler JM, Underwood C. 1989. The use of quality-of-life measures in the private sector. In: Mosteller F, Falotico-Taylor J (eds.). Quality of Life and Technology Assessment. Washington, D.C.: National Academy Press.

Nelson EC, Berwick DM. 1989. The measure of health status in clinical practice. Med Care 27(3, Suppl):S77-S90.

Patrick DL, Bergner M. 1990. Measurement of health status in the 1990s. Ann Rev Public Health 11:165-183.

Patrick DL, Deyo RA. 1989. Generic and disease-specific measures in assessing health status and quality of life. Med Care 27(3, Suppl):S217-S232.

Quevedo S (ed.). 1991. Proceedings of the American Kidney Fund Consensus Conference on "Quality of Life." Seminars in Dialysis (in press).

Rettig RA, Marks EL. 1980. Implementing the End-Stage Renal Disease Program of Medicare. R-2505-HCFA. Santa Monica, Calif.: The RAND Corporation.

Roper WL, Winkenwerder W, Hackbarth GM, Krakauer H. 1988. Effectiveness in health care: An initiative to evaluate and improve medical practice. N Engl J Med 319:1197-1202.

RPA (Renal Physicians Association). 1990. Improving Patient Care: A Quality Agenda. Washington, D.C. September.

Starr P. 1982. The Social Transformation of American Medicine. New York: Basic Books, Inc.

Tarlov AR, Ware JE, Jr, Greenfield S, Nelson EC, Perrin E, Zubkoff M. 1989. The Medical Outcomes Study: An application of methods for monitoring the results of medical care. JAMA 262:925-930.

Temkin NR, Dikmen S, Machamer J, McLean A. 1989. General versus disease-specific measures: Further work on the Sickness Impact Profile for head injury. Med Care 27 (3, Suppl):S44-S53.

USRDS (U.S. Renal Data System). 1990. Annual Data Report. National Institute of Diabetes and Digestive and Kidney Diseases, Bethesda, Md.

APPENDIX 1

QUALITY OF CARE IN ESRD:
AN EXAMPLE OF A PROXIMATE CLINICAL INDICATOR

The control of anemia is presented here as an example of a proximate clinical indicator. The clinical literature is briefly summarized as to its acceptance or rejection of this formulation as a quality indicator. The discussion includes the acceptable rates or levels of treatment; appropriate time intervals between measurement; the validity (or sensitivity-specificity) of the indicator relative to prior treatment; and pertinent modifying or adjusting factors.

Treating Anemia in Dialysis Patients[1]

Anemia is nearly universal in ESRD and results primarily from impaired erythropoietin production by diseased kidneys (Haley et al., 1989; Paganini, 1989). Anemia appears to be responsible for many of the symptoms that patients, nurses, and physicians associate with kidney failure despite apparently adequate dialysis.

Over the past 25 years, the initial treatment of anemia in dialysis patients has included increased dialysis, diagnosis and repair of iron and vitamin deficiencies, and diagnosis and treatment of aluminum intoxication (Korbet, 1989; Paganini, 1989). Patients who remain unacceptably anemic (the threshold varies from patient to patient and from physician to physician) have been treated with androgens. There is substantial variability in the efficacy of androgen therapy reported by different investigators; this variation may reflect differences in the patient populations studied (Korbet, 1989). Androgens clearly do not work for all patients, perhaps not even for most. Furthermore, their administration is accompanied by frequent adverse effects, including virilization and hepatic toxicity. In some patients, side effects prompt discontinuation of androgen treatment.

Until recently, nearly one-quarter of dialysis patients required red cell transfusion as treatment for anemia (Eschbach et al., 1987). Transfusion carries risks of acute transfusion reactions, of infection with viruses causing hepatitis and with retroviruses, of iron overload, and of immunologic sensitization of individuals who are or may become transplant candidates. There is evidence that repeated red cell transfusion can suppress residual endogenous erythropoietin production, making the patient transfusion-dependent (Watson, 1989).

On June 1, 1989, the Food and Drug Administration licensed recombinant human erythropoietin (rHuEpo) for treatment of anemia associated with chronic renal failure (FDA, 1989). With the advent of rHuEpo, the routine treatment of anemia in dialysis patients has changed dramatically. The results of three clinical trials suggest that rHuEpo reverses uncomplicated anemia of renal failure within months, with predictable dose-response curves (Casati et al., 1987; Korbet, 1989; Winearls et al., 1986). However, superimposed red cell destruction or loss, marrow suppression by inflammation, aluminum toxicity, poorly controlled hyperparathyroidism, and inadequate iron or folate stores will counter or even overcome the therapeutic effect of rHuEpo.

Absent one of these comorbid conditions, rHuEpo raises the hematocrit to 30-35% in more than 95% of patients (Eschbach et al., 1989). The dose of rHuEpo required to achieve this goal varies substantially from patient to patient. The requirement for transfusion wanes correspondingly. Within 3 months of beginning rHuEpo, transfusion frequency drops almost a factor of 10; within the subsequent 3 months, transfusion frequency declines more than 40-fold (Mohini, 1989).

The benefits of rHuEpo treatment include elimination of the adverse effects associated with androgens and transfusion, and potentially a long-term reduction in cardiovascular morbidity and mortality. One study of dialysis patients has shown an inverse correlation between hemoglobin and left ventricular mass index as estimated by echocardiography (Silberberg et al., 1989). Other studies have shown improved exercise tolerance and decreased left ventricular volume in patients whose anemia was treated with rHuEpo (Lundin, 1989).

Exercise testing before and after one year of rHuEpo treatment of 10 hemodialysis patients showed that as the average hematocrit rose from 19.8% to 34.3%, duration of exercise increased in all patients, maximum oxygen consumption increased in 7, and the anaerobic threshold increased in 8 of 9. Before treatment, 8 of the 10 electrocardiograms had some areas of ST depression; 7 of 8 normalized. Left ventricular mass, as measured by echocardiography, decreased significantly (Macdougall et al., 1990a). Long-term studies will be required to determine whether, as seems almost certain, these changes outweigh the consequences for vascular disease of the increase in blood pressure associated with rHuEpo treatment.

The most prominent immediate consequence of rHuEpo treatment appears to be on the quality of life of dialysis patients. The recent open-label study of 333 patients concluded that rHuEpo "greatly enhances the quality of life of anemic patients who receive maintenance hemodialysis" (Evans et al., 1990). Areas of improvement included energy, activity, functional ability, sleep and eating, disease symptoms, health status, satisfaction with health, sex life, well-being, psychological affect, and happiness. This conclusion supports a widespread clinical impression.

On the other hand, a double-blind, placebo-controlled study found that fatigue and physical symptoms and exercise tolerance were substantially improved in patients receiving rHuEpo, but that "the effect on psychosocial function was less impressive" (Canadian Erythropoietin Study Group, 1990). A questionnaire tailored to the problems of patients with ESRD showed some improvement, but psychosocial scores on the Sickness Impact Profile were not significantly different. Patient utilities, as measured by the time trade-off techniques, were not different on rHuEpo.

Important adverse effects of rHuEpo treatment include development or exacerbation of hypertension (about 30-50% of patients) and seizures that sometimes appear to be related to severe hypertension. Iron deficiency can impair the effectiveness of treatment if iron stores are not monitored closely and repleted orally or parenterally. Serum potassium rises slightly (Eschbach et al., 1989). Although any diminution in hemodialyzer clearance that has occurred is unlikely to be clinically important (Eschbach et al., 1989: FDA, 1989), reports regarding a possible increase in the rate of venous access thrombosis are inconsistent (Canadian Erythropoietin Group, 1990; Eschbach et al., 1989; FDA, 1989).

Further investigation will be required to identify and measure the long-term consequences of erythropoietin treatment. These may influence conclusions regarding therapeutic goals. In particular, it will be important to determine the form of the relationships between (1) functional status and red cell mass and (2) improvement in cardiopulmonary function and red cell mass. Are these functions continuous? Where are their maxima? Further investigations of the optimal frequency and route of rHuEpo delivery are also indicated. Some studies suggest that daily subcutaneous administration may achieve the same increment in red cell mass with a smaller total weekly dose (Macdougall et al., 1990b).

Potential Use as an Outcome Indicator

Using rHuEpo or androgens, maintain mean hematocrit equal to or greater than 30% in the absence of causes of anemia other than ESRD. Use transfusion only to replace acute blood loss or for immunologic modulation before transplantation.

Potential Use as Process Indicators

1. In patients who do not achieve or maintain a mean hematocrit equal to or greater than 30%, exclude other causes of anemia. These should include blood loss, hemolysis, aluminum toxicity, uncontrolled hyperparathyroidism, vitamin deficiency, inflammatory states, and other causes of bone marrow disease.

2. Measure iron stores before rHuEpo therapy and at regular intervals during treatment.

3. Attain a mean diastolic blood pressure of 95 mmHg or lower before beginning rHuEpo treatment; reevaluate antihypertensive regimen weekly during treatment until stable rHuEpo dose, red cell mass, and blood pressure are achieved.

Note

1. Prepared by Klemens B. Meyer, M.D., and Sheldon Greenfield, M.D., New England Medical Center, Boston, Mass., 1990.

References

Canadian Erythropoietin Study Group. 1990. Association between recombinant human erythropoietin and quality of life and exercise capacity of patients receiving haemodialysis. Br Med J 300:573-578.

Casati S, Passerini P, Campise MR, et al. 1987. Benefits and risks of protracted treatment with human recombinant erythropoietin in patients maintained by chronic hemodialysis. Br Med J 295:1017-1020.

Eschbach JW, Egrie JC, Downing MR, et al. 1987. Correction of anemia of end-stage renal disease with recombinant human erythropoietin. N Engl J Med 316:73-78.

Eschbach JW, Abdulhadi MH, Browne JK, et al. 1989. Recombinant human erythropoietin in anemic patients with end-stage renal disease: Results of a phase III multicenter clinical trial. Ann Intern Med 111:992-1000.

Evans RW, Rader B, Manninen DL, et al. 1990. The quality of life of hemodialysis recipients treated with recombinant human erythropoietin. JAMA 263:825-830.

FDA (Food and Drug Administration). 1989. Summary Basis of Approval: Drug License name: Epoetin alfa; Brand name: EPOGEN. June 1.

Haley NR, Adamson JW, Schneider GL, Eschbach JW. 1989. There are no uremic inhibitors to erythropoietin (EPO) in chronic renal failure (CRF). Abstract 319A, American Society of Nephrology.

Korbet SM. 1989. Comparison of hemodialysis and peritoneal dialysis in the management of anemia related to chronic renal disease. Semin Nephrol 9(Suppl 1):9-15.

Lundin AP. 1989. Quality of life: Subjective and objective improvements with recombinant human erythropoietin therapy. Semin Nephrol 9(Suppl 1):22-29.

Macdougall IC, Lewis NP, Saunders MJ, et al. 1990a. Long-term cardiorespiratory effects of amelioration of renal anaemia by erythropoietin. Lancet 335:489-493.

Macdougall IC, Hutton RD, Cavill I, Coles GA, Williams JD. 1990b. Treating renal anaemia with recombinant human erythropoietin: Practical guidelines and a clinical algorithm. Br Med J 300:655-659.

Mohini R. 1989. Clinical efficacy of recombinant human erythropoietin in hemodialysis patients. Semin Nephrol 9(Suppl 1):16-21.

Paganini EP. 1989. Overview of anemia associated with chronic renal disease: primary and secondary mechanisms. Semin Nephrol 9(Suppl 1):3-8.

Silberberg JS, Rahal DP, Patton DR, Sniderman AD. 1989. Role of anemia in the pathogenesis of left ventricular hypertrophy in end-stage renal disease. Am J Cardiol 64:222-224.

Watson AJ. 1989. Adverse effects of therapy for the correction of anemia in hemodialysis patients. Semin Nephrol 9(Suppl 1):30-34.

Winearls CG, Oliver DO, Pippard MJ, et al. 1986. Effect of human erythropoietin derived from recombinant DNA on the anemia of patients maintained by chronic hemodialysis. Lancet 2:1175-1178.

APPENDIX 2

EXAMPLES OF ESRD QUALITY ASSURANCE

Dialysis Clinic, Inc., Cincinnati (DCI-C)

DCI-C, affiliated with the University of Cincinnati Medical Center (UCMC), opened in July 1977. It has 24 to 27 stations, a home training program (since 1978), a CAPD training program (since 1980), and a strong commitment to transplantation. Its stated philosophy is: Excellent patient care requires an able concerned team of professional staff, who function as independent professionals, and are well informed about their patients and the details of their medical condition(s). Patients should be as well informed as possible and be encouraged to participate as actively as possible in their care.

Central to implementing the unit's philosophy is a patient-centered electronic Medical Information and Quality Assurance System (MIS), introduced in March 1976 when the unit was still part of UCMC. This provides a clinical data base that is available to staff on each patient at all times. The MIS staff interact on a daily basis with physicians, nurses, and other professionals to provide relevant clinical information for decisions about patient care. For medical as well as administrative purposes, these information professionals are counted as patient-care staff.

The MIS links medical information with administrative, cost, and billing data. This has enabled DCI-C to examine the safety of dialyzer reuse during 1978-79, investigate the effect of reuse on patient well-being and the costs of supplies, and study the enhanced safety and cost-effectiveness of automated dialyzer reprocessing. Patient-specific, dialyzer-specific analysis permitted an increase of average dialyzer uses from 6 to 12, and subsequently to 36. Each improvement in number of uses was accompanied by an improvement in patient well-being.

A key benefit of the MIS is the capacity to analyze many types of patient medical information with very little delay. This has facilitated the incorporation into individual patient care of an iterative, day-by-day or month-by-month, sequential process of action, feedback, and correction, which is the essence of continuous quality improvement. In individual patients, the MIS is used daily to assess hypotension during dialysis and to modulate "target weight" and blood pressure; it is used monthly to evaluate adequacy of dialysis, nutrition, calcium and phosphate control, and anemia and its response to treatment; and it is used yearly to examine survival rates. Applied to groups of patients, the MIS is used regularly to assess dialyzer performance, to detect infection and pyrogenic reactions, and to monitor the quality of the water supply. It is also used to transmit full knowledge about the patient's condition whenever an unexpected event occurs, such as admission to hospital or consultation with other physicians. This process has had a favorable effect on patient well-being and survival.

Greenfield Health Systems

Greenfield Health Systems (GHS), a division of Henry Ford Health System, Detroit, operates 10 dialysis facilities in three states. Since 1978, a clinical management computer system has been in place to monitor and evaluate the dialysis therapy and clinical status of ESRD patients. Data elements of the QA program include dialysis treatment, medications, routine laboratory studies, urea kinetic modeling results, and dialyzer reprocessing parameters.

The QA program involves a monthly review of "key results" for established outcome measures by the multidisciplinary team of each treatment unit. The program generates summary data about patients who fail to meet established outcome targets. The clinical team can then modify treatment for those patients as appropriate. The standard for hyperphosphatemia, for example, is that the mid-week predialysis serum phosphorous level be less than 6.0 milligrams per deciliter. Corrective action for patients falling below this would include nutrition and medical counseling and review of phosphate binders.

Parameters measured against a target outcome include dialysis efficacy (Kt/V, protein catabolic rate); a wide range of intradialytic symptoms and signs (nausea, vomiting, cramps, hypotension); calcium; phosphorus; ferritin; potassium; blood urea nitrogen; interdialytic blood pressure control; interdialytic weight gains; and treatment problems (poor blood flow, clotted needles, clotted dialyzers). Mortality and morbidity are monitored monthly; direct causes of hospitalization are reviewed.

The QA program also involves a "discipline audit" of everyday practice for consistency of performance of routine procedures. The results may lead to education of personnel or reevaluation of a procedure. On a quarterly basis, the GHS Medical Advisory Board reviews trends within and across treatment units. The program provides a monitoring capability that is used for outcome-oriented patient management, that supports clinical research, and that creates a setting for formal discussion of unit and system performance. The system has provided the data for numerous publications, book chapters, abstracts, and presentations. It has also been adapted for use by the Division of Nephrology and Hypertension of the Beth Israel Medical Center in New York City.

National Medical Care, Inc. (NMC)

NMC, the largest proprietary dialysis chain in the country with over 300 units, has quality assurance programs both for its manufacturing division, regulated by the FDA's Good Manufacturing Practices, and its health services (dialysis) division. For several years, NMC has collected summaries of laboratory test values; these have allowed unit medical directors to assess a unit's performance against the averages for the entire organization, and to compare the values for an individual patient against those for both the unit and the entire patient population.

Recently, prompted by data showing a relationship between dialysis time and mortality and by laboratory data implicating serum albumin (as a nutrition marker) and other clinical variables in mortality, a program of testing and monitoring of urea reduction and the effective dialysis prescription (expressed as urea reduction ratio) has been introduced. A pre- and postdialysis blood urea nitrogen test is made monthly of each patient, concurrent with monthly chemistries, to measure the fractional reduction of urea during a dialysis procedure. Quarterly summaries of data on each patient are being provided to units on serum albumin and selected clinical variables as well as urea reduction ratio. NMC requires that these reports be reviewed as part of unit QA meetings.

The purpose of this NMC action is to provide a clinical management tool to assist physicians and medical teams with the routine evaluation of treatment intensity, both for the assessment of individual patients and for the evaluation of treatment patterns within and between facilities. NMC officials expect that the testing, reporting, and summarizing of URR and *Kt/V* values will help achieve that goal (Lowrie and Lew, 1991). Forthcoming steps in the NMC quality assurance effort will involve calculating risk-adjusted mortality, and using clinical and laboratory data as specific quality indicators.

Reference

Lowrie EG, Lew NL. 1991. The urea reduction ratio (URR): a simple method for evaluating hemodialysis treatment. Contemporary Dialysis and Nephrology 12(2):13-20.

PART V
Data and Research

The final portion of the report addresses data system and research needs of the ESRD program. Chapter 13 deals with the evolution of ESRD data systems in the Health Care Financing Administration, as well as the more recent development of the U.S. Renal Data System and the scientific registry of the United Network for Organ Sharing.

Chapter 14 addresses ESRD-related research needs, emphasizing the importance of a comprehensive approach that spans laboratory and clinical research, epidemiology, and health services research. Clinical studies of the adequacy of dialysis also receive attention.

13

Data Systems

The OBRA 1987 charge asked that the IOM assess the adequacy of existing data systems to monitor epidemiology, access, quality, and reimbursement effects on quality on a continuing basis. In this chapter, three major sources of information about ESRD patients and the ESRD program are described: the HCFA data systems, the U.S. Renal Data System (USRDS), and the United Network for Organ Sharing (UNOS). The adequacy of these data systems is addressed, as are some of their specific deficiencies, and the committee makes recommendations for their improvement. The committee[1] also evaluates how these data systems fulfill the respective legislative requirements: OBRA 1986 and the National Organ Transplant Act of 1986.

HEALTH CARE FINANCING ADMINISTRATION

From 1973 until mid-1977, the ESRD program was administered jointly by the SSA Bureau of Health Insurance (BHI) and the PHS Bureau of Quality Assurance (BQA). BHI was responsible for monitoring Medicare entitlement, utilization, and reimbursement; BQA was responsible for developing quality assurance standards and the medical information system for dialysis and transplant patients. Divided management resulted in continuing data-system chaos. As a consequence, data about the ESRD patient population and the ESRD program are incomplete for the 1970s.

After HCFA was established in 1977, the monitoring of Medicare program management and ESRD patient information was consolidated in HCFA's Bureau of Data Management and Strategy (BDMS). Following enactment of Public Law 95-292 of 1978, the ESRD Program Management and Medical Information System (PMMIS) was developed to provide medical and program information for ESRD program analysis, policy development, and epidemiologic research. A precursor of the current ESRD, PMMIS was implemented by HCFA between 1978 and 1980. Data forms were collected through the Medicare intermediaries and Medicare central office. No measures were used to enforce compliance, and the completion rate was as low as 50 percent for some information. In 1981, adjustments were made in the data collection process: Reporting of the onset of ESRD was tied to the entitlement; a new Medical Evidence Form was introduced, consolidating the previous form and the request for entitlement form, and reducing the content of information collected. Since that time, there has been continuous improvement in the quality and completeness of these HCFA data.

HCFA data bases containing ESRD financial data include provider cost reports as well as beneficiary medical utilization records with Medicare Parts A and B billing information. No charge or payment information is included in PMMIS. The relevant data forms and data files for financial information are shown in Table 13-1. Cost reports are now submitted electronically, an improvement that will facilitate program analysis and research. Previously, facilities had submitted paper copies of these reports and ensuing data entry and analysis were lacking.

PMMIS assembles information on Medicare ESRD patients and Medicare-approved ESRD hospital-based and independent dialysis facilities. Major PMMIS statistical files and the relevant data forms are indicated in Table 13-1. These include the Medical Evidence File, the Patient Identification File, the Transplant File, the Transplant Follow-up File, the Quarterly Dialysis File, the Hospital Inpatient Stay Record File, and the Facility Survey.

A new transplant form, developed jointly by the American Society of Transplant Surgeons and HCFA, was introduced in 1983, providing more clinical data about transplants. Compliance in reporting increased substantially: More than 91 percent of the transplant information forms were received for kidney transplants performed during 1985-86.

ESRD Facility Survey data present state- and network-specific data and treatment modality statistics and includes Medicare and non-Medicare patients. Data from the Facility Survey are complete at the time of reporting (3 months after the year for which data are reported) in contrast to most other PMMIS data which are largely complete after 15 months but continue to be reported for several years. Facility Survey data are a resource for evaluating trends in treatment modality as well as ESRD network- and state-specific incidence, prevalence, and treatment data.

The 1978 legislation required that HCFA submit an annual report to Congress on the ESRD program. Three reports were published (HCFA 1979, 1980, 1982). Given the burden of many related reports, Congress, at HCFA's request, rescinded the requirement and permitted the agency to report on the ESRD program in its annual report on the Medicare program. HCFA now publishes an annual series, *Health Care Financing Research*

TABLE 13-1 Medicare Data Sources and Data Files for ESRD Patients and Providers

Form	Name	HCFA Statistical Files
Patient-Specific Information:		
1450	Uniform Bill (UB-82) Part B Medicare Annual Data (BMAD)	Utilization records with Medicare Parts A and B billing information for beneficiaries including ESRD patients
		Hospital Inpatient Stay Record File, PMMIS
2728	Chronic Renal Disease Medical Evidence Report	Medical Evidence File, PMMIS
2742	ESRD Patient History and Treatment Plan	PMMIS
2745	ESRD Transplant Information	Transplant File, PMMIS
a	ESRD Transplant Follow-up	Transplant File, PMMIS
2746	ESRD Death Notification	Patient Identification File, PMMIS
Provider-Specific Information:		
	Medicare Certification Approval Notice	PMMIS
2744	ESRD Facility Survey	Provider File, PMMIS
2552	Cost Report Information System	Outpatient dialysis facilities' cost reports

a Not applicable.

NOTE: The ESRD Program Management and Medical Information System has 6 statistical files; 5 of these files are mentioned above; the 6th file is the Quarterly Dialysis File.

Report: End Stage Renal Disease, which provides statistical information on incidence and prevalence of currently entitled Medicare patients stratified by age, gender, race, and primary disease as well as survival analyses on patients who have ever had Medicare entitlement. Separate analyses are presented for dialysis, cadaver transplant, and living-related-donor transplant patients.

HCFA has made substantial progress in ESRD data collection since 1977, largely due to the efforts of BDMS and the Office of Research and Demonstrations. HCFA has made ESRD data increasingly available to researchers and others, consistent with a general HCFA policy to make Medicare data available for research purposes. PMMIS and other Medicare data files, although not without problems, have provided practically all the data for analysis of the ESRD program, whether by HCFA, other federal government agencies, or nongovernmental organizations. Indeed, this committee benefited from HCFA data sharing.

U.S. RENAL DATA SYSTEM

The USRDS originated from discussions during 1984-85 involving the renal community, Congress, and the National Institute of Diabetes and Digestive and Kidney Diseases (NIDDK). These discussions led in two diverging pathways. First, Congress, in OBRA 1986, passed in October, directed the Secretary to establish a National End-Stage Renal Disease Registry (discussed below).

Independently, but proceeding from the same discussions, NIDDK issued a Request for Proposals (RFP) in November 1986 for a renal data system. This reflected an internal decision that epidemiologic research was needed in the context of NIH-sponsored kidney research. In May 1988, NIDDK awarded a contract to the Urban Institute to establish the USRDS, with a subcontract to the University of Michigan.[2] The USRDS receives funds and management control from NIDDK; routine HCFA data from the PMMIS Annual Facility Surveys, the ESRD Master Provider File, as well as data from the Transplant Follow-up File, BMAD, and other files; and special studies data from the ESRD networks. In addition, Department of Veterans Affairs (DVA) data not previously reported to HCFA have been added in a PMMIS-like format, but are separate from PMMIS.

The mission of the USRDS is primarily epidemiologic, focusing on the causes of ESRD, the effective care of ESRD patients, and other related research of interest to NIDDK and the renal community. Specifically, NIDDK defined four goals for the USRDS:

(1) Design and implement a consolidated renal disease data system to provide the biostatistical, data management, and analytical expertise necessary to characterize the total renal patient population and describe the distribution of patients by sociodemographic variables across modalities;

(2) Report on the incidence, prevalence, and mortality rates and trends over time by primary diagnosis, treatment modality, and other sociodemographic variables;

(3) Develop and analyze aggregate data on the effect of various modalities of treatment by disease and patient group, including examination of the prevention and progression of renal disease with special emphasis on mortality, morbidity, and quality-of-life criteria; and

(4) Identify problems and opportunities for more-focused special studies of renal research issues currently unaddressed by the consolidated data system (USRDS, 1990a).

In addition to data drawn from PMMIS, the USRDS incorporates annual census population estimates and data about population characteristics of ZIP codes (USRDS, 1990a). The USRDS also works with HCFA to collect additional data through the 18 national ESRD networks. The structure and contents of the USRDS data base are described in annual data reports (USRDS, 1990a, pp. 81-99).

The USRDS issued its first major report in 1989 (USRDS, 1989). That report contains extensive data on incidence, prevalence, patient and graft survival, and institutional providers. It also includes preliminary data from several special studies on the transplant process. The USRDS reports data for all patients who are included in the PMMIS data base, regardless of whether they have current Medicare entitlement (in contrast to the HCFA reports which include only currently entitled patients in incidence and prevalence analyses). The second annual report was published in August 1990 and is substantially expanded from the initial volume.

Numerous studies using existing data have been approved by NIDDK. Of 30 reviewed (USRDS, 1990a), eight are under way or have been completed:

(1) effect of HLA matching on kidney graft survival;

(2) use of Cox's proportional hazards model for observational data;

(3) racial differences in incidence of treated ESRD, 1982-87;

(4) influence of donor and recipient gender and age in parent-child transplantation;

(5) compilation of a national ESRD atlas by county;

(6) carpal tunnel syndrome;

(7) trends in mortality among dialysis and transplant patients in the United States; and

(8) hospitalization among dialysis patients and transplant recipients in the United States.

In addition to these eight, 11 studies have been approved for implementation once resources become available.

The USRDS also has six special studies under way that involve the collection of new data (USRDS, 1990a):

(1) measurement of case-mix severity and its effect on mortality and morbidity (described in Chapter 12);

(2) data validation, comparing USRDS data with their sources in the field;

(3) renal biopsy as an indicator of specific renal diagnoses and subsequent outcomes;

(4) EPO use and quality of life;

(5) CAPD and rates of peritonitis; and

(6) developmental growth of pediatric patients.

Three additional studies have been approved by NIDDK for possible implementation during 1990-93: EPO, hypertension as a cause of ESRD, and prospective mortality comparisons by treatment modality. This sampling approach via special studies is well ahead of schedule and is only beginning to be exploited. Resources are needed to facilitate the collection and analysis of additional new clinical and epidemiologic data in this regard.

The establishment of the USRDS represents a major, and long-overdue, step by the NIH into kidney disease-related epidemiologic research. The committee commends NIDDK for taking this step; it also acknowledges the substantial contribution that the USRDS has made in the brief period since its creation. Its effect is already being felt as researchers and clinicians begin to use its published data to explore a variety of questions.

The committee notes a tendency among renal providers to urge that USRDS assume quasi-operational roles in the Medicare ESRD program, especially in the quality assurance area. The committee believes that USRDS should be limited to registry and research functions and that operational responsibilities of HCFA in quality assessment and assurance, for example, should properly be exercised by it.

UNITED NETWORK FOR ORGAN SHARING

UNOS was created in 1978 as a subsidiary organization of the Southeast Organ Procurement Foundation (SEOPF). SEOPF, a regional organ-sharing entity established in 1973, took this step to expand participation by transplant centers across the country in its organ-sharing activities. In 1986, UNOS was formally separated from SEOPF as an independent nonprofit corporation in anticipation of bidding on the contracts for the Organ Procurement and Transplantation Network (OPTN) and the scientific registry of the recipients of organ transplant called for in the National Organ Transplant Act of 1984. UNOS was awarded both the OPTN and the registry contracts by the DHHS Health Resources and Services Administration (HRSA).

The OPTN contract includes the responsibility to develop an equitable, scientific, and medically sound organ allocation system in the United States. In addition, OPTN has been charged with developing policies to promote maximum utilization of organs and with developing standards of quality for acquisition and transportation of donated organs.

UNOS implements the registry contract through four subcontracts for organ-specific registries—kidney, heart, liver, pancreas. UNOS and HCFA, in cooperation with HRSA, NIH, and the transplant community, developed common forms by which transplant centers report kidney transplant data to both organizations as well as to USRDS. An annual report is compiled by UNOS and by each subcontracting registry. In late 1990, UNOS published its first scientific registry report on 1988 and 1989 data (UNOS, 1990).

The UNOS report includes statistics on donor demographics (age, gender, race, and ABO blood group); transplant recipient demographics; waiting-list demographic information including age, race, blood group, prior transplants, urgency category, and panel reactive antibody[3]; organ procurement and disposition; and outcome statistics. Each UNOS participating transplant center receives a semi-annual report that includes national, regional, and center-specific data. The latter includes a list of patients (for review and verification) on whom data were submitted. All UNOS members receive the national data, which is also made available to the public.

UNOS is currently conducting a number of research studies. These include the effect of six-antigen HLA matching on renal transplantation outcome, examination of outcomes among Native Americans, and a comprehensive study of waiting-list data. The waiting-list study has recently been completed and submitted for publication. UNOS is developing plans for additional studies.

UNOS has relatively few personnel directly responsible for the analysis of its own data, as distinct from personnel who operate the four registries. Although analyses are now beginning to be performed, budgetary constraints may limit the issuance of research reports by UNOS itself.

NATIONAL END-STAGE RENAL DISEASE REGISTRY

The progress of ESRD data systems under HCFA during the 1980s and the development of USRDS and UNOS are beginning to change the amount and quality of ESRD data available to analysts and others. Unresolved, however, are several issues raised by the OBRA 1986 requirement for a national ESRD registry.

Congress, in OBRA 1986, directed the Secretary of DHHS to establish a National End-Stage Renal Disease Registry in order to "assemble and analyze the data reported by network organizations, transplant centers, and other sources on all end stage renal disease patients." This registry was to (1) prepare an annual ESRD report to Congress; (2) identify "the economic impact, cost-effectiveness, and medical efficacy of alternative modalities of treatment"; (3) evaluate "the most appropriate allocation of resources for the treatment and research into the causes of end-stage renal disease"; (4) determine "patient mortality and morbidity rates, and trends in such rates, and other indices of quality of care"; and (5) conduct other analyses to "assist the Congress in evaluating the end-stage renal disease program."

The implementation of this statutory requirement has been a matter of confusion and controversy. Many providers mistakenly assumed that the NIDDK's establishment of the USRDS represented implementation of the registry requirement of OBRA 1986. The NIDDK RFP, issued in November 1986, had called for "a consolidated registry . . . to meet the needs of the nephrology and transplant communities concerning the genesis, complications and treatment of End Stage Renal Disease in the United States." It appeared to most careful observers that this action responded to the statute. NIDDK later argued that since an RFP requires 9 to 12 months to prepare, review, and issue, the RFP and the statute were independent events, although close in timing. During this time, however, NIDDK was party to the discussions that led to the legislation and was aware of its progress through Congress. The language of the RFP was similar to the language of OBRA 1986; the term "registry," for example, was used at several key places in the RFP. NIDDK was also in a position in November, following enactment of the statute, to delay issuance of the RFP and remove any ambiguity about the relationship of the RFP to the statute. It did not do so.

Moreover, NIDDK prepared the progress report that DHHS submitted to Congress in April 1987 on the implementation of the registry (DHHS, 1987). NIDDK and HCFA were identified as having ongoing activities antedating the law "and that are responsive to the requirements of this law." Reference was made to an "Interagency Agreement to Collaborate in the National End-Stage Renal Disease Patients Registry" and to the fact that NIDDK was in the process of awarding a contract for a "Coordinating Center" for a Consolidated ESRD Data Base for the Epidemiological Surveillance, Genesis, and Complications of ESRD in the United States."[4] The report stated: "Under this contract, data will be collected in a manner that will enable a variety of organizations to perform most of the types of analyses mentioned in P.L. 99-509 (OBRA 1986). Data collection and analysis with respect to economic and cost-effectiveness issues will, however, continue to be performed by the HCFA." The report to Congress, itself a requirement of the 1986 law, explicitly interpreted the NIDDK efforts that led to the USRDS as responsive to OBRA 1986.

The view that the USRDS was implementing the registry called for in the statute, then, is an impression derived from NIDDK's initial representation of its actions as responding to the act. On the other hand, the NIDDK RFP referred primarily to epidemiologic purposes and made no mention of economic analyses as called for by OBRA 1986. It did refer, however, to studies of relative efficacy of ESRD treatments "in terms of criteria ranging from mortality rates to quality of life," which might easily be construed as consistent with the statute's expressed concern for mortality, morbidity, and "other indices of quality." Controversy has focused on one substantive issue. Subsequent to the contract award, NIDDK barred USRDS from linking epidemiologic and economic data on the grounds that it (NIDDK) lacked the experience and professional competence to oversee such research and that this type of research is not consistent with the role of NIH. This action was taken, even though the USRDS data base is derived from HCFA administrative data, the contractor has extensive experience in economic analyses of ESRD data, and no technical barrier exists to linking economic and epidemiologic data.[5]

HCFA, in response to this limitation of USRDS activity, and under pressure to implement the economic analyses called for by OBRA 1986, issued an RFP in 1990 for studies of the cost-effectiveness of ESRD treatment modalities and of reimbursement for EPO. The Renal Physicians Association argued that these one-time-only studies did not respond to the statute's implied function of continuing studies and should have been assigned to the USRDS as implementing the registry function. The HCFA Administrator, Gail Wilensky, replied that these studies were "intended to be the first, but not the only" HCFA studies directed to responding to the legislative mandate. In fact, in late September 1990, HCFA awarded the economic and cost-effectiveness studies contract to the Urban Institute and the EPO study to investigators at the Johns Hopkins University Schools of Medicine and Public Health.

Appointment of the professional advisory group called for in the statute to assist the Secretary in formulating policies and procedures for the registry was long delayed. However, it was chartered in January 1990, and its members were appointed in October 1990.

The committee concludes that DHHS is currently engaged in a complicated search for a satisfactory way to implement the 1986 statute. With respect to the registry functions, the status is as follows:

• Epidemiologic analyses are being performed by USRDS and currently are based on HCFA data. Special studies are under way using data collected through the ESRD networks and other sources (e.g., National Medical Care).

• NIDDK has barred USRDS from conducting analyses that link epidemiologic and economic data. HCFA has recently awarded a contract to the Urban Institute which responds, in part, to the OBRA 1986 call for cost-effectiveness studies.

• Analyses of mortality and morbidity are being performed by USRDS. Data collection for a retrospective study of patient case-mix complexity has been completed by USRDS, and a prospective study of case mix has been recommended by its Scientific Advisory Committee. The development of "other indices of quality" has been barred by NIDDK.

OBRA 1986 is quite cryptic about quality studies, implied by the last point above. The quality-related activities of USRDS are very important. However, they do not respond adequately to all the quality assurance (QA) needs of the Medicare ESRD program, which this committee has emphasized strongly in the previous chapters. The ESRD program QA function involves more than data. It includes the development of measures and instruments specific to the ESRD setting and the conduct of supporting research. These activities are not a registry function. They require the active involvement of physicians trained analytically in health services research, especially quality assessment, functional- and health-status assessment, severity-of-illness adjustment, and related fields. This argues for augmenting the expertise of the nephrology community with that of the health services research community.

The ESRD program QA function, moreover, is appropriately a government responsibility. The authority for its exercise with respect to Medicare and the ESRD program clearly resides with HCFA. It is essential that HCFA, in concert with the renal community, develop this QA function. Moreover, with respect to the registry, it is important that the respective roles of government agencies and private contractors be recognized and that the registry not be expected to assume quasi-operational responsibilities better performed by the government.

> **The committee concludes that the Secretary of DHHS should fully implement the three OBRA 1986 registry functions of epidemiologic research, economic and cost-effectiveness studies, and the development of measures of quality.**

The options facing DHHS relative to the implementation of the registry provision of OBRA 1986 are these: (1) agree to a joint NIH and HCFA effort by which USRDS fulfills all registry functions; (2) have HCFA conduct the economic analyses internally or through an outside research organization; and (3) authorize USRDS to fulfill the QA data function as long as HCFA undertakes a broader QA effort that includes the development of measures and instruments and the conduct of supporting research.

At a minimum, the renal data system should be continued another 5 years beyond the USRDS contract expiration in 1993. Second, in the next 2 years, the unresolved issues of the relationship of USRDS to all of the OBRA 1986 registry requirements should be clarified, and ways should be found to fully implement the statute. If registry functions cannot be performed under existing arrangements, it may be appropriate to consider a transfer of the data system from NIDDK to another agency, perhaps the Agency for Health Care Policy and Research or the Centers for Disease Control, either at the time of the contract renewal or earlier. Third, a broader agenda of research in epidemiology, economic analysis, and quality assessment and assurance should be undertaken, along lines set forth in Chapter 14.

ADEQUACY OF DATA SYSTEMS

Medicare's data systems (billing and payment records, cost reports, and PMMIS) provide information for examining most ESRD policy questions. In comparison to Medicare in general, the ESRD program is rich in data.

There remains, however, a continuing lack of information necessary to evaluate certain aspects of the ESRD program. This is especially true regarding the clinical and functional status information to assess and ensure quality: primary diagnosis of renal failure, secondary diagnosis, comorbid conditions, and initial functional status. It is necessary to replace the existing medical evidence form with a new form that systematically captures these data.

For primary diagnosis, the care and accuracy with which these data are recorded can be improved by means of a checklist with clear guidance to clinicians regarding its use. Differentiation of Types I and II diabetes mellitus, not currently recorded, is especially needed, perhaps in conjunction with a measure of functional status.

In addition, ethnicity data are not adequate, especially for the Hispanic population. HCFA purged the data collection forms of any question about Hispanic patients a few years ago largely because few data were being reported. This occurred at a time when the Census Bureau projected that the Hispanic population would grow from 14 percent of the U.S. population today to 20 percent by the year 2000. Furthermore, epidemiologic evidence suggests that Hispanics have a higher incidence of renal failure than non-Hispanic whites. The ability of HCFA and the federal government to track this population group should be vastly strengthened.

Similarly, the demographic and epidemiologic characteristics of ESRD patients not eligible for Medicare coverage are not known. Data do not exist on the economic status of ESRD patients, including the availability of private health insurance, the effect of the Medicare-as-secondary-payer provision on patient coverage, and the effect on individuals and families of loss of kidney function.

Regarding providers, more detailed information is needed about hospital units (backup units versus the equivalent of freestanding units), exceptions status, and ownership and chain affiliation.

RECOMMENDATIONS

The committee recommends that:

• **With respect to ESRD data, HCFA maintain a strong ESRD data acquisition and analysis capability; modify the patient medical evidence form to collect data on comorbid conditions, risk factors, functional status, and other factors bearing on treatment and outcomes; identify data needs for systematically analyzing the relationships between resource use, treatment, and patient outcomes; fund research pertinent to these questions; and provide publicly available tapes for research on all aspects of the ESRD program to the interested research community.**

• The U.S. Renal Data System be authorized to conduct research linking epidemiologic and economic data on the ESRD patient population, and that the special-studies sampling approach be exploited to its full potential.

• With respect to the United Network for Organ Sharing, resources be provided to sustain and strengthen its data analysis capability; that UNOS continue, as planned, to collect follow-up data on transplant patients who lose Medicare eligibility after 3 years; and that the collaboration in generating common data forms between the transplant community, HRSA, HCFA, NIH, and UNOS be seen as a possible model for emulation in the dialysis area.

• With respect to the National ESRD Registry, the Secretary of DHHS take all steps necessary within the next 2 years to fully implement all functions of the National ESRD Registry called for in OBRA 1986; that the renal data system be continued another 5 years when the current USRDS contract expires and that the contract be recompeted at that time; and that consideration be given at the time of such contract renewal to the transfer of the data system function to another agency if jurisdictional disputes continue to hamper implementation of the statute.

• With respect to the ESRD program quality assessment and assurance efforts called for by this committee, USRDS efforts be augmented by an appropriate HCFA effort to develop or adapt QA measures and instruments for the ESRD setting and that the necessary related research be supported.

NOTES

1. Dr. Philip J. Held, a member of the IOM ESRD committee and Director of the U.S. Renal Data System Coordinating Center, was not present at the committee meeting of October 4, 1990, at which this chapter was discussed, and he did not participate in the discussion leading to the recommendations that were adopted.

2. Both the Urban Institute and its USRDS subcontractor, the University of Michigan, conduct ESRD research independent of the USRDS.

3. The waiting-list data are subgrouped by time on the waiting list. Thus one can compare time on the waiting list between various age groups, by race, gender, and so on.

4. The cooperative agreement between NIH and HCFA remained unsigned at the time this report was written in October 1990.

5. In fact, the economic and epidemiologic data transmitted by HCFA to USRDS must be separated before being entered in the renal data system, a step that actually impedes the epidemiologic analyses.

REFERENCES

DHHS (U.S. Department of Health and Human Services). 1987. Report to Congress on National End-Stage Renal Disease Patient Registry Required by P.L. 99-509. Washington, D.C.: April.

HCFA (Health Care Financing Administration). 1979. End-Stage Renal Disease Program: Annual Report to Congress, 1979; P.L. 95-292, 1881(g). Washington, D.C.

HCFA. 1980. End-Stage Renal Disease Program: Second Annual Report to Congress, FY 1980. Washington, D.C.

HCFA. 1982. 1981 End-Stage Renal Disease Annual Report to Congress. Washington, D.C.

UNOS (United Network for Organ Sharing). 1990. Annual Report on the Scientific Registry for Organ Transplantation and the Organ Procurement and Transplantation Network, 1988 & 1989. U.S. Department of Health and Human Services. Washington, D.C.

USRDS (U.S. Renal Data System). 1989. Annual Report. National Institute of Diabetes and Digestive and Kidney Diseases, Bethesda, MD, August.

USRDS. 1990a. Annual Report. National Institute of Diabetes and Digestive and Kidney Diseases, Bethesda, MD, August.

USRDS. 1990b. Gold Notes. Washington, D.C. March 30.

14

Research Needs

Many questions remain unanswered regarding treatment of ESRD. The committee believes that a comprehensive research program related to renal disease is essential. This research program should include basic and applied medical research, epidemiologic research, and health services research.

There are near-term and long-term benefits of such an effort. In the near term, the effective management of a large and growing ESRD patient population requires that the scientific foundations of treatment be strengthened, that clinical practice be improved, that innovation be stimulated, that renal disease-specific measures and instruments be developed to assess and ensure quality, and that patient well-being be enhanced. In the long term, research is absolutely essential to the search for effective means of preventing ESRD.

Recently, the National Kidney and Urologic Diseases Advisory Board (NKUDAB, 1990) published a long-range plan for kidney and urologic diseases. The scope of its report includes nephrology, kidney transplantation, and urology and thus is broader than, but inclusive of, ESRD. The NKUDAB identified several objectives that are consistent with this IOM committee's effort. It identified improved access to and quality of care as important objectives, the subjects of Chapters 7, 8, and 12 of this report. It drew attention to the need for expanded data collection and analysis to facilitate the understanding of kidney and urologic diseases, consistent with the general concern of this committee expressed in Chapter 13. It highlighted the need for patient, professional, and public education about opportunities for prevention, early detection, and rehabilitation, themes reiterated throughout this report.

The NKUDAB made numerous recommendations regarding basic research, clinical research, and clinical trials, as well as epidemiology. These recommendations included the expansion of current NIH research grant programs and the training of research investigators in several important fields of renal and urologic research. The Board also recommended a separate NIH institute for kidney and urologic diseases. Readers are referred to the NKUDAB report for additional discussion of its important recommendations.

This committee has focused more sharply on the research issues that pertain to ESRD and, potentially, to its prevention. In the judgment of the committee, a serious need exists to reestablish a program of clinical studies on dialysis treatment. The termination of the Artificial Kidney/Chronic Disease research program of the National Institute of Arthritis and Metabolic Diseases (predecessor to NIDDK) left major gaps in clinical studies of dialysis. NIDDK, in the period from 1984 to 1989, supported basic research on transplantation and cellular and subcellular studies of the kidney, but made no awards for clinical dialysis studies (Levin et al., 1990).

Other sources of support for clinical research in dialysis have declined. The Department of Veterans Affairs supports practically no clinical dialysis studies in its internally funded research programs (Levin et al., 1990). Baxter Healthcare recently launched an important research program (Baxter, 1990), but the private sector in general has funded little clinical research. Perhaps reflecting declining research support, the number of clinical dialysis papers presented at the annual meetings of the American Society of Artificial Internal Organs and the American Society of Nephrology has declined (Maher, 1989).

Overall, the decline in dialysis research has two primary effects. First, it reduces the rate at which new clinical research is generated and thus restricts the flow of scientific information to dialysis clinicians. This may have been costly in the past decade during which the clinical community was placed under increasing financial stress by Medicare reimbursement reductions at a time when it was perhaps in greatest need of the benefits of clinical research. In particular, the discussion among clinicians of unresolved issues regarding the adequacy of dialysis, the effective delivery of the dialysis prescription, the effects of short treatment time on patient outcomes, and the relationship of nutrition to outcomes highlights the need for sustained clinical research.

Second, without clinical studies, the reservoir of scientific ideas necessary to stimulate innovation in treatment technology is not replenished. Without public support for research on underlying issues, private commercialization of new products is dampened. Economic studies have shown that the societal benefits from research exceed the private return on research, thus resulting in underinvestment by the private sector in the socially optimal level of research and strongly arguing for public support (Mansfield et al., 1977).

Research on the prevention of permanent kidney failure is essential to reduce the anticipated growth of the ESRD patient population. Recent laboratory investigations indicate that progression of established kidney disease can be slowed or possibly even prevented by various techniques. These include alterations in certain dietary constituents (protein, phosphate) and reduction in blood pressure, especially in the glomeruli (blood filtering elements) of the kidney. Early clinical studies suggest that these techniques may be effective in patients. This area of investigation holds great promise as a means to reduce both the human and the economic cost of ESRD. The effects of pre-ESRD interventions such as blood pressure control and glycemic control on the incidence and progression of renal disease must be evaluated. Effective prevention may require substantial behavioral change in activities as fundamental as diet, exercise, and smoking. Thus, research on behavioral change should be part of the program.

Epidemiologic research on kidney disease has been greatly strengthened by the NIDDK support of USRDS. Epidemiology needs to become a more integral part of kidney disease research, as it has been in heart disease, cancer, and aging research. In particular, there is a need to identify and measure with greater specificity the major risk factors causing chronic kidney failure, for prevention as well as patient management purposes. Special attention should be given to racial and ethnic differences in the incidence and causes of renal failure and in strategies for prevention.

The Transplant Amendments Act of 1990 expands the authority of the Health Resources and Services Administration to make grants related to organ procurement to entities other than organ procurement organizations. This opportunity should be seized to support well-designed research and demonstration projects that are promising with respect to increasing organ donation. Factors affecting access, outcomes, and organ donation for renal transplantation for minorities, females, and lower-income groups should be addressed. Hypotheses-generating medical anthropology studies may be appropriate ways to probe the social, cultural, and religious values that influence organ donation. The issues surrounding equitable access to organ transplantation require clarification and, where equity is not achieved, efforts should be made to identify remedies.

The range and magnitude of the economic effects of kidney failure on the patients and their families, although known to be substantial, have not been adequately addressed. Data are needed on the extent of insurance coverage for ESRD patients by Medicare, private health insurance, and Medicaid. This concern about insurance reflects the growing awareness that private insurance correlates positively with health and functional status and may affect access to transplantation and other therapies. The effects of the Medicare-as-secondary-payer provision on patients' ability to obtain health insurance should be carefully examined. Studies of the economic effects of kidney failure should be designed to illuminate issues related to other chronic disease patients.

A variety of methods are used for analyzing mortality, and these have led to some confusion and misinterpretation. A methodological working group, whether internal to HCFA or an external advisory body, is needed to deal with methodological problems on a continuing basis. A standard protocol for calculating mortality should be developed for use by HCFA, USRDS, UNOS, treatment facilities, and ESRD networks.

Health services research, which deals with the organization, financing, and delivery of health care, has laid the foundation for linking clinical and expenditure data, nurtured the development of functional- and health-status assessment, promoted the concern for outcomes and effectiveness research and quality assessment, and been responsible for advances in measurement, methodology, and data-base development.

Kidney disease research should embrace health services research as an integral part of a larger research strategy. Research should be supported to determine which components of medical care lead to better outcomes and to identify and validate quality measures for structure, process, and outcomes. Measuring the severity of illness of ESRD patients, including primary diagnosis, comorbid conditions, and functional status, and determining the relationship of these measures to treatment processes and patient outcomes should be central concerns of such research. Research related to functional- and health-status assessment should be directed to the adaptation of these tools for patient management.

Research on the relationships of reimbursement (to physicians and facilities), patient characteristics, and treatment modalities to patient outcomes is sorely needed. During its work, the committee received numerous analyses that documented these interactions and indicated that a potential exists among nephrologists to generate a literature on these issues that would be useful to clinicians and policy makers alike.

REFERENCES

Baxter Renal Division. 1990. Extramural Grant Program. Deerfield, Illinois.

Levin NW, Keshaviah P, Gotch FA. 1990. Effect of reimbursement on innovation in the ESRD program. Paper prepared for ESRD Study Committee, Institute of Medicine. New York: Beth Israel Hospital.

Maher JF. 1989. The decline in dialysis research in the United States. Semin Dialysis 2:203-206.

Mansfield E, Rapoport J, Romeo A, Wagner S, Beardsley G. 1977. Social and private rate of return from industrial innovations. Quarterly J Econ 91(May):221-240.

NKUDAB (National Kidney and Urologic Diseases Advisory Board). 1990. 1990 Long-Range Plan: Window on the 21st Century. NIH Publ. No. 90-583. Washington, D.C.: U.S. Department of Health and Human Services.

APPENDIXES

A

Glossary

Access Potential and actual entry of a population into the health care delivery system; the ability to obtain needed medical care.

Access Device A piece of equipment or a surgical adaptation for access to the patient's bloodstream (for hemodialysis) or to the peritoneal membrane (for peritoneal dialysis).

Activities of Daily Living Basic self-care activities, including eating, bathing, dressing, transferring from bed to chair, bowel and bladder control, and independent ambulation. These activities which are widely used as a minimal basis for assessing individual functional status.

Adjustment A procedure (such as age adjustment) used to remove the influence of the differences in the (age) distribution of populations being compared for some factor, for example, mortality. Usually, the method involves applying rates (such as mortality rates) calculated for subgroups of each comparison population to the comparable subgroups of the standard population. Then, using the distribution of the standard population, a corrected (adjusted) rate is computed for each comparison population.

Advance Directives Directives about a person's preferences concerning medical treatment in the event of future incapacity to decide or communicate. These can be oral or written and can concern any aspect of medical treatment, although such directives usually focus on life-sustaining treatments in critical or terminal illness. Written, legally sanctioned advance directives include living wills and durable powers of attorney for health care.

Agreement A written document executed between an ESRD facility and another facility in which the other facility agrees to assume responsibility for furnishing specified services to patients and for obtaining reimbursement for those services.

Allowable Costs   Costs of operating a facility, which are accounted as reimbursable under the federal Medicare or the state Medicaid program.

Ambulatory Peritoneal Dialysis   A treatment where the patient is ambulatory at least part of the time while dialyzing. (See Continuous Ambulatory Peritoneal Dialysis.)

Automated Peritoneal Dialysis Method   A method where fluid exchanges are performed by a preset peritoneal dialysis cycling machine after connection by the patient or other operator.

Backup Dialysis   A dialysis session furnished to an ESRD patient which is outside the patient's routine dialysis setting, e.g., a home patient dialyzing in the facility or an in-facility patient transferred to a backup (usually hospital) facility.

Backup Hospital   A hospital with whom a dialysis facility has a written agreement under which inpatient hospital care or other hospital services are available routinely and promptly to the dialysis facility's patients when needed.

Cadaveric Kidney Transplant   The surgical procedure of removing a kidney from a cadaver and implanting it into a suitable recipient.

Capitation   1. The method of paying for medical care by means of a prospective payment per patient or treatment that is independent of the number of services received.   2. A contractual agreement between the federal government and an organized health plan such as a health maintenance organization, whereby Medicare pays the plan a fixed prepaid amount per enrolled beneficiary.   In return, the plan is responsible for providing all appropriate entitled health services for some specified period of time.

Case Mix   1. The combination of diagnoses, medical care, and social care needs present in the population of a health care facility.   2. The relative frequency of admissions of various types of patients, reflecting different needs for hospital resources. Some ways of measuring case mix are based on patient diagnoses or the severity of their illness, some on the utilization of services, and some on the characteristics of the hospital or area in which it is located (this is measurement by proxy rather than actual measurement).

Certificate-of-Need   A certification made by a state that a certain health service is needed and authorizes a specific operator, at the operator's request, to provide that service.

Charge   The amount of money billed by a seller in return for a product or a service.   A hospital's charge is equivalent to its list price for a service. Medicare, Medicaid, most Blue Cross plans, and some other payers, however, do not pay charges, but pay another rate, variously determined, for inpatient hospital services. Thus, the charge is not the price from Medicare's or certain other payers' perspectives.

Chronic Maintenance Dialysis Dialysis that is regularly furnished to an ESRD patient in either a hospital-based, independent (non-hospital-based), or home setting.

Claim A request to a third-party payer (e.g., private insurer, government payment program, or employer payment program) by a person covered by the third-party's program or an assignee (usually a provider of service) for payment of benefits.

Classification The act or process of systematically arranging in groups or categories according to established criteria. Under the Prospective Payment System (PPS), hospital patients are classified into disease categories using the ICD-9-CM diagnostic classification system and then clustered into diagnosis-related groups (DRGs).

Cohort A population group that shares a common property, characteristic, or event, such as a year of birth or year of marriage. The most common one is the birth cohort, a group of individuals born within a defined time period, usually a calendar year or a 5-year interval.

Coinsurance The portion of the balance of covered medical expenses that a beneficiary must pay after payment of the deductible. Under Medicare Part B, after the annual deductible has been met, Medicare will generally pay 80 percent of approved charges for covered outpatient services and supplies; the remaining 20 percent is the coinsurance, for which the beneficiary is liable.

Comorbidity For the purposes of the Prospective Payment System (PPS), a preexisting condition (disease, disorder, disability, or other risk factor) that will, in the opinion of clinical experts, increase length of stay by at least one day in approximately 75 percent of cases with a specific diagnosis.

Continuous Ambulatory Peritoneal Dialysis (CAPD) A type of peritoneal dialysis whereby the patient dialyzes at home, being continuously filled with dialyzing fluid and making three to five exchanges of fluid per day.

Continuous Cyclic Peritoneal Dialysis (CCPD) A continuous, ambulatory automated method for nightly fluid exchanges, and one exchange indwelling throughout the daytime.

Cost Actual expenses incurred for inputs. For example, the cost of nursing home care includes direct costs such as staff salary, facility, equipment, supplies, and indirect costs such as mortgage, general and administrative fees, and cost of capital.

Cost-Based Reimbursement A method of paying for services based on the costs incurred by a provider to furnish those services.

Cost Sharing Financing arrangements whereby the consumer pays some out-of-pocket cost to receive care.

Coverage (Medicare) The range of services authorized for entitled beneficiaries.

Current Procedural Terminology 1. Coding system for physician services developed by the American Medical Association; basis of the HCFA Common Procedures Coding System. 2. Coding system for procedures performed by physicians that is used in Medicare Part B billing.

Customary, Prevailing, and Reasonable (CPR) Method (Medicare) The method used by Medicare carriers to determine the approved charge for a particular Part B service from a particular physician or supplier; based on the actual charge for the service, previous charges for the service by the physician or supplier in question (customary), and previous charges by peer physicians or suppliers in the same locality. (See Usual, Customary, and Reasonable Charges.)

Deductible A form of cost sharing in which the insured incurs an initial expense of a specified amount within a given time period (e.g., $250 per year) before the insurer assumes liability for any additional costs of covered services.

Diabetes Mellitus A constitutional disorder of carbohydrate metabolism that is characterized by inadequate secretion or utilization of insulin, by excessive amounts of sugar in the blood and urine, and by thirst, hunger, and loss of weight. Frequent complications include damage to the heart, circulation, eyes, and kidneys.

Diagnosis-Related Groups A classification system that groups patients according to diagnosis, type of treatment, age, and other relevant criteria. In October 1983, Medicare instituted a prospective reimbursement system based on 467 DRGs. Under this system, hospitals are paid a set fee for treating patients in a single DRG category, regardless of the actual cost of care for the individual.

Dialysis A process of maintaining the chemical balance of the blood when the kidneys have failed; specifically, a process by which dissolved substances are removed from a patient's body by diffusion from one fluid compartment to another across a semipermeable membrane. The types of dialysis currently used are hemodialysis and peritoneal dialysis (CAPD and CCPD are peritoneal dialysis techniques).

Dialysis Center A hospital unit that is approved to furnish the full spectrum of diagnostic, therapeutic, and rehabilitative services required for the care of ESRD dialysis patients, including inpatient and outpatient dialysis.

Dialysis Facility   A unit (hospital-based or freestanding) which is approved to furnish dialysis services directly to ESRD patients.

Dialysis Station   The single functional unit of a dialysis facility which is needed to provide therapy to one patient.

Durable Power of Attorney for Health Care   A form of advance directive by which an individual delegates, in a legally valid document, decision-making authority to some other person to act in his or her behalf regarding medical care when the individual has lost the capacity to decide or to communicate especially regarding life-sustaining treatment.

Eligibility Requirements   To qualify for Medicare under the renal provision of the Social Security Act, a person must have ESRD and either be entitled to a monthly insurance benefit under Title II of the Social Security Act (or an annuity under the Railroad Retirement Act), or be fully or currently insured under Social Security (railroad work may count), or be the spouse or dependent child of a person who meets at least one of these last two requirements (there is no minimum age for eligibility). In addition, an application for Medicare beneficiary status must be filed (effective October 1, 1978).

End-Stage Renal Disease (ESRD)   Advanced destruction of the kidneys by disease resulting in chronic, irreversible, near total loss of kidney function.

ESRD Network   A legally authorized regional organization, consisting of ESRD providers in a designated geographic area, which collects data for HCFA, conducts medical reviews, and supports patients and providers.

Epidemiology   The scientific study of the distribution and occurrence of human diseases and health conditions and their determinants.

Federal Prospective Payment Amount   The portion of the hospital prospective payment rate derived from national and regional standardized prospective payment amounts. During the transition period of Medicare's Prospective Payment System, hospitals are paid at a rate that blends the federal and hospital-specific portion. After the transition period, the payment rate is based entirely on the federal standardized payment amount. From April 1, 1988, through September 30, 1990, the federal rate will be based on the national average standardized amount, or a blend of 85 percent national and 15 percent regional amounts, whichever is higher.

Fee for Service   Refers to paying physicians for individual medical services rendered, as opposed to paying them with salaries or under capitation. Customary, prevailing, and reasonable (CPR), usual, customary, and reasonable (UCR), and fee schedules are examples of fee for service.

Hemodialysis A method of dialysis in which blood from a patient's body is circulated through an external device or machine and thence returned to the patient's bloodstream. Such an artificial kidney machine usually is designed to remove fluids and metabolic waste products from the bloodstream by placing the blood in contact with a semipermeable membrane which is bathed on the other side by an appropriate chemical solution resembling normal plasma water referred to as dialysate.

Home Dialysis Patients Medically able individuals who maintain their own dialysis equipment at home and, after proper training, perform their own treatment alone or with the assistance of a helper.

Hypertension Persistently high blood pressure. The chief importance of hypertension lies in the increased risk it confers of illness and death from cardiovascular, cerebrovascular, and renal disease.

In-Unit (In-Facility, In-Center) Patients Individuals whose dialysis is performed in a dialysis unit or facility.

Incidence The frequency of new occurrences of a condition within a defined time interval. The incidence rate is the number of new cases of specific disease divided by the number of people in a population over a specified period of time, usually 1 year.

Intermittent Peritoneal Dialysis A technique where dialysis solution is infused and dialysate is drained through a single catheter. During a fluid exchange (cycle) three distinct periods occur: inflow, dwell, and outflow. After the outflow, before the next inflow, and during the dwell, the flow of fluid is interrupted, hence the term intermittent.

Living Related Donor Transplant The surgical procedure of removing a kidney from a living relative of the patient and implanting it in the patient.

Living Will A form of advance directive by which an individual expresses, in written legal instructions, his or her preferences for medical treatment if he or she becomes incompetent to decide or unable to communicate at the end of life. There are general forms for living wills and specific forms sanctioned by law in most states.

Manual Peritoneal Dialysis Method A method where fluid exchanges are performed manually with active participation of a person (patient, partner, or nurse) during each exchange procedure.

Margins Percentage of Medicare payments remaining after accounting for Medicare costs. The aggregate margin for a group of outpatient dialysis facilities is defined as total Medicare payments for the group minus total Medicare costs for the group, divided by total Medicare payments for the group.

Market Basket Forecasts the change in the hospital industry's price; an input index reflecting changes in hospital labor markets and nonlabor-related expenses.

Medicaid A federal/state health insurance program, authorized in 1965 as Title XIX of the Social Security Act, to provide medical care for low-income individuals. Federal regulations specify mandated services, but states can expand services and eligibility standards at their cost. The federal government's share of costs ranges from 50 to 78 percent and is based on per-capita income in the state.

Medicare A nationwide, federally administered health insurance program authorized in 1965 as Title XVIII of the Social Security Act, to cover the cost of hospitalization, medical care, and some related services for most people over age 65, people receiving Social Security Disability Insurance payments for 2 years, and people with ESRD. Medicare consists of two separate but coordinated programs — Part A (Hospital Insurance) and Part B (Supplementary Medical Insurance). Health insurance protection is available to Medicare beneficiaries without regard to income.

Medicare Carriers Fiscal agents (typically Blue Cross or Blue Shield plans or commercial insurance firms) under contract to HCFA for administration of specific Medicare tasks. These tasks include computing reasonable charges under Medicare Part B, making actual payments, determining whether claims are for covered services, denying claims for noncovered services, and denying claims for unnecessary use of services.

Medicare Cost Report (MCR) An annual report required of all institutions participating in the Medicare program that is used to identify Medicare-reimbursable costs. The costs are defined and reported following guidelines established by the Medicare program. The 1981 MCRs were used to develop both the Federal standardized amounts and the original diagnosis-related group (DRG) weights for the Prospective Payment System.

Medicare Provider Analysis and Review File (MEDPAR) HCFA data file that contains billed-charge data and clinical characteristics, such as principal diagnosis and principal procedures, for Medicare hospital discharges during a fiscal year. Before 1984, the MEDPAR file contained only a 20 percent sample of inpatient bills submitted by hospitals. Since 1985, it has included those bills as well as bills on all Medicare inpatient discharges. For 1984, the comparable file is called the PATBILL file.

Monthly Capitation Payment A predetermined reimbursement amount per patient per month that is paid for physician outpatient dialysis-related services under Medicare.

Morbidity A diseased state; often used in the content of a "morbidity rate," i.e., the rate of disease or proportion of diseased people in a population. In common clinical usage, any disease state or complication is referred to as morbidity.

Morbidity Rate   The rate of illness in a population. The number of people ill during a time period divided by the number of people in the total population.

Mortality Rate   The death rate, often made explicit for a particular characteristic, e.g., gender, sex, or specific cause of death. Mortality rate contains three essential elements: (1) the number of people in a population group exposed to the risk of death (the denominator); (2) a time factor; and (3) the number of deaths occurring in the exposed population during a certain time period (the numerator).

Organ Procurement   The process of acquiring donor kidneys.

Organ Procurement Agency   An organization that performs or coordinates the performance of all the following services: acquisition and preservation of donated kidneys, and maintenance of a system to locate prospective recipients for acquired organs.

Outcome   The consequences related to a specific medical intervention for an individual or a group of patients.

Panel Reactive Antibody (PRA)   A value, expressed as a percentage, that indicates a person's sensitivity to various antigens. It is determined by mixing a sample of an individual's blood with blood samples from a large number of people considered to be representative of the general population. The number of reactions between the patient's blood and this cell panel is converted to a percentage. The greater the PRA value, the greater the likelihood that existing antibodies will cause a positive crossmatch reaction, preventing the transplant.

Part A (Medicare)   Medicare's Hospital Insurance program, which covers specified hospital inpatient services, posthospital extended care, and home health care services. Part A, which is an entitlement program for those who are eligible, is available without payment of a premium, although those not automatically eligible for Part A may enroll in the program by paying a monthly premium. The beneficiary is responsible for an initial deductible and/or copayment for some services.

Part B (Medicare)   Medicare's Supplementary Medical Insurance program, which covers physician services, hospital outpatient services, outpatient physical therapy and speech pathology services, and various other limited ambulatory services and supplies such as prosthetic devices and durable medical equipment. This program also covers home health services for Medicare beneficiaries who have Part B coverage only. Enrollment in Part B is optional and requires payment of a monthly premium. The beneficiary is also responsible for a deductible and a coinsurance payment for most covered services.

Peritoneal Dialysis A procedure that introduces dialysate into the abdominal cavity to absorb and remove waste products through the peritoneum (a membrane which surrounds the intestines and other organs in the abdominal cavity). It functions in a manner similar to that of the (artificial) semipermeable membrane in the hemodialysis machine. Two other forms of peritoneal dialysis are continuous ambulatory peritoneal dialysis and continuous cycling peritoneal dialysis.

Physician Payment Review Commission The commission reviews physician payment in the Medicare program, describing a comprehensive proposal for reform of Medicare payment to physicians including a Medicare fee schedule, balance-billing limits, expenditure targets, and a program of effectiveness research and development of practice guidelines.

Prevailing Charge One of the factors determining a physician's payment for a service under Medicare. It is currently set at the 75th percentile of customary charges of all physicians in the community. Since 1976, its growth has been limited to the increase in the Medicare Economic Index. (See Customary, Prevailing, and Reasonable Method.)

Prevalence The number of existing cases of a disease or condition in a given population at a specific time.

Professional Standards Review Organizations (PSROs) Community-based physician-directed, nonprofit agencies established under the Social Security Amendments of 1972 (Pub. L. No. 92-603) to monitor the quality and appropriateness of institutional health care provided to Medicare and Medicaid beneficiaries. PSROs have been replaced by Professional Review Organizations (PROs—utilization and quality control peer review organizations).

Program Management and Medical Information System (PMMIS) A system that contains, in part, medical information on patients and the services that they have received during the course of their therapy. The HCFA ESRD PMMIS is an automated system of medical records that deals primarily with current Medicare-eligible ESRD patients but also maintains historical information on people no longer classified as ESRD patients by reason of death or successful transplantation. In addition, it contains information on ESRD facilities and facility reimbursement.

Prospective Payment 1. A method of payment for health care services in which the amount of payment for services is set before the delivery of those services and the hospital (or other provider) is at least partially at risk for losses or stands to gain from surpluses that accrue during the payment period. Prospective payment rates may be per-service, per-capita, per-diem, or per-case rates. 2. Payment for medical care on the basis of rates set in advance of the time period in which they apply. The unit of payment may vary from individual medical services to broader categories, such as hospital case, episode of illness, or person capitation.

Prospective Payment Assessment Commission   The commission reviews the goals, principles, rates, and major design features of the Medicare PPS, and it advises the Congress and the Secretary of DHHS.

Quality Assessment   Measurement and evaluation of quality of care for individuals, groups, or populations.

Quality Assurance   1. Process of measuring quality, analyzing the deficiencies discovered, and taking action to improve performance, followed by measuring quality again to determine whether improvement has been achieved. It is a systematic, cyclic activity using standards for measurement.   2. Activities to safeguard or improve the quality of medical care by assessing quality and taking action to correct any problems found.

Quality of Medical Care   The degree to which actions taken or not taken increase the probability of beneficial health outcomes and decrease risk and other untoward outcomes, given the existing state of medical sciences and art.

Rate Setting   A method of payment for health care services in which a state (or other) regulatory body decides what prices a hospital, for example, may charge in a given year.

Reasonable and Necessary (Medicare)   Criteria used by HCFA or Medicare contractors to determine which services are eligible for Medicare coverage. Coverage is distinguished from payment in that coverage refers to services available to eligible beneficiaries, and payment refers to the amount and methods of payment for coverage. The criteria used to determine whether a service is reasonable and necessary are (1) general acceptance as safe and effective, (2) not experimental, (3) medically necessary, and (4) provided according to standards of medical practice in an appropriate setting.

Rebasing   Method for calculating the base payment rate using most recent cost and charge information.

Renal Dialysis Center   See Dialysis Center.

Renal Dialysis Facility   See Dialysis Facility.

Renal Transplant Center   See Transplant Center.

Resource-Based Relative Value Scale   An index that assigns weights to each medical service, representing the relative amount to be paid for each service based on resources consumed or required to produce the service.

Risk A measure of the probability of an adverse or untoward outcome and the severity of the resultant harm to health of individuals in a defined population and associated with the use of a medical technology for a given medical problem under specified conditions of use.

Self-Care Services Services provided by a dialysis facility or center in which patients who have been trained to perform self-dialysis do so with little or no professional assistance.

Self-Dialysis Patients Patients who have been trained in dialysis techniques and dialyze themselves in a dialysis facility with minimal staff assistance or at home without professional assistance. Patients who are entirely responsible for administering their own dialysis treatments without professional support (except in emergency situations) are in this category.

Special-Purpose Facility A renal dialysis facility that is approved to furnish dialysis at special locations on a short-term basis to a group of dialysis patients otherwise unable to obtain treatment in the geographical area. The special locations must be either special rehabilitative (including vacation) locations servicing ESRD patients temporarily residing there, or locations in need of ESRD facilities under emergency circumstances.

Staff-Assisted Dialysis Dialysis performed by the staff of the renal dialysis center or facility.

Supplemental Security Income A federal income support program for low-income, disabled, aged, and blind people. Eligibility for the monthly cash payments is based on the individual's current status without regard to previous work or contributions to a trust fund. Some states supplement the federal benefit.

Supplementary Medical Insurance A voluntary insurance program (also known as Medicare Part B) that provides insurance benefits for physician and other medical services in accordance with the provisions of Title XVIII of the Social Security Act, for aged and disabled individuals who elect to enroll under such program. The program is financed by premium payments by enrollees, and contributions from funds appropriated by the federal government.

Survey Period The period January 1 through December 31 of each year for which all ESRD facilities must complete Form HCFA-2744, ESRD Facility Survey.

Tax Equity and Fiscal Responsibility Act (Pub. L. No. 97-248) (TEFRA) Legislation enacted in 1982 that initiated the shift in the Medicare program away from cost-based reimbursement for hospitals toward prospective payment. TEFRA made other major changes in audit, medical claims review, and utilization and peer review. The most significant was to establish the PRO program as a substitute for the PSRO program.

Third-Party Payment Payment by a private insurer or government program to a medical provider for care given to a patient.

Tidal Peritoneal Dialysis A technique where, after an initial fill of the peritoneal cavity, only a portion of dialysate is drained and replaced by fresh dialysis fluid with each cycle, leaving the majority of dialysate in constant contact with the peritoneal membrane until the end of the dialysis session, when the fluid is drained as completely as possible.

Transfer For the purposes of PPS, a movement of a patient (1) from one inpatient area or unit of the hospital to another area or unit of the hospital; (2) from the care of a hospital paid under prospective payment to the care of another such hospital; or (3) from the care of a hospital under prospective payment to the care of a hospital in an approved statewide cost-control program.

Transient ESRD Patients Patients who are treated by ESRD facilities episodically (less than 51 percent of the survey period), e.g., vacationers.

Transplant The surgical procedure that involves removing an organ from a cadaver or a living donor and implanting it in another individual.

Transplant Center A hospital unit that is approved to furnish direct transplantation and other medical and surgical specialty services for the care of the ESRD transplant patient, including inpatient dialysis furnished directly or under arrangement.

Updating Method of inflating a base payment rate for years in which the rate is not recalculated using more recent data.

Usual, Customary, and Reasonable Charges (UCR) In private health insurance, a basis for determining payment for individual physician services. "Usual" refers to the individual physician's fee profile, equivalent to Medicare's "customary" charge screen. "Customary," in this context, refers to a percentile of the pattern of charges made by physicians in a given locality (comparable to Medicare's "prevailing" charges). "Reasonable" is the lesser of the usual or customary screens. (See Customary, Prevailing, and Reasonable Method.)

Waivers Exemption from meeting a particular regulatory requirement. Waivers of certification requirements may be given by states to facilities. Waivers of program requirements may be given by the federal government to states.

B

Acronyms and Initialisms

AAMI	Association for the Advancement of Medical Instrumentation
AAPCC	Average adjusted per capita cost
ADL	Activities of daily living
AHA	American Hospital Association
AHCPR	Agency for Health Care Policy Research (formerly NCHSR & HCTA), PHS
ALOS	Average length of stay
AMA	American Medical Association
ANNA	American Nephrology Nurses Association
ASTS	American Society of Transplant Surgeons
BDMS	Bureau of Data Management and Strategy, HCFA
BERC	Bureau of Eligibility, Reimbursement, and Coverage (now BPD), HCFA
BHI	Bureau of Health Insurance, SSA
BLS	Bureau of Labor Statistics, Department of Labor
BMAD	Part B Medicare Annual Data
BONENT	Board of Nephrology Nurses and Technicians
BPD	Bureau of Policy Development (formerly BERC), HCFA
BQA	Bureau of Quality Assurance, PHS
BUN	Blood urea nitrogen
CAPD	Continuous ambulatory peritoneal dialysis
CBO	Congressional Budget Office, U.S. Congress
CDC	Centers for Disease Control, PHS
CFR	Code of Federal Regulations
CNSW	Council of Nephrology Social Workers

COBRA	Consolidated Omnibus Budget Reconciliation Act of 1985 (Public Law 99-272)
CON	Certificate-of-need
CPR	Customary, prevailing, and reasonable
CPT-4	Current Procedural Terminology, 4th Edition
CY	Calendar year
DCI-C	Dialysis Clinic, Inc.-Cincinnati
DHHS	U.S. Department of Health and Human Services
DRG	Diagnosis-related group
DVA	Department of Veterans Affairs (formerly the Veterans Administration)
EDTA	European Dialysis and Transplant Association
EPO	Erythropoietin
ESRD	End-stage renal disease
FASB	Financial Accounting Standards Board
FDA	Food and Drug Administration, PHS
FFS	Fee for service
FI	Fiscal intermediary
FTE	Full-time equivalent
FY	Fiscal year
GAAP	Generally accepted accounting principles
GAO	General Accounting Office, U.S. Congress
GHS	Greenfield Health Systems
GNP	Gross national product
HCFA	Health Care Financing Administration, DHHS
HCRIS	Hospital Cost Report Information System, HCFA
HIC	Home Intensive Care, Inc.
HMO	Health maintenance organization
HRSA	Health Resources and Services Administration, PHS
HSQB	Health Standards and Quality Bureau, HCFA
ICD-9-CM	International Classification of Diseases, 9th Revision, Clinical Modification
IHS	Indian Health Service
IOM	Institute of Medicine
JCAH	Joint Commission on the Accreditation of Hospitals (now JCAHO)
JCAHO	Joint Commission on the Accreditation of Healthcare Organizations (formerly JCAH)
LOS	Length of stay
LPN	Licensed practical nurse

LRD	Living related donor
MAAC	Maximum allowable actual charge
MADRS	Medicare Automated Data Retrieval System, HCFA
MCP	Monthly capitation payment
MEDPAR	Medicare Provider Analysis and Review, HCFA
MEDTEP	Medical Treatment Effectiveness Program, PHS
MFS	Medicare fee schedule
MIS	Medical Information and Quality Assurance System, HCFA
MMACS	Medicare/Medicaid Automated Certification System, HCFA
MOS	Medical Outcomes Study
MSA	Metropolitan statistical area

NAMCS	National Ambulatory Medical Care Survey, NCHS
NAS	National Academy of Sciences
NCDC	North Central Dialysis Centers
NCDS	National Cooperative Dialysis Study
NCHS	National Center for Health Statistics, PHS
NCHSR & HCTA	National Center for Health Services Research and Health Care Technology Assessment (now AHCPR), PHS
NIDDK	National Institute of Diabetes and Digestive and Kidney Diseases, NIH, PHS
NIH	National Institutes of Health, PHS
NKF	National Kidney Foundation
NMC	National Medical Care, Inc.
NMCES	National Medical Care Expenditure Survey, AHCPR, PHS

OBRA	Omnibus Budget Reconciliation Act (1981: Public Law 97-35; 1986: Public Law 99-509; 1987: Public Law 100-203; 1989: Public Law 101-239; 1990: Public Law 101-508)
OHTA	Office of Health Technology Assessment, AHCPR, PHS
OIG	Office of the Inspector General, DHHS
OPTN	Organ Procurement and Transplantation Network
ORD	Office of Research and Demonstrations, HCFA
OTA	Office of Technology Assessment, U.S. Congress

PATBILL	Medicare Inpatient Bills File
PD	Peritoneal dialysis
PHS	Public Health Service, DHHS
PMMIS	Program Management Medical Information System
PMP	Per million population
PPCIS	Physicians Practice Cost and Income Survey
PPI	Physician Performance Index
PPO	Preferred provider organization

PPS	Prospective Payment System
PRA	Panel reactive antibodies
PRO	Utilization and Quality Control Peer Review Organization
ProPAC	Prospective Payment Assessment Commission
PRRB	Provider Reimbursement Review Board
PSRO	Professional Standards Review Organization
QA	Quality assurance
QRO	Quality Review Organization
R&D	Research and development
RFP	Request for proposal
RKDP	Regional Kidney Disease Program
RN	Registered nurse
ROE	Return on equity
SEOPF	Southeast Organ Procurement Foundation
SIP	Sickness Impact Profile
SMSA	Standard metropolitan statistical area
SNF	Skilled nursing facility

C

Commissioned Papers and Contractor Reports

Feldman HI. 1990. End-stage renal disease in U.S. minority groups. Philadelphia, Pennsylvania: University of Pennsylvania School of Medicine.

Fine RN. 1990. The effect of the End-Stage Renal Disease program on the pediatric patient. Los Angeles, California: University of California, Los Angeles.

Hawthorne VM. 1990. Preventing kidney disease of diabetes mellitus. Ann Arbor, Michigan: University of Michigan.

Klag MJ. 1990. The patient with hypertensive end-stage renal disease. Baltimore, Maryland: The Johns Hopkins University Hospital.

Levin NW, Keshaviah P, Gotch FA. 1990. Effect of reimbursement on innovation in the ESRD program. New York, New York: Beth Israel Medical Center.

Pollack VE, Pesce A. 1990. Analysis of data related to the 1976-1989 patient population: Treatment characteristics and patient outcomes. Cincinnati, Ohio: Dialysis Clinic, Inc.-Cincinnati.

Sehgal A, Rennie D, Showstack J, Amend W, Lo B. 1990. Chronic end stage renal disease in the elderly. San Francisco, California: University of California, San Francisco.

Wolfe RA. 1990. Survival analysis methods for the End-Stage Renal Disease (ESRD) program of Medicare. Ann Arbor: University of Michigan.

Intergovernmental Health Policy Project, George Washington University

Laudacina SL. 1990. Medicaid coverage and payment of ESRD services. Washington, D.C., 1990.

Laudacina SL, Donohoe E. 1989. The Medicaid experience with end-stage renal disease: Findings of a national survey. Washington, D.C.: Intergovernmental Health Policy Program, George Washington University.

Thomas CS. 1989. Certificate of need (CON) regulation of ESRD services: Findings of a 50-state survey. Washington, D.C.: Intergovernmental Health Policy Project, The George Washington University.

Medical Media Associates, Inc.

Oberley ET. 1990. A patient review of the ESRD program: A focus group study. Madison, Wisconsin: Medical Media Associates, Inc.

Urban Institute

Garcia J, Held PJ, Cahn MA, Pauly MV. 1990. Staffing of dialysis units and the price of dialysis. Washington, D.C.: The Urban Institute.

Held PJ, Garcia JR, Pauly MV, Wolfe RA, Gaylin DS, Cahn MA. 1990. The impact of the price of dialysis on mortality and hospitalization: An overview. Washington, D.C.: The Urban Institute.

Held PJ, Garcia JR, Pauly MV, Wolfe RA, Gaylin DS, Cahn MA. 1990. Mortality and the price of dialysis. Washington, D.C.: The Urban Institute.

Held PJ, Garcia JR, Wolfe RA, Gaylin DS, Pauly MV, Cahn MA. 1990. The price of dialysis and hospitalization. Washington, D.C.: The Urban Institute.

D
Survival Analysis Methods for the End-Stage Renal Disease (ESRD) Program of Medicare

ROBERT A. WOLFE, Ph.D.*

This document addresses two specific areas related to survival analysis of Medicare ESRD data. The first focus is a critical review of methods of survival analysis for Medicare ESRD data, including methods used in the past by HCFA and the USRDS, methods that have been proposed by other members of the renal community, and methods that are potentially useful for future analyses. The second focus is a review of the results of international comparisons of mortality rates with the objective of determining what conclusions can be drawn from such comparisons.

While this paper gives a critical review of methods of analysis of ESRD mortality data, it does not report the results of any new analyses of empirical data. Instead, this paper is intended to help in the interpretation of the results of previous data analyses and to give directions for future analyses and data collection that address some of the limitations of the research carried out to date. Although a review of statistical methods must unavoidably involve some degree of abstraction, I have tried to tie abstract concepts to specific issues whenever possible.

The analysis of mortality among ESRD patients is complicated by the nature of the data available for analysis and by the heterogeneity of the patients receiving therapy. These issues are addressed in some detail in this paper in order to show how to avoid potential limitations of analyses and errors in their interpretation. Some of the specific issues are listed below.

The data for ESRD patients are complicated because they are collected over time and involve a sequence of events for each subject being studied. The sequence of relevant medical information for some of the subjects in

*Department of Biostatistics, University of Michigan, Ann Arbor, Michigan

the data set may be incompletely documented. For example, patient follow-up of younger ESRD patients is not typically tracked in the Medicare data system until 90 days after first therapy for ESRD. Analyses of such incomplete data are susceptible to subtle forms of bias.

Patients with treated ESRD exhibit a wide variety of characteristics that influence mortality patterns. An evaluation of the importance of any one of these characteristics must also account for the potential impact on the results of the other characteristics.

The Medicare data collection system was designed primarily for reimbursement purposes and, consequently, has some limitations for research purposes. Some patient characteristics related to mortality, such as previous medical history, are not regularly recorded in it. Other characteristics, such as patient treatment history, are derived from billing records rather than from dedicated data collection instruments and, consequently, are subject to error.

Interpretation of the results of mortality analyses is complicated by the variety of analytical methods and types of numerical summaries that can be reported. Analytical methods include adjusted and unadjusted results, cross-tabulations and multiple regression models, parametric and nonparametric methods, Cox models and logistic regression models, and other methods discussed below. The results of statistical analyses can be summarized as death rates, death proportions, mortality ratios, and expected lifetimes.

An overview of several crucial issues central to the analysis of mortality data is presented in the first section as a series of questions. Each question is followed by some of the issues that should be addressed when answering the question. These issues recur in more specific forms in subsequent sections of the document.

In the second section, general strategies for adjusting statistical analyses for patient characteristics are discussed. Patient characteristics that are currently measured or that would be useful to measure are examined, and two approaches toward adjusting statistical analyses for patient characteristics are provided.

In the third section, several methods of survival analysis that are relevant to ESRD data are reviewed with the intent of showing how to compare, interpret, and synthesize the results of survival analyses. Most of the methods reviewed in this section have been used, or proposed for use, by other members of the renal research community. Each method has qualities that make it appropriate for specific purposes. Some proposals are also made in this section for analysis methods that have not yet been widely used in renal research. In addition, several different numerical parameters that are used to summarize the results of survival analyses are discussed.

The fourth section reviews several problems associated with the interpretation of international comparisons of mortality rates. Although this section focuses on the analysis recently reported by Held et al. (1990), the issues are largely relevant to any international comparisons.

GENERAL ISSUES IN SURVIVAL ANALYSIS

Overview

Survival analysis of ESRD patient data can help to identify factors, such as etiology, that are related to differences in patient mortality. For example, a comparison of the one-year survival proportions for diabetic and nondiabetic patients shows that mortality rates differ by etiology. With the identification of such factors, survival analysis also yields estimates of the magnitude of the differences in survival associated with those factors. Although the comparison of mortality figures for two groups of patients gives a direct evaluation of the importance of the factor distinguishing the two groups, it seldom leads to a complete understanding of the mechanisms causing the difference. Since any two groups of patients may differ with respect to several factors simultaneously, it is of some interest to determine how much effect any one factor would have on mortality, if all other factors were held constant. For example, the average age among diabetic and nondiabetic patients is different, so we want to know by how much the mortality rates would differ for diabetic and nondiabetic patients, if the ages were similar in the two groups. Survival analysis can help to answer hypothetical questions such as "By how much would the mortality patterns in two groups of patients differ, if they were to differ from each other with respect to only one characteristic at a time?" Although much this appendix describes examples related to the study of mortality differences for several treatment groups, the concepts and statistical methods that are presented apply equally well to the comparison of outcomes for groups of patients defined by other characteristics, as well.

Survival analysis can only yield results concerning factors that are measured and recorded in the available data. Unfortunately, some of the most important determinants of survival may not be recorded in the Medicare data base. Survival analysis cannot account for the potential effect of unmeasured or unmeasurable factors on patient mortality. Many of the important questions related to policy and scientific research involve factors that have not or cannot be measured. In such cases, expert opinion blended with indirect or imperfect evidence must be relied upon. Although decisions that are based on inconclusive evidence can be wrong, the available data still should be evaluated and weighed carefully when making policy decisions.

Sir Ronald Fisher, one of the great statisticians and scientists of this century, argued throughout much of his life that there was no definitive evidence showing that tobacco smoking causes lung cancer. He argued that there could be an underlying factor that caused certain individuals both to smoke and to be more susceptible to lung cancer. Although his reasoning was correct (the evidence is not conclusive unless a randomized controlled clinical trial is performed), the resulting policy decision based on his reasoning would undoubtedly have been a poor one.

Statistical analysis is just one tool used in the weighing of empirical evidence. The process involves the formulation of a question, the assembling of relevant data to address the question, and careful interpretation of the results of analysis of the data. An evaluation of the strengths and weaknesses of the conclusions derived from the analysis sometimes leads to a reformulation of the question, collection of new data, or reanalysis of the data. The choice of appropriate method of statistical analysis cannot be discussed in isolation. Just as the specific question that we want to answer determines the way in which we try to answer it, the choice of appropriate statistical methodology depends strongly upon the specific purposes that motivate the analysis.

Examples

Several major types of research objectives and questions can be addressed through the collection and analysis of national ESRD data. The examples listed below were selected to highlight specific issues in the appropriate interpretation of survival analysis results. Some of the examples are based on hypothetical or simplistic situations but illustrate fundamental issues that arise in more realistic situations, as well.

The examples show that statistical comparisons are central to the interpretation of statistical analyses. Reduction and avoidance of bias, through the selection of appropriate comparison groups and the control of confounding factors, are fundamentally important to most analytic research. Minimizing and evaluating the impact of random variability on the results of research is also important. The selection of methods that yield interpretable numerical summaries is an essential aspect of the dissemination of results.

Identification of the Study Population

What is the death rate among ESRD patients? The death rate among untreated ESRD patients is very high; with no kidney function, they will surely die within days. Data are available in the Medicare system for treated ESRD patients after they become eligible for Medicare payments. However, victims with undiagnosed kidney disease are not counted in the Medicare data base. Further, because of eligibility requirements, the first 90 days of ESRD therapy for many younger patients in the United States are not captured by the Medicare data system. Among the elderly, the fraction of deaths attributable to withdrawal from therapy can be substantial (10 percent or more), but these deaths are included in most reports of ESRD mortality. Even among treated ESRD patients, the length of survival of patients with some residual kidney function is likely to depend upon the amount of impairment and the rate of progression of the disease.

If the deaths of never-treated ESRD victims were included in reported mortality rates, then the death rates likely would be elevated above those currently reported. In contrast, if the deaths among those withdrawing from treatment were excluded, then the death rates would likely be substantially lower than those currently reported. Different definitions distinguishing between reduced kidney function and ESRD could also have a substantial effect on reported death rates among the ESRD population.

Thus, any evaluation of mortality rates among ESRD patients must identify which patient population is being considered. Without such identification, it is difficult to compare different mortality results.

Evaluation of the death rate in a group can depend strongly upon who is included in the group and which period of patient follow-up is included in the evaluation.

The Importance of a Comparison Group

Are mortality rates among treated ESRD patients very high? Mortality rates among dialyzed ESRD patients in the United States are typically 24 percent per year (USRDS, 1990, p. E.31). Although of some value in isolation, this fact is of most interest when compared to other death rates.

For example, the 24 percent annual death rate among dialyzed ESRD patients is exceptionally high in comparison to that of a non-ESRD population with the same age distribution (approximately 2 percent per year). However, the discrepancy would be somewhat smaller if the comparison were made to a non-ESRD population with the same history of diabetes and hypertension as is found among incident ESRD patients. This comparison would be especially useful for the evaluation of programs designed to prevent the progression of hypertension and diabetes to ESRD.

Although death rates among treated ESRD patients are high relative to those in a healthy population, they are low compared to those among untreated ESRD victims.

Furthermore, the comparison of death rates among ESRD patients receiving different forms or amounts of therapy would be useful for comparing the relative efficacy of the various therapies.

When evaluating ESRD death rates, it is useful to make comparisons to other death rates.

Biased Comparisons

Spurious Differences   Is the death rate for dialyzed ESRD patients higher with continuous ambulatory peritoneal dialysis (CAPD) or with center hemodialysis (CH)?   CAPD was preferentially given to insulin-dependent diabetic ESRD patients in some regions of the United States in the early 1980s because it offers a convenient method for administration of insulin to the patient. Because of this, diabetes is more prevalent among CAPD patients than among CH patients in the United States. Thus, even if CAPD and CH were inherently equally efficacious therapies for ESRD (analyses to date have been inconclusive), then the high death rate among diabetic ESRD patients and the higher prevalence of diabetes among CAPD patients would cause unadjusted death rates to be higher among CAPD patients than among CH patients. Comparison of crude (unadjusted for patient characteristics) death rates for CAPD and CH patients would not account for this fact and would erroneously lead to the conclusion that death rates were higher among CAPD patients than among CH patients.

Observed differences in outcome may be due entirely to differences in patient characteristics.

Biased Comparison and Age-Specific Comparisons and Inappropriate Comparison Group   How much lower are death rates among transplant patients than among dialysis patients?   The annual death rate is typically 6 percent per year among ESRD patients with transplants (USRDS, 1990, p. E.40) and is typically 24 percent per year among dialysis patients (p. E.32). The death rate among transplant recipients is much lower than among dialyzed ESRD patients. However, transplant recipients are also younger, on average, than dialyzed patients. Comparison of the age-specific 5-year survival probabilities for dialyzed patients and transplant recipients indicates a substantial variation in death rates with the age of the patient (p. E.32, E.40). Thus, a large part of the difference in overall (crude) death rates between transplant recipients and dialyzed patients is due to the difference in ages between the two groups.

Part of an observed difference in outcomes may be due to differences in patient characteristics. Comparison of specific mortality rates for homogeneous subgroups of patients yields a less biased evaluation.

In addition to the effect of age, which is known and recorded for each patient, other differences between dialyzed patients and transplant recipients may account for part of the difference in death rates for these two treatment modalities. Dialyzed ESRD patients who are on the transplant waiting list are distinguished, in a variety of ways, from dialyzed ESRD patients who are not on the waiting list. Some of these distinctions may be difficult to identify or measure. Therefore, in order to compare the death rates of dialyzed patients and transplant recipients, it would be more appropriate to use the survival experience of dialyzed patients who are on the waiting list rather than that of all dialyzed patients.

Comparison groups should be similar in all aspects other than the characteristic being studied, especially in those other aspects that cannot be measured.

Bias Due to Unobserved Factors How can a new therapy for ESRD patients be evaluated without bias? The ultimate evaluation of a treatment protocol should be based upon how well it works and how much it costs in comparison to other protocols. Specific outcomes (mortality is an overriding outcome) can be selected as the basis for comparison of two protocols, and the outcomes can be evaluated for two series of patients treated according to the two protocols. Quantitative comparison of the outcomes for the two protocols leads to conclusions about the size of the difference in patient outcomes, which then can be evaluated in comparison to the relative costs of the protocols.

An observed difference in outcomes cannot be ascribed to the difference in treatments unless the two patient groups are equivalent in other major regards. The interpretation of the differences should account for any preexisting differences between the two groups of patients.

Ideally, evaluation of a new treatment should be based on the comparison of patient outcomes under the new and old treatment regimens, all else equal. This ideal can never be realized because it would require two identical series of patients for study. In practice, during patient enrollment, the two treatment groups can be deliberately balanced for important factors that are likely to have substantial effects on patient outcome. However, in order to ensure balance with respect to unknown factors, the only practical solution is randomization (Campbell and Stanley, 1963).

Randomization can be used to control for unforeseen differences between patient groups. The controlled randomized clinical trial offers the only study design that can be guaranteed (with high probability) to be free of bias. All other study designs are subject to potential bias because the groups being compared may differ with respect to several factors that affect patient outcome.

Interpreting Standard Errors for Population Data

When there is no sampling error because a statistic is reported for all ESRD patients, how should the standard error be interpreted? The standard error does not reflect uncertainty about the specific population being described, since the statistic precisely summarizes the experience of the whole population. However, results from apparently similar populations do vary from each other, and this variability is reflected in the standard error. For example, even in an apparently stable population, the number of deaths varies from day to day. There is a corresponding variability in the number of events that occur each year as well. The amount of variability in the number of certain types of events, such as ESRD incidence and death, is closely approximated by the Poisson distribution. The standard error of the statistic reflects the amount of variability that typically occurs in the value of the statistic upon repeated observations of similar populations.

The value of the standard error of a statistic measures the typical amount of variability due to random causes that occurs in the value of the statistic.

Accounting for Random Variation

Among ESRD patients over age 65, the proportion of patients surviving for 4.75 years decreased from 20.6 percent to 16.3 percent between 1982 and 1983 (USRD, 1989, p. D.21). Does this signify a trend for this age group? Even in otherwise similar populations, incidence counts and death counts vary from year to year apparently because of random variation. A calculation using the standard errors (USRDS, 1989 p. D.22) indicates that, even in two stable populations with identical death rates, a difference in survival proportions bigger than 4.3 percent would be likely to occur frequently just by chance. The expression $P > .20$ indicates that a difference as large as that observed could occur between successive years more than 20 percent of the time, just by chance, for two groups of patients with identical death rates. When a difference could plausibly occur by random chance, the difference is called insignificant. A difference that would not likely occur by chance is called a significant difference. The probability that a difference as big as or bigger than the one observed could occur by chance is called the P-value of the difference. (P-values less than 5 percent are labeled as significant whereas those greater than 5 percent are labeled as insignificant.) Using this criterion, the difference reported above is insignificant.

The reported difference could represent a trend, or it could represent random variability. In this case, the change was noted for a single age group between two consecutive years. On the basis of those limited data, there is no way to know whether it is a trend or a chance occurrence. However, if the trend persisted in subsequent years, or was also seen in other age groups, then the P-value could be recomputed taking into account all the evidence. If the resulting P-value was small, then it would be unlikely that the difference had occurred by chance, so it would be more plausible that the difference represented a true trend. If the evidence from other age groups and years was inconsistent with the trend noted previously, then the recomputed P-value would tend to remain large and the difference could plausibly be attributed to chance.

When a large change is noted that can be plausibly ascribed to chance, it is prudent to look for further evidence in order to determine whether the change represents a true trend. If a trend over time has been found to be significant, then the next step would be to try to determine what was causing the trend.

Random occurrences can lead to apparently substantial differences in outcomes, especially with a small, narrowly defined study group. Statistical and probabilistic evaluation of the chances of such differences can help to distinguish unimportant random fluctuations from more persistent patterns.

Important Versus Significant

Is it important that the difference between 5-year survival probabilities of 0.388 for females and 0.411 for males (averaged for 1977-83; see USRDS, 1989, p. D.21) is not likely to have occurred by chance (approximate $P < .10$)?

The difference (2.1 percent) is small relative to the survival probabilities (average 40 percent) and is therefore uninteresting. Even a small difference will be statistically significant if there are enough data documenting the consistency of the difference. In this case, the difference is statistically significant because the sample size is so large (all ESRD data for patients incident between 1977 and 1983).

Although the difference reported here is not significant at the 5 percent level ($P < .05$), it is significant at the 10 percent level ($P < .10$). Such a difference is often called marginally significant.

When a difference is significant, it is appropriate to interpret the difference as a real one rather than one that was likely to have occurred by chance. Once found to be significant, the importance of the difference must be evaluated.

The decision process about the importance of a significant difference is largely subjective. A 2 percent difference is small in comparison to other differences that have been found between patient subgroups, but it still represents a substantial number of individuals and consequently might be judged to be important. For example, a treatment change that lengthens life by 3 months for 4,000 patients yields a numerical benefit of 1,000 person-years of extra life. In contrast, special therapy that extends the life of a single person for 10 years is of special significance to the individual involved, but the numerical benefit is 10 person-years of life.

A statistically significant result is not always an important one if it is small. However, a small difference can be important if it affects a large number of individuals.

Analysis of Provider Versus Patient

Suppose that the annual death rate is 15 percent at institution A and 25 percent at institution B, that the difference is significant ($P < .001$), and that the patient characteristics are similar at the two institutions. Institution A reuses dialyzers while institution B does not. Does this prove that all institutions should reuse dialyzers?

The statistical significance reported from the analysis was based on the sample size of patients at each institution. Thus, the difference in mortality rates for the two groups of patients is unlikely to have occurred by chance. That is, there is a true difference in mortality between the two institutions. The appropriate generalization is to patients at the two institutions. However, we cannot generalize reliably to other institutions because the sample size of institutions is only two. When the P-value is calculated on the basis of an analysis of the institutional data, with a sample size of 2, the P-value is 0.50, which is not significant. Differences between institutions A and B other than in dialysis reuse may be responsible for the reported difference in death rates (Donner and Donald, 1987.

The statistical significance of an analysis based on patients should not be used to make conclusions about the population of providers.

Choice of Parameter for Mortality Summaries

If one study reports a 50 percent increase in death rates for one group relative to another group, whereas another study reports that the fractions surviving at 12 months differ by only 8.9 percent, which is right?

The results might be entirely consistent with each other. Monthly death rates of 2 percent and 3 percent will lead to surviving fractions of 78.7 percent and 69.8 percent, respectively, at 12 months. A death rate of 3 percent is accurately described as being 50 percent higher than a death rate of 2 percent. The difference in surviving fractions is accurately summarized as 8.9 percent. Note that the fractions dead in this example would be 21.3 and 30.2 percent, respectively, corresponding to a nearly 50 percent increase in the fraction dead. Part of the apparent discrepancy between the original reports from the studies was due to the fact that one comparison was made using a ratio whereas the other comparison was made using subtraction. Another, less important, cause of the apparent discrepancy can be illustrated by the analogies of death rates to compound interest rates and of death proportions to simple interest rates.

The proportion of individuals, P, surviving through an interval of time is related to the death rate, R, per unit interval by the equation

$$P = \exp(-R).$$

For example, if the death rate per year is 20 percent, then the fraction that survives through the year is 81.9 percent [= $\exp(-0.2)$]. The fraction that dies during the year is 18.1 percent, slightly less than 20 percent.

The death rate, fraction dead, and fraction surviving are all different ways to summarize mortality experience. Each is useful for particular purposes. Proper interpretation of results requires an understanding of the meaning of each.

Type I and Type II Error Issues

A clinical trial based on 120 patients found no significant difference between two treatment therapies (P > 0.05). Does this prove that the therapies are equally effective?

The only conclusion that should be reached from the insignificant P-value is that the difference between treatment groups seen in the clinical study could have arisen by chance. There may be a substantial difference between the therapies, but there were not enough data in the trial to document the difference.

The results of a comparative study should include, in addition to P-values, confidence intervals for the values of important outcome parameters. The confidence interval helps in the evaluation of the potential importance of the difference between two groups whereas the P-value tells whether the difference could have arisen by chance.

A nonsignificant difference should not be interpreted as a definitive result by itself. Confidence intervals for the size of the difference are more useful for interpretation. If the confidence interval includes large differences, then the true difference might also be large. If the confidence interval includes only small differences, then the true difference is likely to be small.

Projections and Extrapolations

The one-year surviving fraction among cadaveric transplant recipients has been increasing every year since 1977 (USRDS, 1989, p. E.19). Can this trend be extrapolated to give an estimate for 1990?

Extrapolations and projections of trends are very susceptible to bias because circumstances can change over time. Projections work well if the nature of the process that is being predicted does not change over time. The usual standard errors reported in a statistical analysis reflect only the uncertainty due to random fluctuations and measurement error, not the uncertainty due to bias or to change in the nature of the problem. Thus, the trend can be extrapolated but there is no way to evaluate the accuracy of the projection.

Extrapolations and projections of trends are very susceptible to error.

Accuracy of Counts

The counts of incident ESRD patients reported by the USRDS for 1987 (USRDS, 1989, pp. A.1, A.11) do not agree. How can any data analysis from the Medicare data system be trusted?

Data reporting and analysis are based on a sequence of operations and decisions that differs from system to system, from analyst to analyst, and from purpose to purpose. The discrepancy of 611 patients out of close to 33,000 represents less than a 2 percent difference. In many cases, it may not be worth the trouble to find the reason for such a small difference. In this case, the discrepancy is due to the fact that U.S. territories are not included in one of the counts (p. A.11).

Small discrepancies in counts of subjects are to be expected as definitions and methods of data reporting change over time. Interpretations based on percentages are often more useful than those based on counts.

ADJUSTING MORTALITY ANALYSES FOR PATIENT CHARACTERISTICS

A variety of methods have been used to summarize mortality results for the U.S. ESRD population. The summaries produced by HCFA (Eggers, various years) and USRDS (Held et al., 1990) have shown the broad patterns of ESRD mortality in the United States and point out many of the major factors that need to be considered in the design of more focused analyses of specific hypotheses.

The most important aspect of survival analysis is to have the relevant data available for analysis. Several patient characteristics collected by the Medicare system are known to be related to patient survival. Using appropriate methods to compare mortality rates should account for these factors. Other potentially important patient characteristics not currently collected should be investigated in order to determine their importance.

Patient Characteristics Related to Mortality

Several patient characteristics that are, or might be, related to mortality rates among ESRD patients are discussed below. For many of these characteristics, there are difficulties in the appropriate interpretation of their effects on mortality, and these issues are briefly discussed.

Currently Available Data

The Medicare data collection system for ESRD patients includes a wealth of information that is useful for evaluating survival of the ESRD patient population. Several of the most important items of data that are currently collected are discussed below.

Diagnosis This measure is an extremely important predictor of patient mortality. Death rates among diabetic patients are elevated by close to a factor of 2 compared to other diagnoses. Unfortunately, the data for diagnosis have not always been collected reliably. Through the early part of the 1980s, this measure was missing for a substantial number of patients. Since diagnosis is an important determinant of mortality, it is difficult to evaluate trends in mortality before 1982 using national data. There is still a fundamental problem with the interpretation of this measure because it relies heavily upon a subjective evaluation, by the physician, of the patient's medical history. It is often difficult to determine the underlying cause of ESRD for patients who are first diagnosed after their kidney function is already minimal.

Age at First Treatment   Mortality rates generally increase with patient age, except possibly at very young ages. To date, most analyses of mortality rates have accounted for age by assuming that it has the same effect on mortality for all patients. However, there are indications that mortality increases at differential rates with age for different types of patient, especially for patients with different diagnoses. That is, mortality rates increase more quickly with age among diabetic patients than they do among patients with other diagnoses. In addition, most analyses of mortality have accounted for the effect of age at first treatment, but not for the progressive effect as a patient gets older. The impact on mortality rates of 5 years of aging is substantially higher for a patient whose ESRD therapy begins at age 65 than it is for a patient whose therapy starts at age 20. The proportional hazards survival models account for some of these differential effects, but such effects should be carefully accounted for in any analyses used for the formulation of policy.

Year of First Treatment   The year of first ESRD treatment is not of major interest in its own right, but is important because it is a surrogate measure for other important factors that have changed over time. Unfortunately, treatment patterns as well as patient characteristics have changed over the years, and both could affect patient outcomes. Some of the changes, such as the availability of transplantation therapy and the aging of the treated ESRD patient population, are documented in the data and can be adjusted for through statistical analysis. Other changes in patient and treatment characteristics are less well documented in the Medicare data system, so it is difficult to isolate their effects on patient mortality.

• Treatment Methods: The use of cyclosporine for transplant patients has become pervasive, and the technology for CAPD therapy has also changed. New methods of CH, such as high-flux dialysis with shorter dialysis times and reuse of dialyzers, have not been unanimously adopted but may have affected patient survival at specific institutions. The detailed data necessary to evaluate such treatment choices are not readily available in the Medicare data base. Similarly, the effect of EPO on patient outcomes will be difficult to evaluate because the specific measures, such as hematocrit, that are likely to be most affected by EPO have only recently been added to the Medicare data collection forms.

Data collection instruments related to new treatments have historically been introduced in the Medicare system after the new treatment method is in widespread use. This prevents comparison of the new and old treatment methods during the crucial period of transition. If the times of treatment change were known precisely for each patient, or even for each provider, then comparisons could be made of mortality rates before and after the change, and these could be used to evaluate the change during the time of transition while the new treatment is still in its formulative stages. With the current data collection patterns, the comparison of patient outcomes for the new and old treatments is complicated by the fact that data typically are collected only after a consensus has largely been reached concerning appropriate methods of therapy.

• Patient Characteristics: The number of older patients and of diabetic patients accepted in the Medicare ESRD program has increased dramatically in recent years (USRDS, 1990). Both of these characteristics are associated with higher mortality rates. Careful statistical analysis methods can be used to account for such changes in patient characteristics if the characteristics are recorded in the data base. However, there are likely to be other patient characteristics that have changed over the years that are also associated with mortality but which have not been recorded in the Medicare data base. If such characteristics are not recorded in the data base and accounted for in statistical analyses, then their effects would appear as an unexplained general trend in mortality rates over the years. A current special study by the USRDS may help to identify some of the other important patient characteristics that are related to mortality.

Number of Years of Treatment Many of the survival analyses performed to date for ESRD patients have used years since first ESRD treatment as the fundamental measure of time (USRDS, 1990), although some have used the calendar year instead (HCFA, Eggers, 1984, 1987). Typically, analyses based on the years since initiation of ESRD therapy have summarized the experience of a cohort of patients whose ESRD therapy started during a particular year. Analyses based on calendar time have typically summarized the experience of all patients who received any treatment during a particular year. Each method of analysis has specific applications.

Death rates among ESRD patients vary substantially depending upon the time since first treatment. There is a general short-term decrease in death rates as the number of years of therapy increases, although aging has a counterbalancing long-term effect. Such patterns of decreasing mortality rates are to be expected when the population at risk is heterogeneous (Vaupel et al., 1985). It is important to account for such short-term trends in the evaluation of mortality patterns. The prognosis for individual patients is most easily characterized in terms of time since first ESRD therapy.

Norms of treatment patterns are likely to change nationally at a particular calendar time in response to innovations in technology or to changes in policy. A series of analyses, based on all patients receiving treatment during successive years, would be most sensitive for detecting such an effect (National Medical Care, personal communication, 1990). Such a change in treatment patterns would not be detected easily by a series of analyses based on the year of first ESRD therapy, because the treatment change would have different effects at different times relative to first ESRD therapy for the different cohorts of patients.

Multiple Measures of Time Statistical methods cannot isolate the unique effects of each of several factors when they are related to each other by a linear equation. For example, the simultaneous effects on mortality of patient year of birth, current patient age, and current year of therapy cannot be simultaneously evaluated because the following equation holds for all patients:

$$\text{Current Year of Therapy} = \text{Year of Birth} + \text{Current Age}$$

Such limitations of statistical methodology require that choices be made about which factors are to be included in a statistical analysis. Three time measures—current patient age, the number of years since first ESRD therapy, and the current calendar year of therapy—can be evaluated simultaneously because in a given year, there are ESRD patients of various ages who are in their third year of ESRD therapy. That is, age cannot be determined from the current year and the number of years of therapy. In survival analyses, age and current year of therapy are relevant because death rates vary dramatically with both of these measures. Current year of therapy is relevant because it is likely to reflect national norms of treatment practice.

Race For dialyzed patients, mortality rates are generally lower among black ESRD patients than among white ESRD patients for a given age and diagnosis. The reasons for this difference are not well understood. Recent analyses have shown that the difference is not uniform across diagnoses but is prominent only among hypertensive and diabetic patients. Further analyses may yield detail that leads to an understanding of the pathophysiological mechanism for the difference in mortality between races.

Sex Gender does not appear to have a substantial effect on mortality, although treatment patterns are gender related. However, when comparisons are made among treatment groups, adjustment for gender should be made in order to avoid any potential bias in the comparison.

Unavailable or Difficult-to-Evaluate Data

There are several data items that may be related to patient mortality that are not currently collected by the Medicare data system. Other items are collected, but not in an ideal format for analysis. Several of the most important of these are discussed in this section.

Treatment Modality   A national registry for ESRD data offers the potential for a comparison of patient outcomes by treatment modality. Such comparisons would be of substantial utility in determining patterns of optimal care for ESRD patients. A national registry could also offer timely evaluation of outcomes by treatment modality in order to allow monitoring of the quality of care being provided to the ESRD patient population. Both goals require accurate information concerning the pattern of treatment given to each patient.

Currently, the Medicare data system collects information concerning treatment modality through a variety of methods. For transplantation information, a series of dedicated data collection forms are filled out for each transplant patient. Billing information from the providers is the primary data collection instrument for dialysis treatment. Since dialysis is the most common form of therapy, billing data are a key component of the Medicare data base. Unfortunately, the bills are not designed to track patient treatments over time; consequently, it is often difficult to determine treatment histories for each patient. The timing of treatment modality changes can only be approximated from quarterly dialysis reports. It is likely that the current handling of the billing data misses some of the treatment modality changes for some patients.

Such inaccuracies in the treatment history data make it difficult to discern differences in patient outcomes for different therapies. Many of the statistical techniques discussed in this report are designed to yield comparisons of outcomes for groups of patients receiving different treatments. The statistical techniques can account for differences in patient characteristics that might otherwise bias the comparison, but they do not account for errors in the classification of patients into treatment groups.

The weakest link in the current Medicare data system may well be the relatively imprecise data available concerning the timing of dialytic treatment changes for each patient.

Medical History   The medical histories of ESRD patients may have a substantial effect on their subsequent mortality rates. The important aspects of medical histories are only partially measured by the etiology of ESRD; they also include medical events and health practices for which there are little data in the Medicare data base.

Differences in past medical histories should be accounted for when comparing the mortality experience of two or more groups of ESRD patients. The choice of treatment modality for ESRD patients is based on an evaluation, by the physician and patient, of the convenience and efficacy of the therapy. Thus, the choice of therapy may well depend upon the past medical history of the patient. This leads to the assignment of different types of patients to different types of treatments, making the comparison of outcomes for the treatments more difficult to interpret. Data concerning the differences in medical history between groups of patients receiving different therapies could be used in a statistical comparison of outcomes to account for those differences in medical history.

It is useful to attempt to distinguish between the past medical history of a patient and the medical outcomes that are caused by ESRD, although the distinction can be difficult to make in some cases. It is important to distinguish between characteristics that were present when a treatment was begun and those that were caused by the treatment. Differences present when therapy was started should generally be adjusted for when comparing outcomes, whereas those differences that are caused by the treatment are to be evaluated. For example, the frequency of hospitalization prior to the start of a therapy is a measure of the morbidity experienced by the patient and should be adjusted for, if possible, when comparing therapies because it is likely related to subsequent mortality rates. In contrast, the frequency of hospitalization after the start of therapy may well be a result of the inadequacy of the therapy and should itself be analyzed as a patient outcome, but not as a predictor of patient outcomes.

For example, hypertension can be an essential cause of ESRD, but most ESRD patients also exhibit hypertension that has resulted from ESRD. The presence of hypertension after therapy has started should not generally be adjusted for when comparing outcomes of several treatments. However, the presence of essential hypertension should be adjusted for in a comparison of patient mortality because it is likely to be associated with cardiac disease that would occur regardless of which treatment a patient receives for ESRD.

Generally, since many useful summaries of ESRD mortality are based on survival after first treatment for ESRD, data should be recorded at or before the time of first treatment for ESRD.

Social Support Systems (Family Arrangements) There are several aspects of social and family support that are known to be associated with survival in the general population. Both marital status and whether or not a person lives alone have been found to have important relationships with mortality. Since ESRD is a disease that can have substantial burdens on both the time and the financial resources of the patient, it is likely that aspects of family and social support are even more important determinants of mortality for the ESRD patient than for the general population. If two treatment groups differed with respect to social and family support arrangements, then a comparison of mortality for the two groups would be biased unless the analysis could be adjusted for that difference. Such differences are likely to occur when comparing different treatment modalities. Treatment modalities appear to have differential use according to gender, race, and income, all of which are likely to be associated with different patterns of family and social support.

The current Medicare data base does not include data on social and family arrangements. In order to ensure equal access to care, it is unlikely that such factors will be considered in policymaking. However, for the reasons cited above, such measures might be extremely valuable to consider in the evaluation of medical treatment methods. Although such data are not currently available at the national level, they are routinely collected by some providers through the efforts of a social worker. If the data are available at the provider level, including them in the national data base or in a sample from it may not be difficult or expensive.

Multivariable Methods

The examples in the previous sections of this paper have shown that it is important to adjust for differences in patient characteristics when comparing patient survival for several treatment groups of ESRD patients. Without adjustment, the presence or absence of differences in survival might be due to the differing characteristics of the patients rather than to the treatments. Typically, adjustments may have to be made simultaneously for several patient characteristics. Multivariable statistical methods are often used to make such adjustments, and the patient characteristics that are adjusted for in such comparisons are called confounding factors.

Generally, a measure, Z, is potentially a confounding factor in a study of association between two other factors, X and Y, if Z is associated with both X and Y. Often, a study attempts to quantify the amount by which an outcome, Y, is changed if a factor, X, is varied and all other conditions are left unchanged. For example, a study may attempt to quantify the amount of change in survival probabilities (Y) when the treatment method (X) is varied, all else (Z) equal. Except with a randomized trial, it is difficult to design an experiment that involves differences in the study factor, X, without differences in other factors, Z, also being present. If the factors, Z, can cause a change in the outcome of interest, Y, then the differences in Y observed at the end of the experiment could be due simultaneously to differences in both X and Z. One objective of statistical analysis is to attempt to isolate the separate effects of X and Z on the value of Y.

The problem of adjusting for confounding factors is a recurrent issue in statistical comparison of mortality patterns for two or more groups. In comparing mortality rates for two or more treatments, the observed results from the patients receiving the two types of treatment are compared. However, if the characteristics of the comparison groups of patients other than treatment differ (confounding factors), then the results should be adjusted to isolate that component of the difference that is attributable to the treatment alone. In practice, only adjustments for confounding factors that are recorded for each patient in the data base can be made.

Stratification and modeling are two major approaches used to adjust statistical analyses for confounding factors. The stratification approach is based on the principal of "divide and conquer." With stratification methods, patients are classified into subgroups (strata) that are homogeneous with respect to the confounding factors. In a single stratum, any observed treatment difference in patient outcome is attributable to the treatment, since the patients are otherwise similar to each other in each homogeneous stratum. The differences in patient outcome are often not reported for each stratum of patient but are usually summarized with an overall average value.

Modeling is based on the principal of "synthesize and approximate." A statistical model approximates the relationship between patient outcomes and patient characteristics using an equation. Since outcomes vary from patient to patient, individual patient outcomes cannot be predicted precisely with an equation. A statistical model describes the average patient outcome on the basis of patient characteristics. Modeling methods use an equation (model) to summarize the evidence of treatment differences in patient outcomes across various types of patients.

Stratification methods are less prone to bias than are modeling methods, but stratification requires larger amounts of data in order to obtain precise estimates of adjusted rates because many subgroups of patients may be needed in order to form the homogeneous strata. Modeling methods may be biased if the wrong model is used in the analysis, but they usually yield more precise estimates if the correct model is used.

Stratification

Stratification involves tabulating and combining comparative summaries of rates across specific homogeneous subgroups of patients. For any particular patient subgroup, the specific value of the summary for that group can be looked up in the tabulation. Adjusted summaries can then be derived by using a weighted average of estimates in specific cells of the table. Stratification methods work best when there is a substantial amount of data in each cell of the cross-classification of the data.

The tables in the *1989 USRDS Annual Data Report* (USRDS, 1989, p. A.4) give an example of a stratified analysis of incidence rates with direct standardization. A comparison of crude (unadjusted) incidence rates by race does not account for the fact that the black populations and white populations in the United States have different age structures. The table allows a comparison of the incidence rates for both populations in equal age intervals. The specific rates for groups of patients defined by race, age, and gender are reported in one part of the table. The incidence rates can be compared by race for each age-gender subgroup. Since there are many age-gender subgroups, it is useful to derive a single comparison that summarizes the results from the individual comparisons. A weighted average of the specific rates for different age-gender groups is computed for each race by gender group. The resulting adjusted rates allow comparisons across racial groups that are adjusted for age and gender. The age-gender adjusted rates for the two races can be interpreted as though the age-gender distributions for the two races were the same. Even though the age distributions for the two races are not the same in the original data, the age-gender adjusted rates estimate the size of the difference in rates that would have been observed had the age (and gender) distributions been the same.

In the example above, the relationship between race and incidence rates was examined with adjustment for the confounding factors of age and sex. Similar methods could be used to yield adjusted estimates of relationships between any two study factors with adjustment for confounding factors. The same type of cross-classification could theoretically be used for mortality rates, as well. For example, the table presented in the *1989 USRDS Annual Data Report* (USRDS, 1989, p. D.9) is based on direct standardization of one-year death proportions with adjustment for age, race, gender, and primary diagnosis.

Stratified analyses based on indirect standardization use a different computational method to adjust for confounding factors, although the objective of adjustment is the same as it is for direct standardization. The results with indirect adjustment are often similar to those with direct standardization. Indirect standardization can yield more precise summary comparisons when there are not enough data to yield precise results with direct standardization (Breslow and Day, 1987).

Modeling

In survival analysis, a model is an equation that relates the numerical values of a set of patient characteristics to the numerical value of a summary mortality measure for the corresponding group of patients. A hypothetical model for death rates, $h(t)$, based on age (X_1) and race (X_2) could be written as

$$h(t) = 0.05 + 0.004 \; X_1 + 0.14 \; X_2 \qquad (1)$$

Such a simple equation often gives a poor fit to the data for death rates. Models for death rates often use the exponential function (inverse of the natural logarithm) in an equation of the form:

$$h(t) = \exp(-1.95 + 0.008 \ X_1 + 0.15 \ X_2) \tag{2}$$

An important stage of analysis, called identification of the equation, consists of determining which type of equation to use (equations 1 and 2 are two different types) and which measures to include on the right-hand side of the equation (Box and Jenkins, 1976).

The numerical values appearing in the equations above are called coefficients. The values of the coefficients are determined in each analysis so that the equation fits the data as well as possible. The calculated values of the coefficients in the model are called estimates of the coefficients, in recognition of the fact that they only approximate the values that would result if more data were available.

Model building in statistical analysis often involves iterative stages of model identification and estimation. A variety of criteria have been used in order to assess how well an equation fits the observed data. The results of modeling usually include the form of the equation, the values of the coefficients in the equation, and the precision of the estimated coefficients.

The effect on mortality due to changing only one patient characteristic (such as treatment modality) can be estimated by changing the value of only that characteristic on the right-hand side of the equation. The resulting change in the computed value of the summary mortality measure estimates the effect of changing that one factor while all others are held constant.

The detailed interpretation of a model requires an understanding of the form of the equation and knowledge of the units of each measure in the equation. This allows the numerical value of the survival measure to be interpreted for any combination of the characteristics on the right-hand side of the equation. A rough interpretation of a model often involves only the directions of the effects of each factor on mortality and some evaluation of the importance of those effects.

In the hypothetical examples above, the numerical value of the death rate is computed from an equation based on the numerical value of patient age and numerical codings of the race of a patient. The equations can be used to estimate the mortality rate for any type of patient that can be characterized by the variables in the model equation. In equation 2, assume that the units for death rates are per year, that age is given in years, and that race is coded as 0 or 1 if the patient is black or white, respectively. Then the estimated annual death rates for black patients and white patients of age 60 are 0.230 [= exp $(-1.95 + 0.008 \cdot 60 + 0)$] and 0.267 [= $\exp(-1.95 + 0.008 \cdot 60 + 0.15 \cdot 1)$], respectively. According to the hypothetical model, death rates are about 16 percent higher for white patients than for black patients of identical ages.

Simultaneous Effects of Variables

In order to estimate the unique effect of each of several factors on mortality rates when the others are held constant, a multivariable analysis using data for all of the factors must be performed. Results must be simultaneously adjusted for all relevant factors. For example, it is not sufficient to present a set of results that are adjusted for age and another set of results that are adjusted for diagnosis; results must be adjusted for both age and diagnosis simultaneously. As the number of relevant factors increases, the detail needed to summarize the results can increase dramatically.

Research based on data from small sources cannot usually provide the detail that is available from a national registry. Important factors and interactions often appear to be random noise when the sample size is small, and so the results are not reported. Thus, the clinical literature cannot be expected to provide a reliable reference for the level of detail that can be available from a national registry.

Determination of the appropriate level of detail in a statistical summarization requires a balancing of the value of interpretability (the results should not be obscured by the presentation), consistency (broad summaries are more useful than are summaries for each of many subgroups), precision (small standard errors are desirable), and accuracy (the results should not be biased).

Constraints on the Adjustment Process

The major limitation on the adjustment for confounding factors is that the confounding factors must be measured for the patients in the data base. The mortality rates in the USRDS data base cannot be adjusted for patient comorbidity because no such data have been collected. A retrospective collection of such data from patient medical records will allow a study to be performed for some patients, but the validity of the results depends upon the reliability and completeness of the medical records.

A second limitation is specific to the nature of survival analysis. Survival analysis is based on modeling the occurrence of future events (death) on the basis of current patient characteristics. Thus, comparison groups should not be defined in terms of events that occur in the future, but should be defined on the basis of past events. Definitions of patient characteristics cannot be based on the future events for the patients. At any time, the death rates for a group can be modeled in terms of the complete history of the group up to that time, but should not be allowed to depend upon future events.

An example makes the limitations imposed by this second constraint clearer. In order to study the effect of switching treatment modalities on mortality rates, data are needed on the sequence of treatments for a patient. Then, mortality rates at a particular time for patients who have not yet switched are compared to mortality rates for patients who have already switched. Note that the comparison groups are defined in terms of what has already taken place. It is inappropriate to compare mortality rates among patients who do not switch treatment modalities in the future to rates among patients who do switch sometime in the future. The difficulty with the second comparison is that patients who die quickly have less chance to switch treatments than do patients who survive a long time, so the death rate of the nonswitching group would appear to be higher than that of the switching group.

Many attempts have been made to try to make valid comparisons of mortality for groups that are defined in terms of future events. None has been entirely successful.

Case-control studies at first appear to be an exception to the discussion above but are in fact consistent with it. In a case-control study, the comparison groups are defined in terms of the patient outcome itself. That is, survivors are compared to dead patients to see how they differ. This type of study requires great care in its design in order to avoid biased results. Specifically, the controls (survivors) must be selected so that they have been followed for the same length of time as the cases (dead patients). The characteristics of the controls must be evaluated on the basis of their history up to the time corresponding to the death of the case. With this design, the dead patients and the surviving patients are being compared at the same time of follow-up, so their characteristics are effectively being defined on the basis of past (at the time of the dead patient's death) history.

STATISTICAL METHODS OF ANALYSIS FOR
ESRD MORTALITY DATA

Statistical survival analyses are designed to summarize the distribution of lifetimes for a population of patients. The summaries characterize the overall pattern of mortality in the population rather than give details of the individual lifetimes which vary from person to person in the population.

One of the distinctive aspects of survival analysis is that although the lifetimes of individuals in a population are to be summarized, not all of the people in the population have died when the summarization is made. Special methods, derived from actuarial concepts, are used in survival analysis to yield an estimate that summarizes lifetimes even though not all of the lifetimes have been observed. The lifetimes that are not completely observed are called censored data, because they are hidden from the analysis by the nature of the observation process.

There are several ways to summarize patterns of mortality in a population, including death proportions, death rates, survival curves, and average lifetimes. These summaries are discussed in more detail below. Each summary is called a parameter. Survival analysis methods use data from a sample of a population in order to yield estimates of the value of the parameter for the whole population. The word parameter is often reserved for a single numerical value, but its meaning has been extended in this appendix to allow it to encompass a function of time or a curve that is plotted versus time (e.g., survival curve).

Some parameters characterize the way in which mortality patterns differ among subgroups of a population. For example, regression coefficients in a statistical model can summarize the relationship between death rates and patient characteristics.

In addition to parameters that characterize the pattern of mortality in a single population, other parameters measure the difference in mortality for two populations. These include differences, ratios, and log ratios.

Each parameter listed above is a useful summary of mortality and can be used to compare mortality for two or more groups of patients. To appropriately interpret the results of analysis, the meaning of the parameters that are being reported must be understood. Mathematical calculations can sometimes be used to relate the values of different parameters to each other in order to compare results from different studies that have used different sets of parameters.

Descriptive Parameters for One Group

A parameter that summarizes mortality for a single group is measured on an absolute scale, and its numerical value can be interpreted without reference to other values. For example, the fraction of a population that has died after one year (i.e., death proportion) is directly interpretable for that population. Other examples of parameters are death rates, surviving fractions, and expected lifetimes.

Death Proportions

The fraction, or proportion, of a group of individuals who die during a specific interval of time is a widely used summary of mortality.

Since most ESRD survival analyses include censored data (some subjects were withdrawn alive from follow-up before the end of the interval under study), this fraction should be estimated using the Kaplan-Meier method or other actuarial type of estimator. This fraction should not be estimated as a simple proportion if the data include censored observations.

Death proportions should not be compared unless they correspond to equivalent time intervals. Thus, 1-year death fractions can be usefully compared to each other, but 1-year death fractions cannot be compared directly to 2-year death fractions.

In order to be interpretable, death proportions should correspond to a well-defined interval of time. Thus, the beginning and the end of the interval must be well defined. For example, the interval of time could be the first year of ESRD. A death proportion should not be interpreted on the basis of the length of the interval alone because the death proportion during the first year of ESRD is generally higher than it is during subsequent 1-year intervals. Thus, when comparing the death proportion during the first year of renal replacement therapy (RRT) in the United States to that in the first year of RRT in another country, it should be noted that the data for the United States are likely to start only 90 days after first RRT for each patient whereas data from other countries may start on the first day of RRT for each patient. Because of high mortality during the first 90 days of RRT, the mortality during the first 365 days is likely to differ from the mortality between days 90 and 465. Thus, data from the United States may not be directly comparable to data from other countries.

Although the length of the interval used to calculate a death proportion should be specified, there can be exceptions to the rule. One exception is the fraction of transplant recipients who are discharged alive from the hospital after the transplant operation. In this case, the interval of time is appropriately defined by two events (admission and discharge) rather than by the length of the interval. Such proportions cannot be directly compared to proportions that correspond to other time intervals.

Death proportions are defined relative to the population alive at the beginning of the time interval being considered. Thus, a 10 percent death proportion during the second year of RRT means that among those who survive for one year, 10 percent die during the second year, not that 10 percent of those who started RRT will die during their second year. For example, if the death proportion is 10 percent for both the first and the second year of ESRD, then it is not true that 20 percent will die by the end of 2 years; instead, only 19 percent will die during the first 2 years since 90 percent survive the first year and 10 percent of that 90 percent (or 9 percent more) die during the second year.

In order to compare death proportions based on different types of time intervals, it is sometimes possible to compute death rates that correspond to each of the proportions and then to compare the death rates to each other.

Death Rates

The death rate is approximately equal to the fraction dying during an interval of time divided by the length of the interval. The approximation becomes more precise when the length of the interval is made shorter. The numerical value of the death rate usually depends upon the time at which the interval starts. The death rate is thus a function of time and can be represented as a curve plotted against time. The time axis can be chosen from among age, years since first ESRD, or calendar date, depending upon the purposes of the analysis. For example, a plot of death rates versus time since first ESRD would show that the death rate at the beginning of RRT is higher than the death rate in subsequent years. The death rate can be defined as the limiting value of the following equation as the length of the interval declines.

$$h(t) = \Pr(\text{die between times } t \text{ and } t_2 \text{ given alive at } t)/(t_2 - t)$$

Death rates are measured per unit of time and are sometimes called hazard rates. The value of a death rate depends upon the unit of measure of times as shown by the following example: a monthly death rate of 0.01 is equal to an annual rate of 0.12.

The most commonly used estimator for the death rate during an interval of time is equal to the total number of deaths observed during the interval divided by the total length of follow-up during the interval. This is calculated as follows: A series of patients is identified who are alive at the beginning of the interval, and the number who die during the interval is counted. The lengths of time that each patient is observed to be alive during the interval are summed across patients to compute the total length of follow-up. The ratio of the death count to the follow-up time estimates the death rates during the interval. This estimator assumes that the death rate is constant during the length of the interval.

Death rates are *not* proportions, although they are closely related to proportions. They can be greater than 1.0 in value, for example, whereas proportions cannot be. There is a mathematical link between death proportions and death rates that involves a quantity called the cumulative hazard (Breslow and Day, 1987).

The cumulative hazard during a short interval of time is approximately equal to the length of the interval times the hazard at the beginning of the interval. Continuing with the numerical values in the example, the cumulative hazard for death during a 6-month interval would be approximately 0.06, which can be computed as $0.01 \cdot 6$ if the calculations are based on months or as $0.12 \cdot 0.5$ if the calculations are based on years. The cumulative hazard is used to relate death rates to death proportions, as discussed below.

For short intervals of time, the death proportion for the interval is numerically close to the cumulative hazard during the interval. That is, among those alive at the beginning of a short interval of time, the fraction who die during the interval is approximately equal to the cumulative death rate during the interval.

Death proportions and death rates are related mathematically. If the death rate is 0.01 per month, then the death proportion during each month is approximately 1 percent. If a death rate is small during an interval of time, then it is nearly equal to the death proportion per unit of time. The precise relationship involves the exponential function. For example, if the death rate is 0.1 per year, then the proportion surviving for one year is 0.9048. This is calculated as the inverse natural logarithm of the negative of the death rate [inverse $\ln(-0.1) = \exp(-0.1)$]. The death proportion is then calculated as 1 minus the surviving proportion, or 0.0952 in this example. Note that the fraction dead after one year—0.0952—is slightly different from 0.10, the death rate per year.

Survival Curves

Survival curves show the fraction of patients who are still alive at each time of follow-up and the full distribution of lifetimes in a population. They are an excellent graphical tool for summarizing patterns of mortality in a population. The horizontal axis in the survival curve measures time since the start of patient follow-up, whereas the vertical axis measures the fraction of patients who are alive at each time.

Survival curves can be reliably estimated with censored data. The Kaplan-Meier and actuarial methods are usually used to estimate unadjusted survival curves. The Kaplan-Meier estimator is more precise than the actuarial methods but is more difficult to compute. It is preferred for use on small samples of patients, whereas actuarial methods yield excellent approximations with larger data sets. An extension of the Kaplan-Meier estimator based on the Cox model (discussed below) can be used to estimate adjusted survival curves.

The estimated survival curves are composed of a series of horizontal lines, but are sometimes drawn as a smooth curve. Survival curve estimates should not be extrapolated beyond the extent of the data that are used to estimate them. Some statistical packages choose to artificially show the survival curve as dropping to 0 (indicating that everyone has died) after the longest follow-up time in the data set, even though a large fraction of the subjects are still alive at that time. The practice should be avoided.

Expected Lifetimes

The average lifetime is a very interpretable summary of mortality and can be used for making superficial comparisons of the mortality patterns for two or more groups of patients. However, several caveats should be kept in mind when interpreting reported average lifetimes. As discussed in the remainder of this section, the average lifetime gives only a superficial summary of the mortality patterns for a population and is difficult to estimate with censored data. Because of these limitations, and because summaries based on death rates and survival curves are more useful, use of expected lifetimes is not recommended for the routine summarization of survival analyses for ESRD patients.

The average lifetime does not capture the variability in lifetimes in a population. For example, an average lifetime of 5 years results if every person lives for exactly 5 years and also results if half the people die immediately and half live for 10 years. Thus, the average lifetime does not indicate the details of mortality patterns in a population.

There are two major methods for calculating average lifetimes: parametric and nonparametric. Both can be used with censored data. However, both methods can yield unreliable or uninterpretable answers if a large fraction of the population is estimated to be alive at the end of the study. Many statistical packages calculate a nonparametric truncated lifetime with censored data, the truncated point being the time of the longest censored lifetime in the data set. Truncated lifetimes are not comparable to each other unless the truncation times are equal to each other. Parametric models rely on extrapolation to estimate the average lifetime with heavily censored data, but estimates of the average lifetime can be very unreliable if they are based on heavily censored data.

Comparative Parameters

Summaries of individual groups are often compared to each other. Instead of reporting the individual mortality summaries for each of several groups, comparative statistics can be used to summarize just the sizes of the differences between the individual mortality summaries. Important examples include relative death rates (from a Cox or other proportional hazards regression model), differences in death proportions, and relative lifetimes. Comparative statistics cannot be directly interpreted for either of the two groups being compared. However, if a mortality measure is reported for one group and comparative summaries are reported for other groups, then the individual group summaries can usually be calculated for each group.

Two common comparative statistics are often reported: differences (subtraction) and ratios (division). It is crucial to the interpretation of the results to know which is being reported. For example, if the fractions dead in two groups are 10 percent and 20 percent, then the comparison for the second group relative to the first group could be reported as a 10 percent increase (difference), as a 100 percent increase (ratio), or as double the fraction (ratio). In addition, the comparison could be summarized by saying that the surviving fraction in the second group is only 89 percent (100 x 8/9) as high as in the first group.

Several other specific types of comparative summaries are discussed below.

Regression Models

Several different regression models are appropriate for use with survival data, including Cox, Poisson, Weibull, Bailey-Makeham. These are discussed and compared in more detail below. All of these regression models allow multiple patient characteristics to be empirically related to mortality. Since the Cox model is the most widely used method of analysis for survival data and since it has many of the features of other methods, the interpretation of results from the Cox model is discussed in detail here.

The Cox model yields an estimate of the ratio of death rates for two groups of patients and the standard error of the ratio. The ratio represents a single numerical summary of the difference in mortality patterns for two groups. The standard error allows an evaluation of uncertainty of the estimated ratio and can be used to compute the statistical significance of the difference between the groups and a confidence interval for the magnitude of the difference in death rates between the two groups.

In addition, Cox model analyses yield adjusted survival curve estimates for several groups. The adjusted survival curves are a more complete summarization of the comparative mortality patterns among the groups than are death rate ratios. Moreover, the adjusted survival curve estimates are useful for descriptive analyses.

Adjusted Death Rate Ratios The primary results of most Cox model analyses are estimates of death rate ratios. A ratio different from 1.0 indicates that the death rates are different for the two groups being compared. The two groups being compared can be defined in terms of either quantitative (e.g., age) or qualitative (e.g., etiology) characteristics. The model yields adjusted estimates of the ratio of death rates for two groups that differ with respect to one characteristic if all other characteristics included in the model are the same for the two groups. The Cox model regression coefficient is an estimate of the log of the death rate ratio. Thus a coefficient value of 0 corresponds to a rate ratio of 1. The rate ratio corresponding to two groups of patients who differ by 1 unit with respect to the value of a specific characteristic is computed as the exponential function of the coefficient estimate for that characteristic in the regression model.

For example, in order to estimate the ratio of death rates for diabetic and nondiabetic patients, a 0-1 indicator for diabetes would be included in the Cox model. The estimated ratio of death rates would be estimated as the exponential function of the estimated coefficient of the diabetes variable.

If only the diabetes variable were included in the model, then the estimated ratio would be unadjusted and would include the effects of any other differences between the two groups. Part of the difference between the diabetic and nondiabetic patients might be explainable by age differences between the two groups, for example, but this effect would be included in the estimated unadjusted ratio of death rates for the two groups.

By simultaneously including several patient characteristics in a Cox model, the effect on mortality of any one factor can be estimated with adjustment for the other factors in the model. For example, in order to estimate the ratio of death rates for diabetic and nondiabetic patients who are of the same age, both diabetes and age would be included in the Cox model. The resulting coefficient for the diabetes variable estimates the log of the adjusted death rate ratio. This ratio would be adjusted only for age. In order to adjust for other potential confounding factors, they must also be included simultaneously in a Cox model.

In order to adjust appropriately for other factors in a Cox model, they must be included in the model in the correct form. As a first step, many researchers often assume that the effect on mortality of each characteristic in the model is independent of the other characteristics in the model. Such a model is called a main-effects model. However, there is substantial evidence that the effect on mortality of some factors is modified by other factors. For example, white patients have substantially higher death rates than do black patients if their diagnosis is hypertension or diabetes, but not otherwise. Models that account for these more complicated relationships are called interaction models.

The principal value of multiple regression models is to yield estimates of the effect of one factor, with adjustment for other confounding factors. Models that do not adjust for relevant factors, or that adjust for them incorrectly, yield less definitive interpretations than do more complete models. Although no model can adjust for characteristics that are unknown or unmeasured, it is useful to eliminate the effects of known important factors as accurately as possible.

Survival Curves   A qualitative patient characteristic can be included in a Cox model in two different ways. If a characteristic is included as a covariate in the model, then its effect on mortality is summarized by a ratio of rates. If a characteristic is included as a stratifying variable, then its effect on mortality is summarized as a set of survival curves for the different groups that it represents. For quantitative comparisons, a patient characteristic is usually included as a covariate. For descriptive comparisons, a characteristic is usually included as a stratifying factor.

A third method of presentation of comparative results is sometimes used in a Cox model, but it can be deceptive. In that method, a patient characteristic is included as a covariate in a Cox model, and different adjusted survival curves corresponding to different values of the covariate are estimated. Such survival curves are based on the overall experience in the whole data set, which is adjusted up or down, depending upon the value of the covariate. However, it is usually much more informative to estimate the survival curve for each group, based on its own data, through the use of stratification, as described previously.

Specific Models and Methods

A variety of statistical methods have been used or proposed for the analysis of mortality rates among ESRD patients. Several of these methods, all of which are regression models, are discussed below, and include Poisson, Cox, logistic, exponential, Weibull, and Bailey-Makeham. All can yield interpretable summaries of the way in which mortality is simultaneously related to several patient characteristics. All have associated methods of statistical inference that allow confidence intervals and statistical hypothesis tests to be computed.

All statistical methods are based on certain assumptions that must be checked empirically in order to ensure that the methodology is appropriate for the data being analyzed. The methods discussed below differ with regard to the types of assumptions that they make. Methods based upon either Poisson regression or Cox regression models are applicable for a variety of important issues related to the survival of ESRD patients. Methods based on logistic regression models are limited in the types of data for which they are appropriate. Fully parametric methods may prove useful for specific objectives, but they are based on more assumptions than are the Poisson and Cox regression models and therefore require more careful checks of the appropriateness of the model.

The Poisson and Cox regression models are both extremely flexible in the types of models that can be estimated. Both yield estimates of relative death rates. The major difference between them is that Poisson regression models yield direct estimates of death rates whereas Cox models yield direct estimates of survival curves. Both methods can require substantial computing resources if the specification of the model involves patient characteristics that change over time.

The methods discussed below vary according to several dimensions, including the way in which time is accounted for in the analysis, appropriateness, interpretability, ease of implementation, and level of parametrization of the method.

Poisson Regression for Death Rates

A death rate approximates the probability of dying per unit time among those still alive. Death rates among dialysis patients are typically between 3 percent and 60 percent per year for young and old patients, respectively (USRDS, 1990, Table D.29), or approximately 0.25 to 5 percent per month.

It is clear that death rates vary among dialysis patients, depending upon the characteristics of the patients being described. Death rates also vary among ESRD transplant recipients, although they tend to be lower for transplant recipients than they are for dialysis patients. Statistical models as well as cross-tabulations can be used to summarize how the death rates vary according to the characteristics of the patients and their treatment modalities.

A statistical model for death rates uses an equation to summarize the way in which death rates vary according to the characteristics of the patients. Statistical models only approximate the broad patterns of variability in death rates and do not attempt to account for each individual patient death. As an example, Equation 3, below, was estimated using data for black patients (USRDS, 1990, Tables D.28 and D.31):

$$Rate = exp(-3.74 + 0.03518 \times Age)$$

The death rates calculated by this equation agree closely with the observed death rates shown in Table 1, although the agreement is far from perfect. The equation implies that the death rates among black ESRD patients increase by a factor of 1.0358 [=exp(0.03518)] for each 1 year increase in age. The advantage of the equation is that it allows the change in death rates with age to be easily summarized as a 3.6 percent increase per year of age, instead of requiring the full tabulation of observed rates in Table D-1. The lack of agreement between the rates calculated using the equation and the observed rates might be due to random variability in the observed rates or to the fact that the equation is not a perfect representation of the true relationship between age and death rates. However, the discrepancy between the rates calculated using the equation and the observed rates is relatively unimportant compared to the substantial change in death rates with age.

The discrepancies between the rates calculated from the equation and the observed rates may be useful for identifying the exceptions to the general rule given by the equation. For example, the observed rates tend to be higher than the calculated rates at very young ages, indicating that death rates among young patients may follow a slightly different pattern than is apparent among older patients. This process of fitting a model, summarizing the broad features of the model, and then looking for discrepancies between the observed data and the model is very useful in finding a balance between useful generalizations and levels of detail.

Death rates can also be tabulated simultaneously according to several patient characteristics. USRDS Table D.31 reports death rates by age, race, and disease group. The resulting Table D.31 includes a lot of detail that is useful for looking up specific death rates but not for making general conclusions. A statistical model (not presented here) could quantitatively summarize the main features of such a table with just a few broad generalizations.

TABLE D-1 Death Rates and Age Among All Black ESRD Patients in 1988

Age (lower limit)	Death Rate Observed[a]	Model
0	30.6	23.8
5	28.3	28.3
10	51.3	33.7
15	40.9	40.2
20	55.1	47.8
25	64.7	57.0
30	76.2	67.9
35	85.5	80.9
40	91.8	96.3
45	108.7	114.7
50	129.6	136.7
55	154.0	162.8
60	194.1	194.0
65	242.1	231.1
70	299.9	275.3
75	334.3	327.9
80	379.5	390.6
85	461.0	465.3

[a]USRDS, 1990, Table D.31.

Poisson regression models are appropriate for estimating statistical models for death rates using data from a registry such as the USRDS. In its simplest form, this methodology is descriptive; moveover, it can yield estimates of the death rate for any specific combination of patient characteristics. That is, death rates can be estimated for patient subgroups that are defined by a simultaneous specification of several patient characteristics. Poisson regression models can be implemented with GLIM or S-plus statistical packages that are available for many computers.

If the number of characteristics used to classify patients is large, then there may be few patients in any specific cross-classification. Consequently, the data used to estimate death rates for specific groups may be sparse and the resulting estimates are likely to be unreliable. For example, the death rate reported by USRDS (1990, Table D.31) for white diabetic patients age 0 to 4 years in 1988 is 1,500 per 1,000 patient years at risk. This rate is estimated on the basis of two deaths (USRDS, Table D.28) and is likely due to chance events rather than to an important phenomenon. With sparse data, multiple regression models can be used to effectively pool information across various subgroups in order to yield more precise estimates of the true death rate for any particular patient subgroup. In addition, statistical models can be used to summarize the adjusted effect of a single factor on mortality rates.

Death rates of ESRD patients vary with the number of years since first ESRD service, with a general decrease in death rates as the number of years since first service increases. It is speculated that this decrease is due to attrition of the less healthy ESRD patients as time goes on. The death rates discussed in this section ignored this factor and collapsed together patients with differing amounts of time since first service. The time since first service could be accounted for by including it as a patient characteristic that is entered into the Poisson regression model. Alternatively, the Cox model, discussed below, accounts for time since first service explicitly without the need to classify patient follow-up according to this measure of time.

A comprehensive Poisson regression model would include multiple patient characteristics in the estimated equation for death rates. Some of these patient characteristics, such as gender, race, year of first ESRD therapy, and primary diagnosis, do not change with time. Some important patient and treatment characteristics that can change with time include age, years since first ESRD therapy, treatment modality, and treatment facility. Poisson regression models can account for all these characteristics simultaneously, although the data management and analysis costs required to do so would be substantial.

Cox Models for Relative Rates and Survival Functions

The Poisson regression models discussed in the previous section are most appropriate for data based on short intervals of patient follow-up. If long intervals of time are used, then patient characteristics such as age and time since first ESRD service vary during the time interval, and it is less appropriate to ascribe a single death rate to the interval. The Cox models allow the periods of follow-up to be different for each patient and to be arbitrarily long or short. However, instead of yielding estimates of death rates, as with the Poisson regression models, the Cox models yield estimates of relative death rates and of the survival function, i.e., the fraction surviving at various times since entry into study.

The Cox model was designed primarily to estimate relative death rates. Thus, the ratio of death rates for any pair of patient subgroups is estimated directly by the Cox model, whereas survival functions rather than specific death rates are estimated for each patient subgroup.

The survival function gives the fraction of patients surviving at each of several times since entry into study. For ESRD patients incident in 1979, survival functions are reported in Table D-2 for several time points after first ESRD therapy. Mortality among ESRD patients is often described rela-

TABLE D-2 Survival Probabilities for ESRD
Patients Incident in 1979

Years Since 90 Days After First ESRD Service	Fraction Surviving
0	1.0000
1	0.8138
2	0.6786
5	0.4419
10	0.2576

SOURCE: USRDS, 1990.

tive to the number of years since first therapy for ESRD because patient data are entered into the USRDS data base near the time of first ESRD therapy. Since the first 90 days of ESRD therapy is undocumented for many patients in the USRDS, mortality is described subsequent to 90 days after the first service for ESRD in the *USRDS Annual Data Report*. Table D-2 summarizes the fraction of patients still alive for various intervals of time since 90 days after first ESRD service. The data for this table are abstracted from the *USRDS Annual Data Report* Tables E.10, E.12, E.14, and E.16.

The Cox model uses data from patients who have different periods of follow-up. The Cox model uses data from all patients to estimate 1-year survival probabilities. The Cox model then uses only the data from patients with 2 years of follow-up to estimate the probability of survival during the second year, given survival through the first year. The product of these two probabilities yields the overall probability of surviving for 2 years. Although this description of the Cox model is a simplification of the calculations that are actually performed, it captures the essential nature of the concept involved in the survival curve estimates derived from the Cox model. The model also uses data from different periods of patient follow-up to estimate relative death rates.

The ability to utilize data from patients with different periods of follow-up is one of the features that makes the Cox model so useful. Such data are often said to be right censored, and the Cox model is the most widely used method for multiple regression analysis with right censored data. It is adaptable to a wide variety of types of applications and data structures. Moreover, it can be used to evaluate the effect of changing treatment modalities and other time-dependent factors, such as patient age, calendar year, and time since first ESRD therapy. The results of analysis include estimates of relative death rates and survival curves.

The Cox model and the Poisson regression models have similar applications. Both yield estimates of relative death rates. Both yield summaries of overall mortality; the Poisson regression model yields estimates of death rates whereas the Cox model yields estimates of the survival function. The Poisson regression model requires that the data be grouped into relatively short periods of follow-up time, whereas the Cox model allows the follow-up interval for each patient to be arbitrarily long. The calculations for the Cox model tend to be more intensive than for the Poisson regression model, especially if time-dependent covariates are included in the model. The data management costs tend to be higher for the Poisson regression model than for the Cox model.

Estimation for Cox regression models can be implemented with SAS or BMDP computer programs. If time-varying covariates are included, BMDP is preferred, although SAS will soon implement facilities for analyzing time-dependent covariates.

Logistic Regression for the Probability of Death

Logistic regression models can be used to estimate the probability of death during a specified interval of time. Such models are appropriate for analysis of prevalent cohorts and for detecting trends in mortality due to changes in treatment patterns (E. Lowrie, National Medical Care, personal communication, 1990). However, the proposed implementation has serious deficiencies.

The logistic model yields estimates of the probability of death for each set of patient characteristics. Such models must be based on data from a series of patients who are all potentially followed for the same period of time. The follow-up requirement is difficult to ensure with data from a registry such as the USRDS, and it is especially hard to ensure if treatment modality is being studied.

Since mortality patterns change with the length of ESRD treatment, a comparison of mortality proportions for a specific time interval tells only part of the story. The patient characteristics that are most important during the first year of ESRD therapy may be different from the patient characteristics that are most important during the second year of ESRD therapy. A series of probability models, one for each interval of time, would then provide a more complete tool for comparing mortality patterns. This can be more easily accomplished with a single survival analysis model (Cox model), which provides estimates for the probabilities of death at each time interval of follow-up.

Equal intervals of follow-up cannot be ensured when members of the group of interest can leave the study, for example, because of treatment modality changes. As an example of this difficulty, consider the problem of estimating the 1-year survival probability among dialysis patients. In order to estimate this with a logistic regression model, the analysis must be limited to patients who are to be treated for at least 1 year with dialysis. Thus, it is clear that patients who receive transplants during the first year should be excluded from the analysis. The difficulty arises because among the dialysis patients who die in the first year, it is not known which among them would have received transplants had they survived. Thus, there is no way to limit the analysis to patients who would have received dialysis for a full year. Exclusion of the survivors who receive transplants without exclusion of the patients who died before receiving transplants will bias the estimated probability of death and cause it to be higher than it should be.

Models for the probability of death are especially difficult to interpret when the population of interest is defined in terms of the complete treatment history, rather than in terms of the treatment modality at the beginning of the time interval. For example, the 1-year survival probability for all ESRD patients who start on hemodialysis can be estimated as a simple fraction. This probability is based on all patients starting on hemodialysis, regardless of subsequent treatment changes. The 1-year survival probability among those dialysis patients who either remained on hemodialysis for a complete year or who died within one year with no change to another treatment modality is less interpretable. (See the section on Constraints on the Adjustment Process, above.)

The effect of year of current therapy on dialysis mortality rates can be estimated with either Poisson or Cox regression models. A unified analysis would account for the simultaneous effect on death rates of year of first therapy, year of current therapy, patient age, and other patient characteristics. Logistic regression models are not appropriate for this analysis because of the difficulties discussed above.

Conditional Logistic Regression and Sampling from the Risk Set

One of the difficulties with using either Cox or Poisson regression models to evaluate the effect of treatment modality on death rates is that treatment modality changes with time for many patients. The data management efforts required to document all of the treatment changes for all of the patients in the USRDS data base are substantial. For such analyses, the Cox model can be used with a reduced data set to yield results that are nearly as precise as those resulting from analysis of the full data set. The reduced data set is derived by sampling in a specific way from the full data set. The Cox model, then, is equivalent to a conditional logistic regression model. Although the level of detail required to describe this methodology is inappropriate for this document, details of this methodology have been described by Breslow and Day (1987) and are not too difficult to implement.

Fully Parametric Models

Certain specific parametric models have proved useful for answering specific research questions about survival patterns. The major limitation of such models is that they start with the assumption that a particular type of equation is correct for the population being studied. If the assumption is (approximately) correct, then the conclusions based on the model are (approximately) accurate. However, if the assumed equation is incorrectly specified, then the conclusions based on the equation can be inaccurate. Parametric models can sometimes lead to useful qualitative conclusions, even when the quantitative results are inaccurate because the model is incorrectly specified.

Parametric statistical models are based on the choice of a particular type of formula or equation that might plausibly approximate the survival pattern in a population. Such equations are often specified by the numerical values of a few parameters, or coefficients. Once the values of the parameters are known, the equation can be used to compute the value of any other characteristic that can be defined in terms of the equation.

Fully parametric models are based on certain assumptions about mortality patterns which may or may not be true for the ESRD population; thus, the resulting analyses may or may not be appropriate. Nonparametric or semiparametric models are based on fewer assumptions than are fully parametric models, and the results of nonparametric analyses are correspondingly less likely to be biased or incorrect. However, if an appropriate model is used, the results of parametric analyses tend to be more precise than the results of nonparametric analyses.

Exponential Model   The exponential model is based on the assumption that the death rate for a group of ESRD patients does not change with time. If this assumption is correct, then the survival curve for the patients is an exponential function of time and the curve is specified by one parameter: the death rate per unit of time. On the basis of the value of this death rate, other values can be computed, including the median lifetime, the expected lifetime, the probability of surviving for 5 years, and so on.

However, the exponential model is known to be a poor approximator of the long-term survival pattern for people because death rates rise with age. Further, the death rate among ESRD patients tends to decrease with the number of years since first ESRD therapy. Thus, average lifetimes that are calculated on the basis of an assumed exponential distribution are likely to be inaccurate if the calculated lifetime spans a large age or time range.

Weibull Model   This model yields a better approximation of mortality patterns among ESRD patients than does the exponential model. The Weibull model has two parameters that must be estimated from the data, in addition to regression coefficients that relate mortality rates to patient characteristics. These two parameters allow the Weibull model to fit a variety of patterns of mortality. The model yields useful and interpretable summaries of death rates, survival functions, relative death rates, and so on. Estimates of the model can be derived easily using the SAS statistical package. It is not as easy to use the Weibull model with time-varying patient characteristics as it is to use the Cox or Poisson regression models, because the standard statistical packages have not been extended to allow time-dependent covariates with the Weibull model.

One danger in the use of this model, or any other parametric model, is that the model can be estimated on the basis of a short period of patient follow-up and then extrapolated to yield estimates of long-term survival. There is no way to check the assumptions that the model makes for long-term survival on the basis of short-term data, and consequently there is no way to be assured that the long-term extrapolations are correct. The more nonparametric Poisson and Cox regression models naturally limit their predictions to the intervals of time for which data are available and thus are less subject to the abuse of extrapolation.

Bailey-Makeham Model   The Bailey-Makeham parametric model has proved to be very useful for qualitatively distinguishing between predictors of long- and short-term survival. If the model can be shown to yield a good approximation to the survival distribution for ESRD patients, then it may prove to be a particularly important analytical tool. The Bailey-Makeham model is less widely implemented on computers than are the Weibull, Poisson, and Cox models. Although the Bailey-Makeham model can be used to answer the same variety of analytic questions as can other models, it is especially attractive for its ability to quantify the differential effect of patient characteristics on long- and short-term patient survival.

Prevalent Versus Incident Cohort Analyses

In addition to the selection of an appropriate statistical methodology, it is crucial to select the appropriate group of patients to be included in the analysis. The selection depends strongly upon the objectives of the analysis of particular relevance is the distinction between prevalent and incident cohorts of patients. A prevalent cohort includes all patients treated during a specific year, including those whose therapy started prior to that year. An incident cohort includes only patients whose therapy started during a specific year. Many of the analyses performed to date have been limited to one or the other type of study group. Analysis of successive prevalent cohorts is most relevant to detecting trends in mortality over calendar time. Analysis of incident cohorts is more appropriate if the objective is to characterize how mortality changes with the time since first ESRD therapy.

For the purposes of summarizing patient survival after ESRD therapy starts, it is appropriate to classify patients by the year in which their ESRD therapy started. Such classification accounts for the changes in acceptance patterns that might occur over time. By definition, the baseline characteristics of a patient accepted into the Medicare program for ESRD do not change subsequent to acceptance. In such a classification, each patient is in just one cohort. The *USRDS Annual Data Report* (1990) has reported such summaries.

If the objective of analysis is to evaluate changes in therapy that occur with calendar year, possibly in association with changing technology or with program administration, then it is more useful to classify patient follow-up according to the year in which the therapy occurs. A patient contributes information on death rates in the prevalent cohort during each of the years that the patient is treated. Further, a patient is potentially in each of several prevalent cohorts in such a classification. Analysis can be performed either with Poisson regression models or with a Cox model using time-dependent covariates or strata. The analysis is conceptually similar to a series of annual analyses of 1-year survival for all prevalent (new and continuing) ESRD patients in each year. Eggers (various years) has reported such series in some of the HCFA reports.

In order to evaluate the simultaneous effects of both year of incidence and year of treatment, the statistical model used must incorporate both time measures. Tabulation of death rates according to patient characteristic and according to year of incidence and year of treatment would not be useful because the number of cells to be examined would be too large and the data would be too sparse.

Frailty

All of the statistical methods discussed above can account for measured patient characteristics and can summarize the relationship between patient characteristics and mortality. However, none of the models can directly account for patient characteristics that are not measured. There are several unmeasured patient characteristics that are related to mortality, and patients who are at higher risk for these unmeasured characteristics will tend to die sooner than patients who are at lower risk. The ensemble of unmeasured patient characteristics has been given the name *frailty* in the statistical literature (Vaupel et al., 1985), and frailty is known to affect the estimation of death rates. The selection process tends to lead to apparently lower death rates as time goes on because the less frail individuals are those that survive. In counterbalance to the unmeasurable effect of decreasing frailty are the measurable effects of increasing age as time goes on. Several statistical methods are currently being developed to account for frailty.

Treatment Modality

One important objective of survival analysis in the ESRD program is the evaluation of treatment modalities for ESRD. Such analysis is complicated because clinical trials are not commonly used for the evaluation of treatment therapies. Instead, treatment therapies are selected through a highly subjective set of decisions that involve both the patient and the provider of care. Because of this process, it is likely that different therapies have different profiles of patients assigned to them. Thus, any differences noted in patient outcomes could be due either to the different therapies or to differences in patient characteristics.

In order to reach more definitive conclusions, information is needed about the condition of each patient at the time of each therapy change. Using patient condition data collected at the start of each therapy, statistical methods could be used to yield adjusted measures of patient outcomes for a specific therapy. Further, the patient condition at the start of a therapy change could act as a measure of patient outcome for the previous therapy.

It is impractical and unnecessary to collect such detailed data for a census of the ESRD patient population. Instead, statistically valid samples could be drawn from the population of ESRD patients. Such samples could be drawn either prospectively, from newly incident cases, or retrospectively, from patients who have already received ESRD therapy. Prospective samples would be necessary if data collection were to include measures that are not readily available in the medical records. Retrospective samples could be drawn if data collection were to be limited to information that was readily available in existing records.

Publication of Standard Death Rates

The USRDS has started to publish mortality rates that can be used for small data base research. Death rates among prevalent ESRD patients in 1988 have been calculated for each major age-race-disease group classification (USRDS, 1989, Table D.31). These national rates can be used to compute the expected number of deaths for any study group. The ratio of the observed to the expected number of deaths can then be used to evaluate the mortality rates for the study group. Methods for such calculations are reviewed in detail by Breslow and Day (1982, 1987).

The rates published in the *USRDS Annual Data Report* are currently limited to the prevalent cohort of ESRD patients at the start of 1988. If continued for successive years, these rates will be useful for comparing death rates in small study groups to the expected rates based on national data. In addition to the patient characteristics of age, race, and disease group given in the published rates, it would be of value to extend the list of patient characteristics so that more precise comparisons could be made. Other patient characteristics could include gender, comorbidity, treatment, year of current prescription, and year of first prescription.

Institutional Characteristics

Analyses of patient-specific characteristics should be distinguished from analyses of facility-specific characteristics. The effective sample size for patient-specific analyses is related to the number of patients whereas the sample size for facility-specific analyses is the number of facilities studied. These two different types of analyses typically are addressed with different methods. Analysis of facility-specific outcomes should be based on a single observation per facility, as discussed by Cornfield (1978).

The type of institution or treatment protocol at an institution may affect mortality rates. In order to study such relationships, the institution rather than the patient is the unit of analysis (assuming that all patients at an institution receive the same treatment). Factors that could be or could have been studied on the basis of institutional analyses are profit-nonprofit status, dialyzer reuse, length of dialysis, and transplant technique.

Internal and External Standardization

The statistical analyses described here are based on the concept of comparison. For example, the death rates for two groups of patients can be compared. The mortality rate for one group of patients can be compared to that from another group in the same study (internal comparison) or to published mortality rates for another population (external comparison). Death rates published by the USRDS could serve as an external standard of comparison for a series of patients from a small study. In a larger study, there may be sufficient numbers of patients in several patient subgroups that their mortality rates can be usefully compared to each other.

Generally, internal comparisons are more valid than external comparisons, because bias is less likely to be a problem. However, external comparisons can provide indications of trends that may be useful for qualitative comparisons.

Analyses that involve an external comparison or standard may prove useful in understanding the effect of ESRD on mortality rates. ESRD patients with an etiology of hypertension could be compared to the general population with hypertension. Similar comparisons could be made for diabetes. For example, ESRD patients with an etiology of AIDS may have much higher mortality rates than do patients with other etiologies. However, therapy for ESRD may prove to be just as useful in extending the lifetime of ESRD AIDS patients relative to expected lifetimes among non-ESRD AIDS patients, as it is for diabetic ESRD patients relative to non-ESRD diabetic patients.

SURVIVAL ANALYSIS METHODS FOR ESRD PROGRAM

Some of the specific models described previously allow internal as well as external comparisons of mortality rates to be made simultaneously.

International comparisons of mortality among ESRD patients are a form of external comparison in which data from very disparate sources are evaluated. Some of the uses and limitations of such comparisons are discussed in the next section.

INTERNATIONAL COMPARISONS

International comparisons of mortality rates have two major objectives. The first is to document the existence of differences in mortality rates, if they exist. The second is to identify the reasons for the differences, if they exist. Using the currently available data, it is difficult to arrive at a definitive answer to the first objective and it is impossible to arrive at an answer to the second. The current data can give indications, but not proof, of differences in mortality rates for otherwise similar patients from different nations. Expert opinion can then be sought regarding hypotheses about causes of any differences that are thought to exist.

With the current system of separate registries, international comparisons can serve, at best, to point out somewhat crude differences in mortality patterns. Since only rough adjustments are possible across registries, there is no feasible way to isolate the reasons for any observed differences among nations.

The most recent and comprehensive international comparisons of mortality rates have been reported recently by Held et al. (1990). Many of the comments below are specifically motivated by the Held report but are also relevant to the interpretations of any international comparisons. Most of the limitations of international comparisons described below were recognized and acknowledged by Held report but are reviewed here in more detail. The results in the Held report are intriguing and give some indication that ESRD mortality rates are substantially lower in other nations than they are in the United States. Specific hypotheses generated by the Held comparison should be evaluated in more detail in order to determine whether a cause-and-effect explanation can be found for the differences that were found in that study. In addition, mortality rates in the United States should be closely monitored for trends over time.

Limitations

Many of the issues relevant to the use of survival analysis techniques for the analysis of U.S. data are also relevant to the international comparison of mortality rates. However, the problems are compounded in international comparisons because the data bases often have not been analyzed in a consistent way, the data often have not been collected in a consistent way, and there are almost certainly differences in the characteristics of patients from different nations that are not measured in the data bases. Adjustment for confounding factors is more problematical with international comparisons than it is with national analyses because the patient-specific data are not available in a unified structure.

In order to use statistical analysis of international data to determine the reasons for differences in mortality rates, it will be necessary to measure the potential causes of any differences at the national level and to correlate those measures with adjusted mortality rates across the nations.

The level of mortality observed in a national registry is strongly influenced by the criteria for acceptance into the registry. Different acceptance criteria, whether part of stated policy or influenced by the individuals who implement the policies, can have dramatic effects on mortality rates. If only healthy patients are accepted into a treatment program, then mortality rates will tend to be lower than if patients with high levels of comorbidity are accepted into the program. Different rates of diagnosis and treatment of ESRD among various nations gives some indication that acceptance criteria differ among nations, although the direction of the bias, if any, that such differences would cause is unknown. After patient age, the most important patient characteristic for predicting patient mortality may well be comorbidity, which is not recorded at the national level in the United States except for primary diagnosis. Since comorbidity is not currently recorded in the registries, it cannot be currently determined whether differences in patient morbidity are a likely cause of differences in patient mortality.

There are known differences between the types of patient accepted into the U.S. and other ESRD treatment programs. The importance of such differences is documented by the experience in the U.S. alone. The acceptance rate into the ESRD program in the U.S. has increased dramatically over recent years, with the result that the treated ESRD population is substantially older and has many more diabetic patients than it did previously. This has led to an increase in the crude mortality rate in the United States since 1977 (USRDS, 1990, Tables E.10, E.12, and E.14). However, death rates adjusted for age, race, sex, and primary diagnosis have been relatively stable during the same period (USRDS, 1990, Tables E.53, E.55, and E.57). Post hoc adjustments to international comparisons of mortality rates can also be made for known patient characteristics, such as age and etiology, but such adjustments are likely to be less accurate than would be a unified analysis of the combined data from several nations.

Etiology

The adjustments made by Held et al. (1990) to international comparisons have partially accounted for national differences in age and frequency of diabetes in the ESRD population. A more complete adjustment for diabetes would involve information about both the type of diabetes and the respective mortality rates among the non-ESRD diabetic patients in the nations being compared. The frequency of type of diabetes is not accounted for in the current adjustments and may differ across national boundaries. Differences in the management of diabetes may lead to different mortality rates among diabetics from different nations, even if they do not have ESRD.

Other aspects of etiology may also be important. For example, in the United States, death rates are elevated relative to glomerulonephritis if the etiology is hypertension. Since cardiovascular disease is less prevalent in Japan than in the United States, it may also be important to adjust for hypertension.

It is instructive to consider the difference between mortality rates of black patients and white patients as an example of the amount of variability that has been seen in the United States. The 5-year survival probabilities, adjusted for age, gender, and primary diagnosis, for black ESRD dialysis patients and white ESRD dialysis patients incident in 1984 are 36.5 and 30.5, respectively (USRDS, 1990, p. E.73). This unexplained difference of over 6 percentage points in survival probabilities is smaller than some of those reported by Held et al. (1990) for international comparisons, but it indicates that substantial differences can exist between identifiable groups, even within the same data collection system and nation. Other recent analyses (Wolfe et al., 1990) have shown that the difference between the mortality rates of blacks and whites is most substantial for diabetic patients and hypertensive patients, indicating that the impact of these two etiologies can vary substantially across different groups of patients. The existence of substantial differences in mortality between two groups of patients in the United States makes it clear that large differences in mortality rates among nations can be expected.

Age

The adjustment made by Held et al. (1990) for age is in 10-year (Europe) or 15-year (Japan) age groups. These are wide age intervals because the 5-year survival probability decreases dramatically with age after age 20 (USRDS, 1990, p. E.14). Differences of just a few years in the average age of patients in corresponding age groups would cause a substantial difference in the mortality rates for the groups. If patients in one nation are older overall, then they will tend to be older in each age category as well. For example, even if the age-specific death rates were identical in two nations, but the average ages in corresponding age groups were 5 years higher in one nation than in the other, then the two nations would have age-adjusted survival proportions that differed by approximately 5 percent. (The 5-year death fraction decreases by approximately 1 percent per year of age; see USRDS,

1990, p. E.14.) Age differences between patients in the different nations are thus plausibly responsible for at least a portion of the difference in mortality noted by Held et al. (1990).

In addition to factors that are measured across national registries, there are likely to be substantial differences between patients with respect to other characteristics, including past medical history, comorbidity, distance from a treatment center, and level of kidney function at first treatment. These factors cannot be adjusted for with the current data; they would require special studies, but it would be difficult to evaluate the potential impact of such unmeasured factors. However, evaluation of geographic differences in mortality in the United States would give an indication of the amount of variability present nationally that could be compared to the differences seen internationally.

Withdrawal Rates

The rate of withdrawal from therapy among dialysis patients in the United States is not negligible. Port and colleagues (1989) have reported that up to 10 percent of deaths among elderly patients in Michigan follow soon after withdrawal from therapy. Furthermore, at least 8.6 percent of all ESRD deaths in the United States in 1987 can be attributed to withdrawal from therapy (P. Eggers, HCFA, personal communication, 1990). There are large differences in withdrawal rates between groups in the United States, and it is plausible that large cross-national differences in withdrawal rates might also exist. Withdrawal may be a particularly relevant issue in international comparisons because the largest international differences in mortality were reported by Held et al. (1990) in the nonpediatric age groups, the same age range in which withdrawal is common in the United States.

Patient Follow-up

Ascertainment of mortality status by the ESRD data system is largely complete because of the computer links to the Social Security System. Although patients with long-lived transplants may be temporarily lost to the Medicare data collection system, their deaths are recorded when they occur so that overall mortality rates can be accurately estimated. It would be useful to have information from other nations concerning the fraction of the ESRD population that are followed to eventual mortality.

Directions for Further Research

Although the international comparisons in death rates that are reported by Held et al. (1990) indicate that mortality may be higher in the United

States than in some other peer nations, such differences are plausibly attributable to different data collection methods, differences in patient comorbidity and health practices, and differences in patient compliance. However, although international comparisons are not definitive, they still indicate that differences exist, for some unknown reasons. There are several areas of research that could be profitably explored to better our understanding of international comparisons:

• The impact of differential death rates in the general population has been partially addressed by Held et al. (1990). Further study of differential mortality rates in the populations of diabetics and hypertensives from various nations may also be useful.

• The fact that the differences in death rates among nations are largest in the nonpediatric age groups helps give some focus to the search for the reasons for such differences. Further identification of subgroups with differential death rates may help clarify the reasons for differences. Comparison of multivariable models from different nations would be an efficient method for such studies, and cause of death could be a useful measure.

• More international communication on the methods of managing data registries could prove useful for all nations that attempt to maintain ESRD data registries. For example, methods for validation of data registries could be standardized.

• Careful evaluation of different patterns of treatment methods among nations would be useful. Currently, much of the data on treatment patterns are derived from expert opinion rather than through data collection.

• Differences in patient compliance should be studied in order to determine the effect of withdrawal rates.

REFERENCES

Becker RA, et al. 1988. The New S Language, Wadsworth, Pacific Grove, CA.

Box GEP, Jenkins GM. 1976. Time Series Analysis, Holden-Day, Oakland, CA.

Breslow NE, Day NE. 1982 and 1987. Statistical Methods in Cancer Research, Vol I and II, Oxford University Press, Oxford.

Campbell DT, Stanley JC. 1963. Experimental and Quasi-Experimental Designs for Research, Rand McNally College Publishing Co., Chicago.

Cornfield J. 1978. Randomization by group: A formal analysis. Am J Epidemiology 108:100-102.

Cox DR. 1972. Regression models and life tables, JRSSB 34:187-220.

Cox DR, Oakes D. 1984. Analysis of Survival Data, Chapman and Hall, London.

Dixon WJ, et al. 1985. BMDP Statistical Software, University of California Press, Berkeley.

Donner A, Donald A. 1987. Analysis of data arising from a stratified design with the cluster as unit of randomization, Statist Med 6:43-52.

Eggers P. (HCFA). 1990. Personal communication concerning withdrawal rates.

Health Care Financing Research Report (P. Eggers) End Stage Renal Disease HCFA, various years.

Held PJ, et al. 1990. Five-year survival for end stage renal disease patients in the U.S., Europe, and Japan, Am J Kid Dis 15:451-457.

Kalbfleisch JD, Prentice RL. 1980. The Statistical Analysis of Failure Time Data, New York, Wiley.

Lawless JF. 1982. Statistical Models and Methods for Lifetime Data, New York, Wiley.

Payne CD. 1987. The GLIM System Release 3.77, Royal Statistical Society, NAG, Downers Grove, IL.

Port FK, Wolfe RA, Hawthorne VM, Ferguson CW. 1989. Discontinuation of dialysis therapy as a cause of death, Am J Nephrol 9:145-149.

SAS Institute. 1988. SAS/STAT User's Guide, Release 6.03, SAS Institute Inc, Cary, NC.

USRDS (U.S. Renal Data System). 1989. Annual Data Report. National Institute of Diabetes and Digestive and Kidney Diseases, Bethesda, MD.

USRDS. 1990. Annual Data Report. National Institute of Diabetes and Digestive and Kidney Diseases, Bethesda, MD.

Vaupel JW, et al. 1985. Heterogeneity's ruses: Some surprising effects of selection on population dynamics, Am Statist 39:176-185.

Wolfe RA, Port FK, Hawthrone WM, Guire, KE. 1990. A comparison of survival among dialytic therapies of choice: In-center hemodialysis versus continuous ambulatory peritoneal dialysis at home. Am J Kidney Dis 15:433-440.

E
Institute of Medicine
ESRD Study Committee
Public Hearing, May 5, 1989, Chicago, Illinois

List of Participants

American Association of Kidney Patients
  Lou Sand, President
American Council on Transplantation
  Jeptha W. Dalston, M.D.
American Heart Association, Council on Kidney in Cardiovascular
  Diseases
  John Burnett, Jr., M.D.
American Kidney Fund
  Sylvestre Quevedo, M.D.
American Nephrology Nurses Association
  Patricia S. Jordan, B.S.N., R.N., President
American Society for Histocompatibility and Immunogenetics
  Andrea A. Zachary, Ph.D.
American Society of Nephrology
  Wadi N. Suki, M.D.
American Society of Pediatric Nephrology
  Barbara Cole, M.D., President
  Billy S. Arant, Jr., M.D.
American Society of Transplant Surgeons
  J. Wesley Alexander, M.D.
Baxter Healthcare Corporation
  Allison Romer
Board of Nephrology Examiners for Nursing & Technologists
  Douglas L. Vlchek

Dialysis Clinic, Incorporated
  Raymond Hakim, M.D.
  James Perry
Forum of Network Coordinating Councils
  John L. Bengfort, M.D., Chairperson
Health Industry Manufacturers Association
  Susan Hanson
Hennepin County Medical Center, Regional Kidney Disease Program
  Allen J. Collins, M.D.
  Morris Davidman, M.D.
Home Intensive Care, Inc.
  Allan I. Jacob, M.D.
National Association of Nephrology Technologists
  Douglas L. Vlchek
National Dialysis Association
  Myron Nidetz
National Kidney Foundation
  Richard J. Glassock, M.D.
National Kidney Patients Association
  Robert Rosen
National Medical Care, Inc.
  Edmund G. Lowrie, M.D., President
National Organization for State Kidney Programs
  William Ferguson
National Renal Administrators Association
  Maureen Michael, President
Neomedica, Inc.
  Robert Hedger, M.D.
Nephrology Nursing Certification Board
  Janel Parker, R.N.
North American Transplant Coordinators Organization
  Barbara Schanbacher
North Central Dialysis Center, S.C.
  Alan Kanter, M.D., President
Renal Physicians Association
  Nathan W. Levin, M.D., President
Renal Treatment Centers, Inc.
  Robert L. Mayer, President
United Network for Organ Sharing
  Lawrence G. Hunsicker, M.D.

F

Institute of Medicine
ESRD Study Committee
Public Hearing on "Issues in Dialysis Reimbursement Rate-Setting," February 15, 1990, Washington, D.C.

List of Participants

American Nephrology Nurses Association
  Marilyn Neff, R.N., M.B.A.
Central Florida Kidney Center, Inc.
  Maureen Michael, Executive Director
Community Dialysis Center, Inc.
  Peter B. DeOreo, M.D., Medical Director
  Diane P. Wish, Executive Director
Dallas Nephrology Associates
  Alan R. Hull, M.D.
Dialysis Clinics, Inc.
  Ed Attrill, Assistant Treasurer
Greenfield Health Systems Corporation
  Linda L. Donald, Director of Operations
Healthcare Financial Management Association
  Ronald R. Kovener, Vice President
Kidney Center of Delaware County Ltd.
  A. Leo Coyle, Executive Director
Main Line Dialysis Services
  Denise Van Valkenburgh, Administrator
National Dialysis Association
  Myron Nidetz, Board of Directors
National Medical Care, Inc.
  Edmund G. Lowrie, M.D., President
  Edward Berger, Ph.D., Vice President of Government Operations

National Renal Administration Association
    Mardee W. Hagen, President
Neomedica, Inc.
    Gordon R. Lang, M.D.
    P. Kevin Flynn, Vice President, Finance
Nephrology Associates of Tidewater
    Anthony J. Messana
North Central Dialysis Centers, S.C.
    Alan Kanter, M.D., President
Northwest Kidney Center
    Christopher R. Blagg, M.D., Director
    Jeffrey Lehman, Chief Financial Officer

G

Institute of Medicine
ESRD Study Committee
Workshop on ESRD Staffing, November 3, 1989, Washington, D.C.

List of Participants

Carmella A. Bocchino, R.N., M.B.A. *
Christine K. Cassel, M.D. *
Dolph R. Chianchiano
   National Kidney Foundation, Inc.
   New York, New York
Betty I. Crandall, R.N.
   CVPH Medical Center
   Plattsburgh, New York
Marilyn Gammarino, R.D.
   Shady Grove Dialysis Center
   Rockville, Maryland
Margaret Izzo, N.P.
   Buffalo, New York
Susan Jaskula, M.S.W. *
Marjorie Powers, R.N., Ph.D. *
Anita Principe, R.N.
   Montefiore Medical Center
   Bronx, New York

---

* Member, IOM ESRD Study Committee

H
Institute of Medicine
ESRD Study Committee
Workshop on Kidney Transplantation,
December 13, 1989, Washington, D.C.

List of Participants

J. Wesley Alexander, M.D., Department of Surgery
    College of Medicine, University of Cincinnati
Carmella A. Bocchino, R.N., M.B.A. *
Clive O. Callender, M.D. *
Dolph R. Chianchiano
    National Kidney Foundation, Inc., New York, New York
Roger W. Evans, Ph.D. *
Ronald M. Ferguson, M.D., Ph.D. *
Lee A. Hebert, M.D., Professor of Medicine
    College of Medicine, Ohio State University
Philip J. Held, Ph.D. *
Lawrence G. Hunsicker, M.D., Professor of Medicine
    College of Medicine, University of Iowa
Carl Josephson
    Health Care Financing Administration, Baltimore, Maryland
Barry D. Kahan, Ph.D., M.D., Professor of Surgery
    University of Texas Health Science Center at Houston
Carl M. Kjellstrand, M.D.
    Regional Kidney Disease Program, Minneapolis, Minnesota
Norman G. Levinsky, M.D. *
John E. Lewy, M.D. *
Jimmy Light, M.D., Department of Surgery
    Washington Hospital Center, Washington, D.C.
John M. Newmann, Ph.D., Executive Director
    National Disease Research Interchange, Philadelphia, Pennsylvania

---

* Member, IOM ESRD Study Committee

Anita Principe, R.N.
  Montefiore Medical Center, Bronx, New York
John H. Sadler, M.D. *
Fred Sanfilippo, M.D., Ph.D.
  Veterans Affairs Medical Center, Durham, North Carolina
Terry B. Strom, M.D.
  Beth Israel Hospital, Boston, Massachusetts

---

* Member, IOM ESRD Study Committee

I
Institute of Medicine
ESRD Study Committee
Workshop on Black and Other Nonwhite ESRD Patients,* May 15, 1990, Washington, D.C.

List of Participants

Lawrence Agodoa, M.D.
  National Institute of Diabetes and Digestive and Kidney Diseases
Dolph Chianchiano
  National Kidney Foundation
Martin Dillard, M.D., Assistant Medical Director
  Howard University Hospital
Paul W. Eggers, Ph.D., Office of Research and Demonstrations
  Health Care Financing Administration
Carol Lynn Halal
  American Kidney Fund
Michele Hogan
  National Institute of Allergy and Infectious Diseases
Anna Monsef
  American Kidney Fund
Vivian Pinn-Wiggins, M.D., Department of Pathology
  Howard University College of Medicine
Linda Schaeffer, Division of Organ Transplantation
  Health Resources Services Administration,
  Department of Health and Human Services

---

* Held as part of the May 15-16, 1990, meeting of the IOM ESRD Study Committee

J
Institute of Medicine
ESRD Study Committee
ESRD Patient Focus-Group Participants

Washington, D.C.-
Baltimore, Maryland
December 14, 1989

Margaret Barlow
  Arlington, Virginia
James E. Batton
  Baltimore, Maryland
Ed Freeman
  Riverdale, Maryland
Robert V. Jordan
  Glen Burnie, Maryland
Werner Koehler
  Falls Church, Virginia
Patricia A. Krawczyk
  Linthicum, Maryland
Mildred McCoy
  Baltimore, Maryland
Earl Rose
  Baltimore, Maryland
Jill L. Seitz
  Baltimore, Maryland
Judith A. Whitesel
  Springfield, Virginia
Ronald L. Wobby
  Chantilly, Virginia

Irvine, California
February 1, 1990

Patricia Czaja
  Palm Springs, California
Greg Falconer
  LaPalma, California
Jorge Flores
  Los Angeles, California
Marilyn Harris
  Santa Monica, California
Donald Hopkins
  Van Nuys, California
Jeanie Joshua (and spouse)
  Ojai, California
Allen Kensinger
  Garden Grove, California
Mimi Lee
  Hacienda Heights, California
Judy McLaughlin
  Buena Park, California
Lynn K. Moltz
  Agoure, California
Thomas Murdock
  Los Angeles, California
Janice Novikoff
  Encio, California

Eva Ortega
  Thermal, California
David Stapel
  Anaheim, California

St. Louis, Missouri
March 8, 1990

Melinda Angelo
  Belleville, Illinois
James Brennan
  St. Louis, Missouri
Rose Mary Dennison
  Cahokia, Illinois
Bessie Dismukie
  St. Louis, Missouri
Jim Hootselle
  St. Louis, Missouri

Percy Jones
  St. Louis, Missouri
Mike Kern
  Evansville, Illinois
Rosemary Kottmann
  St. Charles, Missouri
Byron Lomax
  St. Louis, Missouri
Frederick Shaw
  Sikeston, Missouri
Houston Stahl
  St. Louis, Missouri
Terrell Stiles
  St. Louis, Missouri
Kathy Wilson
  Manchester, Missouri

Index

A

Abandonment of patients, 58
Access to care
  barriers to, 150–157, 177
  certificate of need and, 10, 158–163
  defined, 335
  dialysis patients, 135–164
  donor organ supply and, 179–182
  education/information and, 150–152
  elderly patients, 150, 175
  exclusion of individuals for medical
    reasons, 178
  geographic variation in, 138–140,
    160–162
  and ineligibility for Medicare
    benefits, 6–7, 136–148
  insurance coverage (private) and,
    152–154, 172–173, 177–178, 330
  magnitude of problem, 138
  Medicare-eligible patients, 148–157
  and payment sources other than
    Medicare, 140–146, 177–178
  pediatric patients, 115, 149–150, 175,
    176
  preventive services, 156–157
  rehabilitation services, 155–156
  state regulations and, 158–163
  transplants, 7–8, 167–185, 187
  transportation and, 154–155

Activities of daily living, 335, 284
Advance directives, 56, 59–60, 335
Age
  and acceptance for treatment, 8, 52–
    53
  and diabetic kidney disease, 90, 93
  and employment of ESRD patients,
    155
  ESRD patient trends, 27, 64, 65, 67–
    68, 70, 91, 100, 150, 216
  and health insurance coverage, 152
  and hypertension, 95
  and hypertensive ESRD, 90, 95–98
  and mortality rates, 72, 74, 76–78,
    213
  and treatment modality, 91, 92, 168
  and transplants, 168, 175, 176
  see also Elderly patients; Pediatric
    patients
Agency for Health Care Policy and
  Research, QA responsibilities, 276,
  287–288
AIDS, 53, 178, 179–180, 184, 252, 286
Albuminuria screening, 94
Alternative Reimbursement Method,
  202–203
American Diabetes Association, 94–95
American Medical Association, 202
American Outpatient Services Corpora-
  tion, 129

American Society of Artificial Internal
     Organs, 329
American Society of Nephrology, 329
American Society of Transplant
     Surgeons, 316
Anemia
     clinical indicators of outcomes and
          process, 19, 281, 307–308
     in pediatric patients, 86, 88
     treatment of, 14, 25, 201, 226, 293–
          294, 305–308
     see also Erythropoietin
Antihypertensives, 88, 142–143
Arkansas, Medicare eligibility status of
     ESRD patients, 138–139
Asians/Pacific Islanders with ESRD
     gender differences in, 101
     incidence and prevalence, 66–67, 70,
          100, 103
Association for the Advancement of
     Medical Instrumentation, 228
Atherosclerotic disease, 53, 79, 80

B

Baxter Healthcare, 329
Baxter Laboratories, 229
Blacks with ESRD
     diabetic, 93, 102
     health insurance coverage, 152
     hypertensive, 97, 102
     incidence and prevalence, 5, 66–68,
          70, 85–86, 99–100, 103, 156
     mortality rates, 74, 76, 78, 105
     pediatric patients, 85–86, 115
     preventive care for, 156
     primary diagnosis, 68–69
     transplant rejection, 104
     treatment modalities, 104, 175, 176–
          177, 183
     see also Race/ethnicity
Blood pressure, and renal disease, 99
Bone abnormalities, 86, 87–88, 149

C

Calcium/phosphorus metabolism
     controllers, 143
Cancer, 53, 79, 80

Cardiac disease, 53
Carpal tunnel syndrome, 319
Case mix
     and composite rate, 252–253
     defined, 336
     in quality-of-life studies, 283, 284–
          285, 294–296, 319
     reimbursement rate-setting and, 252–
          253, 284, 290
Catastrophic Health Insurance Act of
     1988, 172
Catheter declotting, 238
Center hemodialysis, mortality rates, 77
Centers for Disease Control, QA
     responsibilities, 228, 276, 286
Cerebrovascular disease, 53, 79, 80
Certificate of need
     and access to care, 10, 158–163
     constraints on providers, 114
     defined, 336
     elimination of, 160
     survey of programs, 26
Chronic heart insufficiency, 80
Chronic pulmonary disease, 53, 79, 80
Cirrhosis, 80
Clinishare, 129
Community Psychiatric Centers, 129
Comorbidities, 11, 205
     and acceptance for treatment, 8, 53
     defined, 337
     in diabetic ESRD, 94, 97
     in elderly patients, 90, 91
     in measures of quality, 280
     and mortality rates, 72, 80, 94
     in pediatric populations, 86
     and quality of life, 8
     severity assessment, 285
Composite rate
     1983 ESRD, 12, 213–217, 220, 243,
          253
     1986 reduction proposal, 243–244
     audited costs contrasted with, 245–
          246
     and case mix, 252–253
     covered outpatient services, 15–16,
          29, 193, 236–240
     derivation of, 196–199; see also
          Rate-setting process
     dual, 249–251, 253

exceptions and exemptions, 252–253
home dialysis supplies reimbursement, 25, 229
inflation/market basket adjustments, 252, 271
and innovation, 228, 253
labor portion on, 254–255
and mortality, 12
and patient morbidity, 217
and quality of care, 213–217
rebasing and updating, 251–254
reported costs contrasted with, 247–248
and unit staffing levels and composition, 220–221
see also Reimbursement
Conditions of coverage for ESRD providers, 18, 288–290
Congressional charge to IOM, 3–4, 23–24, 62, 133, 212, 274
Connecticut, 158–162
Continuity of care
concerns of patients, 42–43
for problem patients, 57, 58
Continuous ambulatory peritoneal dialysis, 162, 199, 228–229, 279, 283, 284, 309, 319, 337
Continuous cycling peritoneal dialysis, 201, 337
Continuous quality improvement, 19, 276, 297–300
Corticosteroid therapy, 88
Counseling, 46, 239
Cox proportional hazards model, 74, 319
Cox regression model, 77
Criteria screens, 253
Cushingoid facies, 88
Cyclosporine, 14, 143, 170, 172, 226, 230

D

Data systems
artifacts of, 73
National End-Stage Renal Disease Registry, 21, 25, 296, 321–324
needs, 20, 230
provider, 309–311

see also Health Care Financing Administration; Program Management and Medical Information System; United Network for Organ Sharing; United States Renal Data System
Dementia, 53
Demonstration project, 25, 155, 201
Department of Veterans Affairs, 29
data reported to HCFA, 318
dialysis program, 6, 63, 65, 139, 140, 146
ESRD expenditures, 33, 147, 148
financial problems of patients, 136
research in dialysis, 329
Diabetes mellitus, 5, 12, 102, 338
Diabetic ESRD patients, 28, 29
age differences, 90, 93
albuminuria screening, 94
comorbidities, 94, 97
employment of, 155–156
gender differences, 68–70, 93
incidence and prevalence of ESRD, 29, 52, 63, 65, 66–68, 70, 93, 106
insulin-dependent, 93
mortality rates, 74–76, 78, 79, 81, 92, 94
non-insulin-dependent, 93–94, 101, 102
prevention, 94
protein intake, 94–95
quality of life, 283
racial differences, 68–70, 93–94, 102
risk factors, 94
transplants, 168
treatment of, 92–93
Diagnosis-related groups, 268, 270
Dialysis
access problems, 135–164
and anemia, 14, 25, 201, 226, 293–294, 305–308
appropriateness of, 53
backup, 251, 259, 336
characteristics of patients, 52
costs of, 6, 14, 29, 135, 168, 226, 228, 254–255
covered services/allowable costs, 237, 242, 256
defined, 338
demand for, 10

elements involved in use of, 278–279
equipment and supplies, 45, 226–229,
    244, 252, 253, 286–287
high flux, 45, 227, 253
hostile, abusive patients, 9, 58
infection control program, 286, 287
innovations, 45, 226–229
mortality rates, 82, 87, 105
noncompliant, self-destructive
    patients, 9, 57–58
patient population increases, 111
prescription, 253, 311
price level and hospitalization rates
    and length of stay, 13
processes of care, 277–278
reimbursement rate-setting, 27
reuse of equipment and supplies, 45
self-care, 289, 345
state programs, 144
technicians, 13, 43, 161, 218–220,
    222, 223, 230, 277, 290
treatment times, 12–14, 214, 215,
    217, 227, 230, 232, 244, 311
withdrawal from, 53
see also Hemodialysis; Inpatient
    dialysis; Outpatient dialysis;
    Peritoneal dialysis
Dialysis Clinic, Inc., 129, 152, 178,
    216, 218, 224–225, 300, 309–310
Dialysis Management, Inc., 126
Dialysis treatment facilities
capacity, 10, 158–159
conditions of coverage, 288–289
cost reduction measures, 244–245
cost report data, 241
defined, 33–339
for-profit, 111
HCFA state surveys of, 19
number of Medicare-certified, 111
patient concerns about, 43
pediatric, 112
purchase prices of, 130
QA considerations and examples,
    299–300, 309–311
response to economic constraints,
    215–216, 225
rural, 112
staffing in, 13, 14, 43, 218–226, 230,
    244–245, 290

stations/size, 111, 158, 339
utilization, 158–159
see also Outpatient dialysis
Dialyzers, 226–227, 228, 244, 252
Dietitians, 13, 219, 220–222, 225, 230,
    277, 290
Do Not Resuscitate status, 56
Durable power of attorney for health
    care, 56, 57, 339

E

Education and training
and access to care, 150–152
of dialysis technicians, 223, 287
and employment of ESRD patients,
    155
for organ donation, 143
of patients, 41, 44–46, 50, 150–152,
    289
QA-related, 287
Elderly ESRD patients
access to care, 150, 175
causes of death, 92
comorbidities, 90, 91
growth in number of, 27, 29, 56–57,
    89–90, 92, 106
incidence and prevalence of ESRD,
    63, 90
mortality rates, 91
primary diagnosis, 90
treatment modality, 91, 92, 150, 175
see also Age
Employment, barriers to, 48–49, 50,
    155–156, 171, 173
End-stage renal disease (ESRD)
causes of, 5
defined, 339
economic effects of, 47–49, 50, 330
patient experiences with, 40–47
race and, 5
End-stage renal disease patients
acceptance criteria, 8, 52–55, 63, 66
age trends, 27, 64, 65, 67–68, 70, 91,
    100, 150, 216
autonomy model of rights, 41
choice of provider, 10, 162
complexity (case mix), 252–253
composition of population, 5–6, 12,

26, 27–28, 51–52, 65–69, 168,
174–178, 216, 256
conformance with treatment, 41, 42,
57–58, 80
counseling and self-help groups, 46
data sources and data files on, 317
education of, 41, 44–46, 50
effects of erythropoietin, 47, 50
employment problems, 48–49
experiences with renal failure, 40–47
family issues, 44
financial concerns and problems, 44,
47–49, 50, 150
incidence and prevalence of, 3, 5, 27,
30, 62–65, 70, 82
ineligible for Medicare benefits, 6, 7,
136–148
informed consent, 41
participation in care, 39, 276–277
by primary diagnosis, 64, 67–70
projections, 27–28, 30, 63, 66, 81–
83, 90, 256
quality-of-life ratings, 8, 54
relationships with physicians and staff,
40–44, 49–50, 57–58, 151, 282
services important to, 46
types raising problems for providers,
9
see also Elderly ESRD patients;
Focus groups; Pediatric ESRD
patients
End-Stage Renal Disease program
cost control, 6
entitlement under Medicare, 3, 4, 7,
23, 35, 89, 135, 137
expenditures, 26, 28–33
growth of, 31, 65
management of, 4, 24
mortality in, 11–12, 69, 71–72
networks, 19, 24–25, 55–56, 276,
288, 291–293, 296–297, 319, 339
policy concerns, 4, 24, 39
services covered, 29, 32
success of, 3, 23
End-stage renal disease treatment
acceptance criteria, 8
access to, 6–8, 24, 51
conformance with, 41, 57–58
cost-effectiveness studies, 21

costs of, 5–6, 19, 243–244
duration and outcomes, 12–13, 214,
215, 217
initiation of, 8–9, 53–54
limited-treatment plans, 56
modalities, *see* Dialysis; Transplants/
transplantation; Treatment modality
quality of care, 19; *see also* Quality
assessment and assurance
racial differences in, 103–104
technology, 26; *see also* Innovations
and technical change
time-limited trials, 56
withdrawal from, 9, 53–54, 55–57, 91
Epidemiology of kidney disease, 339
hypertensive, 96–98
diabetes, 63, 65, 66–68, 70, 93, 106
elderly, 63, 90
pediatric, 85–86
projections, 63, 66, 81–83, 90
research efforts, 20–21
see also Mortality
Erythropoietin, 281
dosage calculations, 45, 294
clinical trials, 282, 294, 306
costs of, 201–202
effects of, 47, 50, 156, 306–307
injections per year, 239–240
purpose of, 14, 25, 226
and quality of life, 283–284, 294,
307–308, 319, 320
reimbursement policy, 25, 142–143,
193, 196, 201–202, 230, 239–240,
293, 295, 323
self-administration of, 25, 294
Ethical issues
access to treatment, 51
facility ownership by physicians,
129–130
initiation of treatment, 8–9, 53–54
patient acceptance criteria, 8, 52–55
problem patients, 41, 57–58
transplants, 168
withdrawal from treatment, 9, 53–54,
55–57
Europe, survival of diabetic ESRD
patients, 81
European Dialysis and Transplant
Association, 79–80, 149–150

F

First-difference model, 12, 213–214
Focus groups, 26–27, 151
  composition of, 39–40, 409–410
  objective of, 39–40
  see also End-stage renal disease
    patients
Food and Drug Administration, QA
  responsibilities, 229, 276, 286–287

G

Gastrointestinal disease, 80
Gender
  and diabetic kidney disease, 68–70, 93
  and employment of ESRD patients,
    155
  and hypertension, 95
  and hypertensive ESRD, 68–70, 95–
    98
  incidence and prevalence of ESRD,
    66–70, 85, 101
  and mortality rates, 74, 76
  and transplants, 175, 176
Glomerulonephritis, 5
Glomerulonephritic ESRD, 5
  gender differences, 69–70
  incidence and prevalence of, 67, 68, 70
  mortality rates, 75, 94
  racial differences, 69–70, 102
Greenfield Health Systems Corporation,
  129, 300, 310
Growth retardation, 86, 87, 88, 149

H

Health Care Financing Administration
  (HCFA)
  administration of, 315
  annual report on ESRD program,
    316–317
  Bureau of Data Management and
    Strategy, 293, 295, 315, 317
  Bureau of Policy Development, 19,
    293–294, 295
  conditions of coverage for ESRD
    providers, 18, 288–290
  coordination within, 295–296
  cost data, 240–244, 271, 295

data acquisition, analysis, and
    systems, 20, 69, 71, 231, 315–318;
    see also Program Management and
    Medical Information System
  Health Standards and Quality Bureau,
    19, 151, 288, 291–293, 295
  Office of Research and Demonstra-
    tions, 19, 293, 294–295, 295, 317
  patient survival data, 69
  position on social service require-
    ments, 224
  QA responsibilities, 11, 19, 276,
    288–297
  state surveys of dialysis facilities, 19,
    110, 276, 288, 290–291, 316, 318
Health insurance (private)
  and access to care, 152–154, 172–
    173, 177–178, 330
  payment and/or qualification for, 48,
    50, 154, 172–173
  state payments into, 143
  use by Medicare ineligibles, 136
Health Omnibus Programs Extension of
  1988, 173
Health Systems Management, 129
Hemodialysis
  defined, 340
  home, 25
  innovations in, 226–228
  patient distribution, 5
  see also Dialysis
Hemodialysis, Inc., 129
Hepatitis, 286, 305
Hirsutism, 88
Hispanics with ESRD, 5
  access to care, 157
  diabetics, 93
  gender differences in, 101
  incidence and prevalence of, 99, 100,
    102
  non-Medicare dialysis patients, 139
Home hemodialysis
  age and, 91
  defined, 340
  EPO administration, 202
  paid aides for, 25
  and quality of life, 283, 284
  race and, 104
  reimbursement for, 25, 196, 199,
    200–201, 202–203, 229

relationships with providers, 40
training, 196, 309
Home Intensive Care, Inc., 25, 129,
200–201
Hospital Corporation of America, 298
Hospitals
backup dialysis units, 251, 259, 336
organ donation protocols, 182
outpatient dialysis, 116–117, 119–
121, 124, 125, 127, 128, 131, 159,
160
reimbursement of, 13, 29, 205–209
Hospitalization of dialysis patients
reimbursement effects on, 216–217,
230
reimbursement for, 12–13, 205–209
treatment time and, 217
trends, 319
Hypercreatinemia, 99
Hyperlipidemia, 99
Hyperphosphatemia, 310
Hypertension, 5
age and, 95
defined, 95, 340
erythropoietin and, 307
relationship to hypertensive ESRD, 96
in United States, 95–96
Hypertension Detection and Follow-up
Program, 98–99
Hypertensive cardiomegaly, 80
Hypertensive ESRD
age differences, 90, 95–98
and diabetic nephropathy, 94, 97
epidemiology of, 96–98
gender differences, 68–70, 95–98
incidence and prevalence of, 65–68,
70, 95–98, 106, 157
interventions, 98–99
mortality rates, 75–76, 78, 94, 96
racial differences, 68–70, 95–98, 101,
102
relationship to hypertension, 96

I

Illinois, Medicare eligibility status of
ESRD patients, 138–139, 141
Immunosuppressive drugs, 168
Medicare eligibility limitations, 4, 7,
24, 171–172, 174

patient concerns about, 45
reimbursement for, 193
side-effects in pediatric patients, 88
see also Cyclosporine; Imuran
Imuran, 143
Indian Health Service, 6, 103–104, 140,
143, 146, 147
Infection control program, 286
Informed consent, 41, 150
Innovations and technical change
clinical, 14
and composite rate, 253
dialysis research support, 229–220
equipment and supplies, 14, 226–228
hemodialysis, 226–228
labor substitution opportunities, 225
peritoneal dialysis, 228–229
reimbursement and, 13–14, 226–231
Inpatient dialysis, 29
age and, 91
benefit payments, 32, 206
capacity limits, 162
hospital reimbursement, 205–207
physician reimbursement, 208–209
and quality of life, 283, 284
race and, 103, 104
reimbursement for, 205–209

J

Japan, ESRD mortality data, 79–80, 81
Joint Commission on Accreditation of
Healthcare Organizations, 276

K

Kentucky Organ Donation Agency, 179
Kidney Care, 129
Kidney failure, *see* End-stage renal disease
Kidneys
acquisition costs, 191–192
supply of donors, 8, 87, 178–182

L

Licensed practical nurses, 13, 218–220,
290
Limited-treatment plans, 56
Living wills, 56, 57, 340

M

Maryland, Medicare eligibility status of ESRD patients, 138–139
Medicaid, *see* State Medicaid programs
Medical Case Review Procedures, 19, 292
Medical Device Amendments of 1976, 286
Medical Outcomes Study, 277, 278, 282, 285
Medical records review, 292–293
Medical review boards, 291–292
Medical Treatment Effectiveness Program, 288
Medicare
    Automated Data Retrieval System, 35
    conditions of participation, 150, 182
    copayments, 140, 142, 144
    cost data timeliness, 240–241, 271
    data sources and data files of ESRD patients and providers, 317
    data systems adequacy, 324–325
    defined, 341
    eligibility for ESRD program, 3, 4, 7, 23, 149, 166, 339
    ESRD QA function, 18, 19
    expenditures for ESRD beneficiaries, 6, 28–33, 166, 168
    expenses not covered by, 152
    Fee Schedule, 18, 204, 255–256, 259
    Hospital Insurance Trust Fund, 148
    Part A Cost Principles, 241–242, 247, 342
    recertification based on organ donor standard, 182
    as secondary payer, 153–154, 193, 215, 260, 330
    Supplemental Medical Insurance Trust Fund, 148
Medications, 143, 144
    injections per year, 239–240, 254
    reimbursement for, 25, 142–143, 193, 196, 201–202, 239
    transplant-related, 144, 168, 170, 171–172, 174; *see also* Immuno-suppressive drugs
    see also specific drugs
Mexican Americans, 102, 157
Michigan Kidney Registry, 77, 143

Minnesota Regional Kidney Disease Program, 77, 79, 80, 129
Minority patients, *see* Race/ethnicity; *and specific minorities*
Models/modeling
    Bailey-Makeham, 391
    continuous quality improvement, 297–300
    Cox, 74, 77, 319, 386–388
    exponential, 390
    first-difference, 12, 213–214
    logistic regression for probability of death, 388–391
    parametric, 390–391
    Poisson regression for death rates, 383–386
    prescription dialysis, 253
    price-level, 12, 13, 213–214, 217
    regression models, 381–386
    reimbursement effects, 12, 13, 213–214, 217
    statistical methods for ESRD mortality data, 383–389
    survival analysis, 372–373
    Weibull, 390–391
Monthly capitation payment, 18, 202–204, 208, 255–256, 259, 341
Morbidity
    defined, 341–342
    and dialysis treatment time, 14
    measures of, 12–13
    as outcome measure, 279
    see also Hospitalization
Mortality
    adjusted, 74, 75, 91, 94, 212
    age and, 72, 74, 76–78, 213
    analyses, 71, 295–296, 330–331; *see also* Statistical methods for ESRD mortality data; Survival analysis
    defined, 342
    and dialysis treatment times, 12, 14
    in ESRD program, 11–12, 69, 71–72
    factors causing changes in, 71, 72, 80
    international comparisons, 79–81, 395–399
    as outcome measure, 12, 214–216, 279, 294
    private insurance and, 152
    and reimbursement rates, 12, 14, 212–216, 230

source of data, 69
state and regional data, 77, 79
subgroup, 74–78, 88, 91, 94, 103–104
transplants, 75, 77, 82, 87
treatment modality and, 104, 320
treatment time and, 12–13, 214, 215, 221, 222
trend analyses, 21, 71, 319
unadjusted, 72–74, 79, 212
Multivitamin compounds, 143

N

Navajo Indians, 101
National Center for Health Services Research, 288
National End-Stage Renal Disease Registry, 21, 25, 296, 321–324, 318
National Health and Nutrition Examination Survey (II), 95, 102
National Institute of Allergy and Infectious Diseases, 287
National Institute of Diabetes and Digestive and Kidney Diseases, 20–21, 229, 285, 287, 296, 318–323, 330
  Artificial Kidney/Chronic Uremia program, 227, 229, 287, 329
National Institutes of Health QA responsibilities, 287
National Kidney and Urologic Diseases Advisory Board, 328–329
National Kidney Foundation, Council of Nephrology Social Workers, 223–224
National Medical Care, Inc., 126, 129, 300, 310–311
National Medical Enterprises–Medical Ambulatory Care, 129
National Medical Review Criteria Screens, 19, 292
National Organ Transplant Act of 1986, 9, 25, 111, 170–171, 173, 182, 320
National Task Force on Organ Transplantation, 173, 175
Native Americans with ESRD
  gender differences, 101
  incidence and prevalence of, 66–67, 70, 99–100, 103

non-Medicare dialysis patients, 139, 143, 146
  outcomes research, 321
  primary diagnosis, 68, 93, 101
  see also specific tribes
Neomedica Dialysis Centers, Inc., 129
Neurologic impairment, 53, 86, 88
New Mexico, Medicare eligibility status of ESRD patients, 138–139
New West Dialysis, 129
North American Pediatric Renal Transplant Cooperative Study, 149
North Central Dialysis Centers, 218–219, 220
Northwest Kidney Center, 129
Nursing/nurses
  assistants, 13, 218–219
  quality assurance by, 277, 282
  reimbursement effects on, 222–223, 230
  requirements limiting capacity, 161
  shortages, 43
  staffing of dialysis units, 218–223
  standards for, 289–290
Nutrition, parenteral, 238

O

Obesity, 88
Omnibus Budget Reconciliation Act of 1981, 193, 195, 215, 233, 249
Omnibus Budget Reconciliation Act of 1985, 291
Omnibus Budget Reconciliation Act of 1986
  data collection and analysis mandate, 21, 25, 296, 318, 321–323
  ESRD network reorganization, 24–25, 291–292
  quality and appropriateness of patient care, 19
  reimbursement policy, 197, 201, 231–232, 251
  transplant provisions, 172, 173
Omnibus Budget Reconciliation Act of 1987
  charge to IOM, 3–4, 23–24, 133, 135, 212, 274, 283
  composite dialysis rates, 251

Omnibus Budget Reconciliation Act of
    1989
  creation of AHCPR, 287–288
  reimbursement policy, 25, 199, 204,
    251
Omnibus Budget Reconciliation Act of
    1990
  advance directives, 59
  demonstration project, 155, 201
  EPO policy, 202
  OPO performance standards, 182
  reimbursement policy, 25, 153, 193,
    198–199
  research directives, 244, 260
Organ donation, 143, 184, 191–192
  and access to care, 179–182
Organ Procurement and Transplantation
    Network, 25, 171, 174, 182, 320
Organ procurement organizations, 9,
    111, 114
  consolidation of, 174, 182
  grant assistance to, 173
  hospital-based, 111, 114
  independent, 111, 114
  reimbursement of, 192
  staffing considerations, 183
Outcomes
  defined, 342
  measures, 12, 19, 216, 279–280, 294,
    307; see also Morbidity; Mortality
  and QA, 276–277, 279–280, 294
  reimbursement and, 247, 249
  research, 288
  of transplants, 5, 167, 168, 170, 172,
    174, 176
Outpatient dialysis
  advance directives legislation applied
    to, 59–60
  chains, 126, 129, 131, 243, 258
  cost report audits, 241, 245–246,
    262–267
  costs per treatment, 249–250, 296
  covered services, 15–16, 29, 236–240
  expenditures for, 29, 32, 206
  facilities, 10, 112–114, 116–118,
    119–122, 130, 193–202, 244–255
  for-profit, 120–124, 126–129
  hospital backup units, 251
  hospital-based providers, 116–117,

      119–121, 124, 125, 127, 128, 131,
      159, 160, 195, 196, 218, 221–222,
      245–250, 257
  independent providers, 117–119, 121,
      124, 126–128, 131, 159, 160, 195,
      196, 198, 218, 220–222, 245–250
  not-for-profit providers, 119–124,
      127–129
  ownership of facilities, 126, 129–130,
      251, 257
  patient numbers, 116–117, 118–119,
      120–122, 125
  physician reimbursement, 202–205,
      255–256
  rate-setting process, 240–244
  reimbursement for, 6, 11, 13, 15–18,
      193–205, 236–260
  sampling of units, 241
  stations/size, 116–118, 120–129, 131
  structural changes in provider
      community, 116–130
  treatment capacity, 10, 124
  utilization rate, 116–117, 118–119,
      131, 159–160, 162
  see also Home hemodialysis

                              P

Parathyroid gland overactivity, 88
Patient
  characteristics, 277, 285
  complexity, 284–285, 290, 296
  functional and health status, 279–
      283, 284
  satisfaction, 279, 280, 283
  see also End-stage renal disease
      patients
Pediatric ESRD patients, 59
  access to care, 115, 149–150, 175,
      176
  acne, 88
  anemia in, 86, 88
  characteristics of population, 85–86
  clinical trials of pharmaceuticals, 89
  comorbidities, 86
  facilities for, 112, 115–116
  health status assessment, 282
  incidence and prevalence of, 85–86
  ineligible for Medicare, 149

mortality rates, 87, 88
pubertal development delays, 86, 88
quality-of-life factors, 86, 149, 150
special problems and needs of, 85,
    88–89, 106, 149–150, 251, 253,
    259, 319
transplantation in, 86–87, 149, 175,
    176
Peripheral vascular disease, 53, 79, 80
Peritoneal dialysis, 29, 343
age and, 91
innovations in, 228–229
patient distribution, 5
race and, 104
Peritonitis, 319
Persistent vegetative state, 53
Physicians and other health care
    professionals
characteristics, 277
education about ethical issues, 56
education of patients, 44–45, 151
monthly capitation payment, 18, 202–
    204, 208, 255–256, 259, 341
ownership of treatment facilities,
    129–130, 257
pediatric specialists, 89
quality assurance by, 276
reimbursement of, 192–193, 202–204,
    208–209, 255–256
relationships with patients, 40–44,
    49–50, 57–58, 151, 282
supplier services, 29
training of, 43, 150
Pima Indians, 94, 101, 104
Poisson regression, 74
Polycystic disease, 75
Prescription drugs, *see* Medications;
    and specific drugs
President's Commission for the Study
    of Ethical Problems in Medicine
    and Biomedical and Behavioral
    Research, 53
Prevention of ESRD, 156–157, 329–330
Price-level model, 12, 13, 213–214, 217
Primary diagnosis of ESRD
among blacks, 68–69
distribution of patients by, 64, 67–70
among elderly patients, 90
among Native Americans, 68, 93, 101

survival analysis and, 364–365
see also Diabetic ESRD patients;
    Glomerulonephritic ESRD patients;
    Hypertensive ESRD patients
Processes of care, 19, 277–279, 281,
    307–308
Professional Standards Review Organi-
    zations, 276, 288, 343
Program Management and Medical
    Information System, 62, 296, 315–
    318, 343
Prospective Payment Assessment
    Commission, 17, 18, 344, 241, 244
rate updating, 251, 258, 259, 260
Prospective Payment System, 215, 237,
    343–344
inpatient hospital, 193–194, 205
Providers
capacity of, 113, 114
certificate-of-need constraints on, 114
chains, 126, 129, 131, 243, 257, 310–
    311
characteristics, 277
conditions of coverage, 18
data sources and data files on, 317
demand for, 113
defined, 131
kidney transplant centers, 114–115
outpatient dialysis facilities, 10, 112–
    114
patient choice of, 10, 162
pediatric facilities, 115–116
response to economic constraints,
    215–216
size of facilities, 113, 114, 115
staff/patient ratios, 43
structural changes in community, 9–
    10, 110–131, 116–130, 242
utilization of, 113
see also Dialysis treatment units;
    Outpatient dialysis
Proximate clinical indicators, 279, 280–
    281, 305–308
Public Health Service
Bureau of Quality Assurance, 315
dialysis patients, 65
Health Resources and Services
    Administration, 174, 184, 330
QA responsibilities, 276, 286–288

Public Health Service Act, 25, 171
Public hearings, 26–27, 218, 226, 242,
    244, 245, 403–404

Q

Quality assessment and assurance (QA)
    case mix and severity adjustments,
        283, 284–285, 294–296, 319
    conditions of coverage for ESRD
        providers, 18, 288–290
    continuous quality improvement, 19,
        276, 297–300
    data needs, 296–297
    defined, 344
    in dialyzer reuse, 228
    elements of ESRD QA function
        within Medicare, 18
    examples of, 299–300, 309–311
    federal responsibilities for, 276, 285–
        297; *see also specific agencies and
        authorities*
    functional- and health-status
        assessments, 281–283, 284, 294–
        295, 330–331
    HCFA efforts, 11, 19
    infection control program, 286
    internal systems, 276
    Medical Case Review Procedures, 19
    medical review boards, 291–292
    National Medical Review Criteria
        Screens, 19
    obstacles, 274–275
    outcomes and, 275, 279–280
    patient satisfaction and, 283
    principles of, 275–277
    process of care and, 277–279, 280
    proximate clinical indicators, 280–
        281, 305–308
    purposes of, 275–276
    quality of life and, 283–284
    and rate-setting, 258
    state surveys of dialysis facilities, 19,
        110, 290–291
    structure and, 277, 280
Quality of care, 17
    certificate of need and, 10, 162
    composite rate and, 213–217
    cost of treatment and, 19, 244

defined, 275, 344
    measures of, 12–13, 19, 218, 279–
        280, 288
    and provider community structure,
        130–131, 257
    reimbursement and, 11–18, 212–233,
        256–257, 268–269, 272
    standards of care, 237–238, 268–269,
        280
    treatment time and, 221
    treatment unit staffing and, 43, 218–
        225
Quality of life
    comorbidities and, 8
    erythropoietin and, 283–284, 294,
        307–308, 319
    life-sustaining treatment and, 53
    measures of, 54, 283–284
    patient rating of, 8, 54
    of pediatric patients, 86, 149
    research, 294

R

Race/ethnicity
    and age of ESRD patients, 100
    and diabetic ESRD, 68–70, 93–94,
        101, 102
    and eligibility for Medicare ESRD
        program, 139–140
    and ESRD incidence and prevalence,
        5, 66–70, 85–86, 93, 99–103, 106,
        157, 319
    and glomerulonephritic ESRD, 101,
        102
    and hypertension, 95
    and hypertensive ESRD, 68–70, 95–
        98, 101, 102
    and mortality rates, 103–104
    and primary diagnosis leading to
        ESRD, 67–70, 101
    and risk of ESRD, 99
    and treatment modality, 103–105,
        176–177
    see also Asian Americans; Blacks;
        Hispanics; Native Americans
Rate-setting process
    conflicts between HCFA and ESRD
        providers in, 243

cost data timeliness, 240–244, 271
cost-per-treatment calculation, 243–244
defined, 344
dissenting view of, 268–273
generally accepted accounting principles in, 242
goals of, 236
Medicare Part A cost principles in, 241–243, 247, 256
oversight of, 244, 258
procedural issues, 243
public hearings on, 27, 242, 244, 245
and quality assessment and assurance, 251, 258, 290
sampling versus universe, 241, 262–267
Recommendations
access to treatment, 4, 7–8, 24
advance directives, 59
advisory group of nephrology professionals and experts, 20, 301
certificate of need, 11, 162–163
composite rate, 258–259
continuing education in medical ethics and health law, 9, 59
data systems, 19, 20–21, 301, 325–326
entitlement to ESRD treatment, 4, 7, 89, 148
funding considerations, 3, 24, 173
HCFA state survey system, 19, 301
kidney donation, 8, 183, 184, 326
immunosuppressive drug coverage, 8, 173
initiation of treatment, 9, 59
management of ESRD program, 4, 24
Medicare secondary-payer provision, 154
monitoring organizational changes in provider community, 10, 131
National End-Stage Renal Disease Registry, 21, 326
patient acceptance criteria, 9, 59
patient education, 152
quality assurance and assessment, 19–20, 259, 301–302, 326
quality of care, 4, 24, 301
reimbursement policies for dialysis

facilities, 17–18, 19, 257, 258–259, 301
research, 20, 21–22, 59, 301
transplant eligibility limits, 7–8, 173
United States Renal Data System, 21, 326
withdrawal from treatment, 59
Registered nurses, 13, 218–223, 289
Regulations
ESRD network medical review boards, 291–292
interim, of 1983, 227–228
see also Certificate of need; State regulations
Rehabilitation
barriers to, 50, 155–156
reimbursement for physical therapy, 239
Reimbursement
and access to care, 161
Alternative Reimbursement Method, 202–203
appropriateness screens, 291
assessing the effects of, 12, 213, 214–215
case mix and, 252–253, 284, 290
and clinical research, 329
current policy, 198–199
exceptions and exemptions, 194, 199–200, 252–253
facility/center, 191–192, 192–202, 244–255
and hospitalization, 216–217, 230
of hospitals, 205, 207
historical overview, 193–198
home dialysis, 25, 196, 199, 200–201, 202–203, 229
and innovation, 13–14, 226–231, 256
inpatient dialysis services, 205–209
level-of-payment issues, 244–249
for medications, 25, 142–143, 193, 196, 201–202, 230, 239–240, 293–295
monthly capitation payment, 202–204, 208
and mortality, 12, 14, 212–216, 230
from non-Medicare sources, 142, 153
outpatient dialysis, 6, 11, 13, 15–18, 193–205, 236–260

and patient characteristics, 207
of physicians, 192–192, 202–205,
    208–209, 255–256
policy options, 16, 18
and quality of care, 11–18, 212–233,
    247, 249, 256–257, 272
rebasing, 15–18, 194, 344
retrospective, cost-based, 242
staffing in treatment units and, 13,
    14, 218–225, 230, 247, 290
transplant services, 191–193
see also Composite rate; Rate-setting
    process
REN Corporation–USA, 129
Renal biopsy, 319
Renal Physicians Association, 323
Renal Treatment Centers Corporation, 129
Research
    basic, 20, 328
    clinical, 20, 229, 282, 328, 329
    dialysis, 229–230
    epidemiologic, 21–22, 294, 296, 316,
        318, 322–323, 330
    on ethical issues, 59
    health services, 22, 287–288, 324,
        328, 331
    mortality, 319, 330–331, 398–399
    needs, 328–332, 398–399
    outcomes and effectiveness, 288,
        319, 321, 331
    preventive, 20
    treatment modality effectiveness,
        284, 320, 329–330

S

Salick Health Care, 129
San Antonio Heart Study, 157
Satellite Dialysis, 129
Self-help groups, 46
Sickness Impact Profile, 284, 307
Social Security Administration, Bureau
    of Health Insurance, 315
Social Security Amendments of 1972,
    3, 6, 23, 133, 135, 170
Social Security Amendments of 1973,
    137
Social Security Amendments of 1978,
    195

Social Security disability regulations,
    48, 50, 155, 171
Social workers, 13, 218–221, 222–225,
    230, 290, 277
Southeast Organ Procurement Founda-
    tion, 174, 320
State kidney programs, 143–147
State Medicaid programs
    benefits of, 6–7, 142, 146, 155
    defined, 341
    dual eligibles, 142
    expenditures for ESRD patients, 140,
        142
    reimbursement levels and policy,
        142
    use by ESRD patients, 136, 140, 148
State regulations, and access to care,
    158–163
Statistical methods for ESRD mortality
    data
    Bailey-Makeham model, 391
    comparative parameters, 380–383
    Cox models for relative rates and
        survival functions, 386–388
    death proportions, 376–377, 386–388
    death rates, 377–379, 381–388, 393–
        394
    descriptive parameters for one group,
        376–380
    expected lifetimes, 379–380
    exponential model, 390
    frailty, 392
    institutional characteristics, 394
    logistic regression for probability of
        death, 388–391
    models and methods, 383–389
    parametric models, 390–391
    Poisson regression for death rates,
        383–386
    prevalent versus incident cohort
        analyses, 391–392
    regression models, 381–386
    sampling from risk set, 380–391
    standardization (internal and exter-
        nal), 394–395
    survival curves, 379, 382–383, 386–
        388
    treatment modality, 393
    Weibull model, 390–391

Survival analysis
  adjustment for patient characteristics, 364–375
  age adjustments, 358–359, 365, 397–398
  biased comparisons, 358–359
  comparison group, 357
  constraints on adjustment process, 374–375
  counts of patients, accuracy of, 363–364
  data currently available for, 364–367
  data unavailable or difficult to evaluate, 368–370
  diagnosis and, 364–365
  error (types I and II) issues, 363
  etiology in, 396–397
  examples of, 356–364
  inappropriate comparison group, 358–359
  gender in, 367
  general issues in, 355–364
  international comparisons, 79–81, 395–399
  limitations of, 395–398
  medical history, 368–369
  modeling, 372–373
  multivariable methods, 370–374
  overview of, 355–356
  parameters for mortality summaries, choice of, 362–363
  patient follow-up, 398
  population identification, 356–357
  projections and extrapolations, 363
  provider versus patient, 361–362
  race in, 367
  random variation in, 360–361
  research needs, 398–399
  significant versus important differences, 361
  social support systems, 369–370
  spurious differences in, 358
  standard errors for population data, 359–360
  stratification, 371–372
  time in multiple measures, 367
  treatment methods, 365–366
  treatment modality, 368
  unobserved factors, 359
  variables exerting simultaneous effects, 374
  withdrawal rates, 398
  year of first treatment, 365–366
  years of treatment, 366–367
  see also Mortality; Statistical methods for ESRD mortality data
Swedish dialysis centers, 80

T

Tax Equity and Fiscal Responsibility Act of 1982, 137, 345–346
Technicians, *see* Dialysis technicians
Texas Kidney Health Program, 102, 143
Tidewater Nephrology Associates, 129
Time-limited trials, 56
Training, *see* Education and training
Transplant Amendments Act of 1990, 173, 177, 184, 330
Transplant recipients
  access restrictions, 7–8, 167–185, 187
  age and, 168, 175, 176
  characteristics of patient population, 5, 26, 91, 168, 174–178
  compliance with drug regimens, 172
  employment of, 171, 173
  mortality rates, 75, 77, 82, 87
  outcomes, 5, 167, 168, 170, 172, 174, 176
  pediatric, 86–87, 149, 175, 176
  projections, 82
  quality of life, 283, 284
  racial differences in, 104–105, 176–177
  rehabilitation services, 155
  self-destructive, 9, 58
Transplants/transplantation
  access to kidneys, 26, 87, 150, 167, 170, 173–178
  from cadaver donors, 5, 75, 77, 82, 87, 104, 105, 114, 168–170, 175, 176, 182, 336
  conditions of coverage, 288–289
  cost-effectiveness of, 168
  costs of, 6, 29, 115, 135, 168, 192
  covered services, 237

demand for kidneys, 8, 167, 170
distribution of, 173–178
facilities/centers, 9, 111, 114–115,
    191–192, 346
follow-up care, 143, 151–152
HLA matching, 104, 174, 175, 176,
    177, 179, 319, 321
legislation, 25, 170–171
from living related donors, 5, 82, 87,
    168–170, 175, 176, 192, 340, 284
media coverage of, 181–182
Medicare benefit, 29, 170–173
Medicare eligibility limitations, 4, 5,
    24, 171
medications, 144, 168, 170, 171–172,
    174; see also Immunosuppressive
    drugs; and specific medications
number of procedures, 5, 111, 114,
    168–169, 171, 179
parent-child, 319
patient information about, 151
point scoring system, 176–177
registry, 173, 174, 192
reimbursement for, 191–193
rejection of grafts, 40, 88, 104, 105,
    168, 284
state programs for, 144
supply of donor organs, 179–183
survival of grafts, 168, 170, 176
waiting lists, 40, 170, 171, 175–176,
    192, 321
workup procedures, 143
Transportation
and access to care, 154–155
financial assistance for, 143–144, 150
Treatment modality, 23, 44
age and, 91, 92, 168

distribution of patients by, 5
effectiveness research, 284, 320,
    329–330
for elderly patients, 91, 92, 150, 175
and mortality, 104, 320, 368
race/ethnicity and, 103–105, 176–177
in statistical analyses, 368, 393
see also Dialysis; Transplants/
    transplantation

U

United Network for Organ Sharing,
    174, 320–321
United States Renal Data System, 20,
    21, 25, 62, 296, 318–320
mortality analyses, 69, 71, 323
Scientific Advisory Committee, 285,
    323
Utilization and Quality Control Peer
    Review Organizations, 276, 288
Urokinase, 238

V

Vivra, Inc., 129

W

W.R. Grace, Inc., 129
West Suburban Kidney Centers, 129

Z

Zuni Indians, 102